PERIOPERATIVE ASSESSMENT
IN VASCULAR SURGERY

Science and Practice of Surgery

Consulting Editors

John F. Burke

Benedict Professor of Surgery
Harvard Medical School
Massachusetts General Hospital
Boston, Massachusetts

Peter J. Morris

Nuffield Professor of Surgery
University of Oxford
John Radcliffe Hospital
Oxford, England

Additional Volumes in Preparation

PERIOPERATIVE ASSESSMENT IN VASCULAR SURGERY

edited by

D. Preston Flanigan

*University of Illinois College of Medicine
at Chicago
Chicago, Illinois*

MARCEL DEKKER, INC.   **New York and Basel**

Library of Congress Cataloging-in-Publication Data

Perioperative assessment in vascular surgery.

(Science and practice of surgery ; 9)
Includes index.
1. Blood-vessels--Surgery--Evaluation. 2. Blood-
vessels--Diseases--Diagnosis. 3. Therapeutics, Surgical
--Evaluation. I. Flanigan, D. Preston. II. Series.
[DNLM: 1. Intraoperative Care--methods. 2. Postoperative
Care--methods. 3. Preoperative Care--methods.
4. Vascular Diseases--diagnosis. 5. Vascular Surgery.
W1 SC679 v. 9 / WG 170 P445]
RD598.5.P475 1987   617'.413   86-23987
ISBN 0-8247-7632-1

MARCEL DEKKER, INC.
270 Madison Avenue, New York, New York 10016

Current printing (last digit):
10 9 8 7 6 5 4 3 2 1

PRINTED IN THE UNITED STATES OF AMERICA

*To Beth for understanding
and to my mother,
for making it possible*

Preface

The purpose of this book is to assist the vascular surgeon in the perioperative period in making the correct diagnosis, selecting the correct operation (if any), assuring a technically excellent operation, and recognizing impending or actual graft failure.

Tests that assist in diagnosis and in selection of the proper operative procedure are necessarily performed in the preoperative period. Tests that assess the technical results of revascularization are best performed in the operating room, allowing correction of technical errors during the primary procedure. In the postoperative period, tests that determine impending or actual graft failure are important, particularly if impending failure is to be recognized before actual graft failure occurs. Consequently, this book is divided into three major sections, which deal with preoperative, intraoperative, and early and late postoperative assessment.

This is not a book about the treatment of patients, but it *is* about patient management. I believe that the application of the methods of assessment delineated in this volume will allow the practicing vascular surgeon to significantly improve overall patient management and thus the results of treatment.

Vascular surgery has undergone enormous growth in the past three decades. Early growth during this period was meteoric as a result of major developments such as angiography, the use of autogenous saphenous vein, and the manufacture of prosthetic vascular grafts. Recently, growth has been steady but slower as operative techniques, perioperative care, and diagnostic procedures have gradually improved. The recent noninvasive approach to diagnosis has led to the development of numerous types of noninvasive procedures, some more useful than others. Once believed by some to be superfluous, these noninvasive tests have become an integral part of the evaluation and management of vascular patients today. It is my intent in this volume to combine these newer noninvasive modalities with improvements made in the more traditional invasive procedures and to consider them together as modern methods of perioperative assessment in vascular surgery.

It is not intended for this book to be an inclusive work on vascular diagnosis. Rather, emphasis is on recent developments and applications. Thus, no section on history and physical examination, routine angiography, routine noninvasive testing, or other traditional modalities is included. Testing procedures that are not directly aimed at perioperative evaluation are likewise excluded. No attempt was made to include all vascular disease processes. Consequently, for example, there is no chapter on the diagnosis of mesenteric insufficiency, since nothing new has developed in this area over the last several years. The aim was to include only those methods of perioperative assessment that are both new and emerging as standard modalities in modern vascular surgical practice.

No work of this size can be done effectively by one person. I would like to acknowledge the contributors for the timely submission of their high-quality manuscripts and for their scholarly approach to vascular surgery, which has provided for many advances made in the management of patients with vascular disease. Credit also goes to the secretarial staff of the Division of Vascular Surgery at the University of Illinois for their concerted efforts in the preparation and organization of the material, and to the publishers for their expediency and organization in getting the book to press in a timely fashion.

D. Preston Flanigan

Contributors

Gary G. Anderson, B.S.* Biological Laboratory Technician, Department of Vascular Surgery, Veterans Administration Medical Center, Tucson, Arizona

John J. Bergan, M.D., F.A.C.S., Hon. F.R.C.S. (Eng.) Magerstadt Professor of Surgery and Chief, Division of Vascular Surgery, Northwestern University Medical School, Chicago, Illinois

Dale Buchbinder, M.D. Assistant Professor of Surgery, and Chief, Division of Vascular Surgery, University of Health Sciences/The Chicago Medical School, North Chicago, Illinois

John J. Castronuovo, Jr., M.D. Associate Program Director, Department of Surgery, Morristown Memorial Hospital, Morristown, New Jersey

Daniel J. Douglas, M.D. Resident in Surgery, Division of Vascular Surgery, Department of Surgery, University of Illinois College of Medicine at Chicago, Chicago, Illinois

Joseph R. Durham, M.D.[†] Clinical Fellow in Vascular Surgery, Division of Vascular Surgery, Department of Surgery, University of Arizona Health Sciences Center, Tucson, Arizona

D. Preston Flanigan, M.D. Associate Professor of Surgery and Chief, Division of Vascular Surgery, University of Illinois College of Medicine at Chicago, Chicago, Illinois

Present affiliation:
*Research Coordinator, Department of Vascular Surgery, Veterans Administration Medical Center, Tucson, Arizona
[†] Assistant Professor of Surgery, Division of Vascular Surgery, Department of Surgery, University of Illinois College of Medicine at Chicago, Chicago, Illinois

William R. Flinn, M.D. Associate Professor of Surgery, Division of Vascular Surgery, Northwestern University Medical School, Chicago, Illinois

Spencer F. Goodson, M.D. Fellow in Vascular Surgery, Division of Vascular Surgery, University of Illinois College of Medicine at Chicago, Chicago, Illinois

Linda M. Graham, M.D. Assistant Professor of Surgery, Division of Peripheral Vascular Surgery, University of Michigan Medical School; Chief, Vascular Surgery Service, Ann Arbor Veterans Administration Medical Center, Ann Arbor, Michigan

Andris Kazmers, M.D. Assistant Professor of Surgery, Department of Surgery, University of Washington; Assistant Chief, Vascular Surgery Service, Seattle Veterans Administration Medical Center, Seattle, Washington

Walter J. McCarthy III, M.D. Associate in Surgery, Division of Vascular Surgery, Northwestern University Medical School, Chicago, Illinois; Chief, Vascular Surgery, Veterans Administration Lakeside Medical Center, Chicago, Illinois

James M. Malone, M.D. Chief, Vascular Surgery, Tucson Veterans Administration Medical Center; Associate Professor of Surgery, Section of Vascular Surgery, University of Arizona Health Sciences Center, Tucson, Arizona

Allan R. Pasch, M.D. Fellow in Vascular Surgery, Division of Vascular Surgery, University of Illinois College of Medicine at Chicago, Chicago, Illinois

David L. Rollins, M.D. Associate Professor, Division of Vascular Surgery, Department of Surgery, University of Health Sciences/The Chicago Medical School, North Chicago, Illinois

Timothy J. Ryan, M.D.* Assistant Professor of Surgery, Division of Vascular Surgery, Department of Surgery, University of Health Sciences/The Chicago Medical School, North Chicago, Illinois

Gail Sandager, R.N., R.V.T. Assistant Director, Vascular Laboratory, Columbus Hospital, Chicago, Illinois

James J. Schuler, M.D. Associate Professor of Surgery, Division of Vascular Surgery, University of Illinois College of Medicine at Chicago, Chicago, Illinois

---

Present affiliation: Assistant Clinical Professor of Surgery, Department of Surgery, University of Health Sciences/The Chicago Medical School, North Chicago, Illinois

Carolyn Semrow, B.S.E.E.   Research Associate, Division of Vascular Surgery, Department of Surgery, University of Health Sciences/The Chicago Medical School, North Chicago, Illinois

James C. Stanley, M.D.   Professor of Surgery and Head, Division of Peripheral Vascular Surgery, University of Michigan Medical School, Ann Arbor, Michigan

D. Eugene Strandness, Jr., M.D.   Professor of Surgery, Chief, Vascular Surgery Section, Department of Surgery, University of Washington School of Medicine, Seattle, Washington

Brian L. Thiele, M.D., F.R.A.C.S.   Professor of Surgery and Chief, Vascular Surgery, Department of Surgery, The Milton S. Hershey Medical Center, The Pennsylvania State University College of Medicine, Hershey, Pennsylvania

Jonathan B. Towne, M.D.   Professor of Surgery, Department of Surgery, Section of Vascular Surgery, Medical College of Wisconsin, Milwaukee, Wisconsin

Robert L. Vogelzang, M.D.   Assistant Professor of Radiology and Chief, Angiography and Interventional Radiology; Codirector, Division of Body Computerized Tomography, Department of Diagnostic Radiology, Northwestern University Medical School, and Northwestern Memorial Hospital, Chicago, Illinois

Thomas W. Wakefield, M.D.   Assistant Professor of Surgery, Division of Peripheral Vascular Surgery, University of Michigan Medical School, Ann Arbor, Michigan

Larry R. Williams, M.D., M.S.   Assistant Professor of Surgery, Division of Vascular Surgery, University of South Florida, Tampa, Florida; Chief, Division of Vascular Surgery, Department of Surgery, Veterans Administration Medical Center, Bay Pines, Florida

James S. T. Yao, M.D., Ph.D.   Professor of Surgery and Director, Blood Flow Laboratory, Division of Vascular Surgery, Northwestern University Medical School, Chicago, Illinois

Contents

PERIOPERATIVE ASSESSMENT IN VASCULAR SURGERY

Part I
PREOPERATIVE METHODS

1

Noninvasive Arterial Assessment: Differential Diagnosis of Intermittent Claudication

JOHN J. CASTRONUOVO, JR.
Morristown Memorial Hospital
Morristown, New Jersey

INTRODUCTION

The differential diagnosis of intermittent claudication is founded in the history and physical examination. If the clinical presentation of intermittent claudication is atypical, segmental systolic pressures obtained with blood pressure cuff and Doppler ultrasound at rest and after exercise can objectively exclude arterial insufficiency. When it is obvious on physical examination that vascular occlusive disease is present, these same tests can be used to localize the anatomic arterial segment involved. The results can also give some information about the hemodynamic significance of the lesion. If more than one arterial segment is involved, test results can aid in determining the segment primarily responsible for the production of ischemic muscle pain.

DIFFERENTIAL DIAGNOSIS

A significant proportion of patients referred to the vascular surgeon for evaluation of intermittent claudication will not be found to have arterial occlusive disease as the sole cause of their symptoms. A study by Tait found that this was true in 10% of the 456 patients evaluated (1). History and physical examination will identify the majority of these patients.

HISTORY

A patient's young age, variability in the time until onset or relief of claudication, and especially variations in posture required for relief, should alert the clinician to the possibility that atherosclerotic occlusive disease is not the cause of the patient's complaint.

Intermittent claudication is defined as an ischemic muscle pain that occurs after a reproducible period of exercise and subsides after a reproducible period of rest. Warren included the criterion that pain must be relieved by rest in the standing position, to aid in the differentiation of arterial insufficiency from other causes of leg pain occurring in ambulation (2).

PHYSICAL EXAMINATION

The presence of normally palpable pedal pulses with the patient at rest raises the suspicion that the claudication is not vasculogenic. But it must be remembered that subcritical stenosis, that is, a stenosis that is not hemodynamically significant at rest, may become flow limiting with the distal vasodilation caused by walking. DeWeese has pointed out that the pulses must be reexamined after the patient has walked a sufficient distance to reproduce his symptoms (3). The presence of normal pulses after a period of exercise strongly suggests a nonarterial etiology.

NONINVASIVE TESTS

If there is no evidence of a flow-limiting lesion on physical examination, noninvasive tests are used to confirm the examiner's impression. Segmental systolic pressure measurements of the involved extremity with Doppler and appropriately sized blood pressure cuffs will yield normal values when expressed as a ratio (index) of the brachial systolic pressure. Brachial systolic pressures should be measured in both arms and the higher value used if there is a difference in the right and left measurement. The normal ankle brachial index is greater than 1.0. The normal thigh brachial index is 1.1 or greater; values for thigh pressures are affected by the size of the cuff. Normal values given in Table 1 were obtained with a narrow, high thigh cuff 12 cm in width, the low thigh cuff 22 cm, ankle cuff 12 cm, and toe cuff 2-2.5 cm. The pulse volume recorder and mercury-in-silastic strain gauge have also been used to measure segmental systolic limb pressures with the results being applied in the same way.

Stress testing should then be performed. Stress testing eliminates the need to rely on a definition of a normal pressure index determined at rest, in order to exclude arterial stenosis or occlusion. Stress testing is carried out on a treadmill canted at a small grade of 10% at a speed of 1-2 miles per hour. The patient walks

Table 1 Normal values for Doppler arterial examination

Ankle systolic pressure	>Brachial systolic pressure (<40 mmHg = limb-threatening ischemia)
Ankle pressure index (ankle/brachial ratio)	>1.0
Thigh systolic pressure high (narrow cuff) low (wide cuff)	30-40 mmHg > brachial systolic pressure 20-30 mmHg > brachial systolic pressure
Thigh pressure index	>1.1
Pressure gradients	<30 mmHg between adjacent sites
Toe systolic pressure index	0.7 ± 0.19 (0.35 ± 0.15 = claudication), (0.11 ± 0.10 = rest pain)
Penile pressure index	>0.75 (0.60 = vascular impotence)
Finger systolic pressure index	>0.95
Treadmill exercise test (2 mph, 12% grade)	Elevated or no decrease of ankle pressure after 5 min walking time

Source: Reprinted with permission, from Pearce WH, Yao JST, Bergan JJ: Noninvasive vascular diagnostic testing. In Ravitch MM (ed): Curr. Prob. Surg., Vol. 20, No. 8, 1983, p. 480.

for 5 min or until he becomes symptomatic. Ankle systolic pressures are measured immediately and at 1-min intervals for up to 5 min in the supine position. A fall in ankle systolic pressure greater than 20% of the value at rest indicates arterial disease severe enough to cause claudication (4). Results of the postocclusive reactive hyperemia test can be applied in much the same way.

CLINICAL PRESENTATION

The following clinical situations are the most common ones in which noninvasive arterial testing should be used in the differential diagnosis of intermittent claudication. Patients less than 40 years of age, although sometimes found to have atherosclerosis, should be evaluated for popliteal entrapment syndrome. The anomalous course or aberrant insertion of the gastrocnemius compresses the popliteal artery. With ambulation, diminished blood flow to the exercising calf muscle produces claudication. Plantar flexion of the foot will cause a change in the Doppler flow velocity waveform at the dorsalis pedis after this maneuver.

Examination of the pedal pulse with the knee flexed should also be carried out in young claudicants. Adventitial cystic disease of the popliteal artery, usually occurring in males, causes claudication of sudden onset. Knee flexion exacerbates the reduction of luminal diameter caused by the cyst, causing diappearance of the pedal pulse. Noninvasive examination of the popliteal artery with ultrasonic imaging is diagnostic (5). Nonarterial conditions that should be mentioned in the differential diagnosis of intermittent claudication include McArdle's syndrome, venous claudication, peripheral neuropathy (meralgia paresthetica, diabetic neuropathy), vasospastic disorders (especially those resulting from a side effect of medication), and myositis ossificans (6-8).

Muscle phosphorylase deficiency (McArdle's syndrome) causes muscle cramps with exercise. The diagnosis is confirmed by the absence of a rise in venous lactate levels after ischemic exercise of the arm. Severe calf pain on walking can develop after ileofemoral thrombosis. Venous hypertension is the cause of "venous" claudication that is not relieved in the standing position. Myositis ossificans developing after trauma produces pain on ambulation which ceases when the patient stands still. Diagnosis is based on a history of trauma and the presence of soft tissue calcification on X-ray in the affected muscle group. Arthritis usually produces periarticular pain but may be difficult to distinguish from intermittent claudication if the patient has difficulty localizing the pain to the joints. The pain may begin so rapidly after the patient starts to walk that muscle exercise cannot be implicated.

Intermittent claudication caused by arterial occlusive disease usually involves the calf and thigh muscles. Intermittent claudication can also be present in the buttocks (Leriche Syndrome) and the small muscles in the foot (thromboangitis obliterans and tibial vessel occlusive disease).

Buttock and foot pain occurring with ambulation can be confused with intermittent claudication. Morton's neuroma causes foot pain when the patient puts pressure on the foot, but a tender mass between metatarsalphalangeal joints can be identified by palpation. Radiating low back pain can stimulate buttock claudication. When a herniated disk is the cause, the onset of the symptom is typically sudden, often developing after injury and accentuated by flexion of the spine, coughing, and straining. This presentation is not often confused with vasculogenic intermittent claudication, but there is a form of spinal nerve compression with a more insidious onset—spinal stenosis or neurogenic intermittent claudication.

Neurogenic intermittent claudication is caused by narrowing of the vertebral canal. It occurs congenitally, after trauma or surgery, and secondary to degenerative disease of the spine. Compression of the spinal cord, nerve roots, and especially the cauda equina can produce leg pain on ambulation relieved by rest. A number of reports have established neurogenic intermittent claudication as the most difficult diagnostic entity to differentiate from vasculogenic intermittent claudication (9-11).

Patients less than 40 years old with neurogenic intermittent claudication are likely to have a posttraumatic or congenital type of spinal stenosis. The degenerative type of spinal stenosis occurs in patients in their 60s and 70s (12). This population has a higher prevalence of arterial occlusive disease, and the two conditions may coexist, a situation that may be discovered only after the unsuccessful treatment of the vascular or neuroskeletal condition (13). The knowledge that a 20% drop in ankle systolic pressure after treadmill testing is sufficient to produce vasculogenic claudication can be employed in differentiating the relative contribution of each disorder in such patients (4). Noninvasive arterial testing is clearly of value in reaching the proper diagnosis in these patients.

Noninvasive arterial tests are useful, but are not a substitute for a careful history and physical examination in the evaluation of neurogenic intermittent claudication. The quality of the pain, more often described as burning or numbing, with a variable and often short walking distance are in contrast to the claudication caused by occlusive vascular disease. Relief from neurogenic intermittent claudication is not always obtained by standing and the seated or recumbent position may be required. Straight leg raising and hyperextension of the spine may reproduce symptoms but neurologic examination is usually not helpful in the diagnosis of neurogenic intermittent claudication (14). Computerized tomography of the spine is used to make the diagnosis of spinal stenosis (15). Other diagnostic aids are lumbosacral spine films, electromyography, and myelography. We have recommended a schema for the sequence in which these tests should be performed (16) (see Fig. 1).

ANATOMIC AND HEMODYNAMIC EVALUATION OF CLAUDICATION

Although the presence or absence of arterial occlusive disease can accurately be documented by noninvasive arterial assessment, results of the Doppler segmental systolic pressure tests can also be used to localize the lesion to an arterial segment: aortoiliac, femoropopliteal, or tibial. Comparison of the high and low thigh, calf, and ankle pressures will identify the segment that produces the pressure drop. A drop from the thigh to the calf is indicative of femoropoplital occlusion. A drop in pressure from the calf to the ankle indicates tibial disease. When the thigh and calf systolic pressure indices are equally diminished, either femoropopliteal and/or aortoiliac disease may be the cause. Exercise testing will yield abnormal results in both situations.

Noninvasive arterial tests give the most specific results when applied to questions of differential diagnosis because the presence or absence of arterial occlusive disease can be determined accurately. Analyzing the results of resting segmental pressures and indices to localize the involved arterial segment and to characterize the hemodynamic significance of a given segment in multisegmental occlusive disease is more problematic. This is due to several factors, the most significant of which is the fact that arteriographic data itself is subject to interpretation and may not represent the standard against which noninvasive studies should be compared.

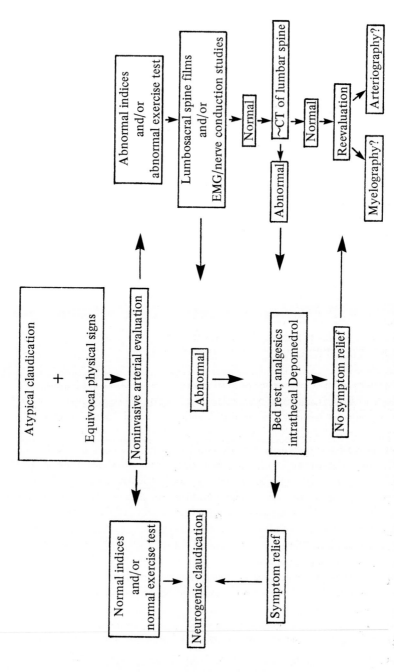

Figure 1   Algorithm for the differentiation of vascular and neurogenic claudication.

Interpretation of segmental pressure measurements is limited by several other factors. Intraindividual variation of segmental pressure values has been studied and is small enough that a change in ankle brachial index of 0.15 is considered significant (17,18). A pressure gradient between two segments of >30 mmHg indicates occlusion in the vessel between those segments. A difference of 15 mmHg between the right and left legs at the same level is also considered evidence of occlusive disease (19).

A significant proportion of diabetic patients will have incompressible vessels due to calcification of the artery wall. Segmental systolic pressures will be spuriously elevated and uninterpretable.

The main limitation of segmental pressures in localizing the diseased segment is caused by the fact that a diminished thigh pressure may reflect either aortoiliac or femoropopliteal (superficial femoral artery) disease. Stress tests are also abnormal in both situations. There is some evidence to suggest that the time taken for the decreased ankle pressure to return to baseline after exercise can be used to differentiate femoropopliteal (5 min), aortoiliac (5-15 min), and multisegment occlusion (>15 min) (20). Common femoral artery waveform analysis can help in identifying aortoiliac lesions. Simple visual inspection of the recording strip can identify loss of the normal triphasic Doppler flow velocity waveform, and should cause suspicion that a decreased thigh pressure is not due to superficial femoral artery occlusion, and that aortoiliac stenosis may be present.

New techniques that evaluate the common femoral Doppler velocity waveform by computerized mathematical analysis are the Pulsatility Index, Laplace Damping Factor, and Principal Component Analysis. Doppler duplex scanning with spectral frequency analysis may also be found to be of help in differentiating aortoiliac from femoropopliteal contributions to the symptom of claudication (19,21,22). Rutherford and others have reported an improved diagnostic accuracy when several methods of noninvasive arterial testing are applied to the common femoral artery to assess aortoiliac disease (23). Our current practice is inspection of the femoral artery flow velocity waveform and segmental systolic pressures to evaluate the aortoiliac segment.

Invasive methods such as intraarterial pressure measurements at arteriography or preoperatively in the context of a Papaverine test are probably the standard against which arteriography and noninvasive test should be compared (21).

Currently available noninvasive tests are of limited value in the assessment of multisegmental occlusive disease. Femoral pulse palpation and auscultation are an essential part of the evaluation of such patients but are also inaccurate, especially in obese patients. The male patient's sexual history is relevant and vasculogenic impotence is an indication of aortoiliac disease. Noninvasive testing with Doppler or photoplethysmography demonstrating a penile/brachial systolic pressure index of less than 0.60 correlates well with internal iliac artery occlusion. Impotence is a presenting complaint of 25% of patients with aortoiliac disease (24).

When more than one arterial segment is involved, noninvasive arterial assessment is used to supplement the interpretation of findings on physical examination and angiography. Fortunately, most patients with intermittent claudication have stenosis or occlusion in a single arterial segment. The femoropopliteal segment is most often the site of the lesion.

The benign course of superficial femoral artery occlusion is well documented (25). The prognosis for limb survival is even more favorable in patients with isolated aortoiliac disease (26). Results of aortoiliac reconstruction, while excellent, are associated with a small but real operative mortality rate. Localization of the diseased segment is essential in defining the risks and benefits of reconstructive surgery to a given patient. If only those patients likely to undergo surgery are to be subjected to arteriography, new methods must be sought to evaluate the aortoiliac segment.

CONCLUSION

Noninvasive arterial testing is a valuable adjunct in the differential diagnosis of intermittent claudication. In patients with occlusive disease limited to a single level, noninvasive tests can often localize the segment, providing anatomic as well as hemodynamic information. In multilevel occlusive disease, noninvasive tests may be of help in evaluating the relative contribution of each segment to the patient's symptoms, but their use is limited and an improved method with a high accuracy is needed to evaluate the status of the aortoiliac segment in patients with superficial femoral artery disease.

REFERENCES

1. Tait WF, Charlesworth D, Lemon JG: Atypical claudication. Br J Surg 72: 315, 1985.
2. Warren R: Two kinds of intermittent claudication. Arch Surg 111:739, 1976.
3. DeWeese JA: Pedal pulses disappearing with exercise: A test for intermittent claudication. N Engl J Med 262:1214, 1961.
4. Yao JST, Hobbs JT, Irvine WT: Ankle systolic pressure measurements in arterial disease affecting the lower extremities. Br J Surg 56:676, 1969.
5. Flanigan DP, Burnham SJ, Goodreau JJ, and Bergan JJ: Summary of cases of adventitial cystic disease of the popliteal artery. Ann Surg 189:165, 1979.
6. McArdle B: Myopathy due to a defect in muscular glycogen breakdown. Clin Sci 10:13, 1951.
7. Bjordal RI: Intermittent venous claudication. Acta Chir Scand 136:641, 1970.
8. Abramson DI, Miller DS: Vascular Problems in Musculoskeletal Disorders of the Limbs, New York, Springer-Verlag, p. 136, 1981.
9. Verbiest H: A radicular syndrome from developmental narrowing of the lumbar vertebral canal. J Bone Joint Surg (Br.) 326:230, 1954.

10. Bergmark G: Intermittent spinal claudication. Acta Med Scand 246 (Suppl): 30, 1950.
11. Evans JG: Neurogenic intermittent claudication. Br Med J 2:985, 1964.
12. Wilson CB, Ehni G, Grollmus J: Neurogenic intermittent claudication. Clin Neurosurg 18:62, 1971.
13. Kirkaldy-Willis WH, Paine KWE, Cauchoix J, McIvor G: Lumbar spinal stenosis. Clin Orthop Rel Res 99:30, 1974.
14. Paine KWE: Clinical features of lumbar spinal stenosis. Clin Orthop Rel Res 115:77, 1976.
15. Landcourt JE, Glenn WV Jr., Wiltse LL: Multiplanar computerized tomography in the normal spine and in the diagnosis of spinal stenosis. A gross anatomic-computerized tomographic correlation. Spine 4:4, 1979.
16. Castronuovo JJ Jr., Flanigan DP: Pseudoclaudication of neurospinal origin. Vascular Diagnosis and Therapy 5:21, 1984.
17. Baker JD, Dix D: Variability of Doppler ankle pressures with arterial occlusive disease: An evaluation of ankle index and brachial-ankle pressure gradient. Surgery 89:134, 1981.
18. Pearce WH, Yao JST, Bergan JJ: Noninvasive vascular diagnostic testing. In Ravitch MM (ed): Current Problems in Surgery, Vol. XX, No. 8, 1983, pp. 468-469.
19. Jager KA, Langlois Y, Roederer GO, Strandness DE: Noninvasive assessment of lower extremity ischemia. In Gergan JJ and Yao JST (eds): Evaluation and Treatment of Upper and Lower Extremity Circulatory Disorders, Grune & Stratton, Orlando FL, 1984, p. 109.
20. Nicolaides AN: The preoperative selection of patients—What must the surgeon know. In Berstein EF (ed): Noninvasive Diagnostic Techniques in Vascular Disease, CV Mosby, St. Louis, 1982, p. 314.
21. Johnston KW, Kassam M, Cobbold RSC: Relationship between Doppler pulsatility index and direct femoral pressure measurements in the diagnosis of aortoiliac occlusive disease. Ultrasound Med Biol 9:271, 1983.
22. MacPherson DS, Evans DH, Bell PRF: Common femoral artery Doppler waveforms: A comparison of three methods of objective analysis with direct pressure measurements. Br J Surg 71:46, 1984.
23. Rutherford RB, Lowenstein DH, Klein MF: Combining segmental systolic pressures and plethysmography to diagnose arterial occlusive disease of the legs. Am J Surg 138:211, 1979.
24. Leriche R, Morel A: The syndrome of thrombotic obliteration of the aortic bifurcation. Ann Surg 127:193, 1948.
25. Imparato AM, Kim GE, Davidson T, Crowley JG: Intermittent claudication: Its natural course. Surgery 78:795, 1975.
26. Juergens JL, Barker NW, Hines EA Jr: Arteriosclerosis obliterans: Review of 520 cases with special reference to pathogenic and prognostic factors. Circulation 21:188, 1960.

2

Prediction of Increase in Distal Perfusion Pressure Following Revascularization

LARRY R. WILLIAMS

University of South Florida
Tampa, Florida

Veterans Administration Medical Center
Bay Pines, Florida

In patients with lower extremity ischemic symptoms due to one hemodynamically significant arterial occlusive lesion, operative treatment is relatively straightforward. Appropriate bypass of the offending lesion results in relief of the hemodynamic abnormality. Distal perfusion pressure returns to normal and relief of symptoms is prompt.

Unfortunately this situation is not commonly the case. Lower extremity atherosclerosis tends to be multisegmental in nature. The development of ischemic symptoms is ordinarily due to the presence of several lesions of varying hemodynamic significance in series. The key to appropriate management of the patient with these multisegmental arterial occlusive lesions thus lies in the ability to determine which lesion or which arterial segment is most responsible for the hemodynamic abnormality. Following this, selection of an appropriate revascularization procedure is required to correct the abnormality.

Advances in investigative methods such as segmental Doppler-derived blood pressure measurements, exercise testing, reactive hyperemia, and pharmacologic vasodilatation with percutaneous arterial pressure measurements have made a significant impact on the hemodynamic evaluation of lower extremity arterial occlusive disease. In addition, multiplanar angiographic techniques have made a significant contribution to the total evaluation of the extremity arterial system.

Although these sophisticated evaluations have proven tremendously important in terms of selecting the appropriate revascularization procedure, determination of the ability of the proposed bypass to correct the hemodynamic abnormality remains of equal importance. This chapter will address some of the many factors that have been utilized to predict the success of lower extremity bypass grafting. In addition, a method for quantitatively predicting the improvement in lower extremity perfusion pressure following arterial bypass will be presented.

PREDICTION OF SUCCESS FOLLOWING ARTERIAL BYPASS

Many different attempts have been made to predict the success of various revascularization procedures. In patients undergoing lower extremity arterial bypass, the usual end points that have been evaluated have been relief of symptoms, limb salvage, or graft patency rates. Symptom relief and avoidance of amputation are ordinarily dependent upon bypass graft patency. Therefore, most authors have focused mainly on factors and methods by which bypass graft patency can be predicted.

Patient Risk Factors

It is generally accepted that multiple clinical factors in any particular patient may, in combination, represent a specific "risk" for lower extremity bypass. Although the overall outcome may at times be predicted on the basis of clinical risk, attempts to classify individuals and predict graft failure by this means have not been possible. Couch et al. (1), in an analysis of femoropopliteal bypasses, suggested that diabetics have unacceptably high graft thrombosis rates. Stipa and Wheelock (2), however, in a series of 73 diabetic and 67 nondiabetic patients, showed no significant difference between the two groups in terms of early graft patency. Several more recent studies on large numbers of patients likewise have failed to demonstrate an ability to predict the success of femoropopliteal bypasses based on the clinical risk factor of diabetes (3,4).

Bouhoutsos and Martin (5), in an analysis of infrainguinal bypass in 300 nondiabetic patients, described patient age as a predictor of bypass graft failure. They found that with advancing age, bypass patency rates increased. They suggested that younger patients might have worse prognoses due to more aggressive atherosclerosis. This trend toward increased patency rates in patients with more advanced age has not been supported by others, and is not felt to be a predictor of bypass success.

Several series of both suprainguinal and infrainguinal bypasses have found higher graft patency rates for patients whose operations were performed for symptoms of claudication when compared with symptoms of more severe ischemia, such as rest pain or gangrene (3,4,6). Miller (7), in an analysis of 156 patients, found no difference between patients treated for complaints of claudication when compared with patients with rest pain or gangrene. DeWeese et al. (8) likewise have shown that the presence or absence of actual tissue loss was not predictive of early graft failure. Whereas smoking and the presence of hypertension have been considered as risk factors by most investigators, controlled studies have failed to demonstrate an ability to predict early graft thrombosis based on these two clinical parameters.

Angiographic Criteria

Angiographic status of the runoff vessels is commonly used as a predictor of lower extremity bypass graft success. DeWeese and Rob (8) evaluated 113 femoropopliteal bypass grafts and found significantly better early and late graft patency rates in patients with two or more patent tibial vessels. Dean et al. (10) likewise documented higher graft patency rates in patients with better angiographic estimation of runoff in a series of 115 femoropopliteal vein grafts. Koontz et al. (9) and Kaminski et al. (10), on the other hand, do not support this concept and have shown no significant difference in patency rates on the basis of the number of outflow vessels.

Imparato et al. (11) have suggested that the presence of a patent pedal arch is a critical factor in predicting femorodistal bypass graft patency. They found that an early graft patency rate of 87% was achieved when the plantar arch, as visualized on angiography, was classified as intact. O'Mara et al. (12) analyzed foot arterial anatomy in detail in 56 distal bypass operations and found that single-plane angiographic views as analyzed by Imparato were inadequate to assess totally the pedal arterial anatomy. Multiple planar views and the demonstration of primary and/or secondary pedal arterial arches were found to be much better prognostic indicators in femorodistal bypass. In 14 of 16 limbs (87.5%) without a patent primary or secondary pedal arch, bypass grafts to the infrapopliteal vessels failed within 30 days. In 40 limbs with intact primary and/or secondary pedal arches, however, only five grafts failed within the first 30 days postoperatively.

Therefore the angiographic delineation of outflow vessels, particularly with regard to pedal arterial anatomy in patients undergoing bypass to the infrapopliteal vessels, may be predictive of early graft patency. It must be kept in mind, however, that the angiographic display of patent vessels is purely anatomic and does not provide information relative to the hemodynamics of distal arterial perfusion. Thus the adequacy of increased distal perfusion is not predicted by angiography. In addition, in patients undergoing more proximal arterial reconstructions the angiographic appearance of the distalmost circulation becomes less important and has not been found to be a significant factor in predicting either patency or hemodynamic success of revascularization.

Graft Material

Although there are many studies comparing the relative merits of various bypass grafting materials, it has not been convincingly demonstrated that early bypass graft patency can be predicted on the basis of the graft material utilized.

Ricco et al. (13) analyzed multiple factors contributing to bypass patency in 204 femorotibial bypasses. They found that the only identifiable predictive factor was the type of graft material utilized. Patients receiving autogenous saphenous vein bypasses had significantly better 1-year patency rates when compared with polytetrafluoroethylene (63% vs. 31%).

Bennion et al. (6) analyzed 102 patients undergoing infrainguinal bypass for advanced ischemia. The overall patency rates for autogenous saphenous vein was slightly better than polytetrafluoroethylene grafts. (6 months: 62.1% vs. 51.4%; 36 months: 50.5% vs. 25.0%). However, in a group of 51 patients who were randomized prospectively to autogenus saphenous vein or polytetrafluoroethylene, there was no statistically significant difference in early or late patency (6 months: 62.1% vs. 51.4%; 18 months: 51.5% vs. 34.3%). Regardless of the influence (or lack of influence) of bypass graft material on eventual patency rates, prediction of the immediate hemodynamic outcome based on graft material is not possible.

Multivariate Analyses

Hiatt et al. (14), in a sophisticated analysis of 34 potential predictive variables on 199 patients undergoing infrainguinal bypass, developed a mathematical model in an attempt to predict bypass graft patency. Multiple patient characteristics, angiographic estimation of distal runoff, Doppler-derived segmental pressure measurements, and physical examination of the limb were analyzed. Stepwise regression analysis allowed the creation of a mathematical model. The six factors that most markedly influenced bypass graft patency, in order of importance, included technical errors at operation, poor angiographic runoff, previous ipsilateral femoropopliteal bypass, clinical estimation of probable amputation level, concurrent proximal reconstruction, and the level of the distal anastomosis. Other variables, including ankle brachial Doppler index, graft material, and the presence of tissue loss, were mildly predictive when analyzed as single variables, however, they did not add to the predictive power of the mathematical model. In an attempt to validate this mathematical model, 67 patients were evaluated prospectively. Thirteen of the 67 patients (20%) had incorrect predictions of eventual outcome. Of eight patients with early graft thromboses, three were predicted; however, five were not. In 59 patients with eventually successful results, eight were predicted preoperatively to fail. Hiatt's conclusions were that there was no way to predict, on the basis of the multiple clinical factors analyzed, which grafts would fail in the early postoperative period. They further concluded that aggressive operative approaches with attempts to perfect technique using complete intraoperative assessments was the key to extending infrainguinal bypass graft patency success.

DOPPLER-DERIVED SEGMENTAL PRESSURES

Thus, a variety of clinical methods for predicting the success of lower extremity bypass based on graft patency have provided conclusions that are at significant variance. A method that would provide a quantitative means of predicting the hemodynamic results of a given bypass would be useful (15). Since lower extremity, Doppler-derived blood pressure measurements are easily obtained and widely utilized as a measure of lower extremity occlusive disease (16-18), this hemodynamic measure may be particularly useful in predicting the outcome of lower extremity bypass procedures.

Method for Aortofemoral Bypass

In patients undergoing aortofemoral bypass, the expected increase in extremity/brachial blood pressure index can be calculated for any particular level of the extremity (high or low thigh, calf, or ankle). This requires preoperative direct percutaneous measurement of the common femoral artery pressure as well as indirect measurement of the extremity pressures at the level of interest with an occluding cuff and sphygmomanometer. This is best accomplished by utilizing Doppler-derived, segmental, lower extremity blood pressures.

A relatively safe assumption is that any hemodynamically significant aortoiliac stenosis will be corrected by the aortofemoral bypass. Thus, the femoral artery/brachial artery pressure index should be elevated to 1.0 postoperatively. If nothing is done to influence any distal hemodynamic abnormality, then the postoperative pressure index at any level in the lower extremity should be increased by the same percentage that the femoral pressure index is elevated. This calculation is illustrated in Figure 1. The simplified equation demonstrates that ankle/brachial indices to be expected following aortofemoral bypass at either the dorsalis pedis or posterior tibial artery can be predicted by dividing the preoperative ankle/brachial index by the femoral/brachial index.

Method for Infrainguinal Bypass

The expected post-bypass ankle/brachial indices in patients undergoing femoropopliteal or femorotibial bypass can be calculated in a similar manner. Assuming that there is no hemodynamically significant aortoiliac stenosis (this can be documented by direct femoral artery pressure measurement), the pressure at the distal end of the bypass should be elevated to systemic (extremity/brachial index = 1.0). In patients undergoing femoropopliteal bypass, calculations for both the dorsalis pedis and posterior tibial arteries can be made by increasing the pre-bypass ankle/brachial indices by the same percentage that the low thigh/brachial index would increase if it were 1.0 post-bypass (Fig. 2). For femorotibial artery bypasses, expected ankle/brachial indices can be calculated only for the bypassed vessel, whereas for femoroperoneal artery bypasses, calculations for both the dorsalis pedis and posterior tibial arteries can be made. As shown in Figure 3, if the below knee/brachial index is increased to 1.0, the same percentage increase should be realized in the ankle brachial index.

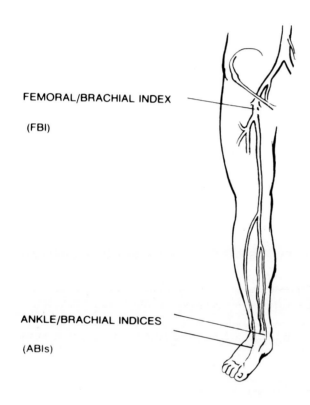

FEMORAL/BRACHIAL INDEX

(FBI)

ANKLE/BRACHIAL INDICES

(ABIs)

$$\text{PREDICTED ABI} = \frac{\text{ABI}}{\text{FBI}} \times 1.00$$

Figure 1 Illustration of the method for calculating the expected increase in ankle/brachial index following aortofemoral bypass.

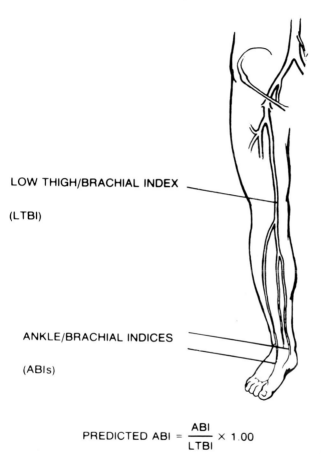

LOW THIGH/BRACHIAL INDEX

(LTBI)

ANKLE/BRACHIAL INDICES

(ABIs)

$$\text{PREDICTED ABI} = \frac{\text{ABI}}{\text{LTBI}} \times 1.00$$

Figure 2 Calculation of the predicted ankle/brachial index in patients undergoing femoropopliteal bypass.

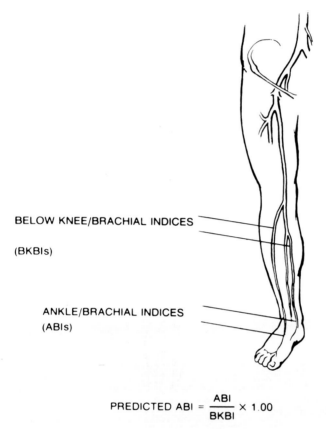

$$\text{PREDICTED ABI} = \frac{\text{ABI}}{\text{BKBI}} \times 1.00$$

Figure 3 Calculation of the ankle/brachial index to be expected following femorotibial or femoroperoneal bypass.

THE UNIVERSITY OF ILLINOIS EXPERIENCE

In an attempt to validate the calculation for prediction of improvement in ankle blood pressures, an analysis of patients undergoing lower extremity arterial bypass was performed. Two-hundred sixty-six patients with complete lower extremity, segmental, Doppler-derived blood pressure measurements pre- and postoperatively were analyzed. Seventy-seven patients underwent aortofemoral bypass and 149 patients underwent infrainguinal bypass grafting. In all patients undergoing aortofemoral bypass, preoperative evaluation included direct femoral artery pressure measurements either percutaneously or under direct vision in the operating room. All pressures were recorded as ratios of the systemic pressure, which was estimated by brachial cuff pressure measurement.

Expected increases in ankle/brachial indices were calculated as described previously in this chapter. The expected ankle/brachial indices were then compared with the ankle/brachial indices actually obtained postoperatively for both aorto-femoral and infrainguinal bypass groups.

In patients undergoing aortofemoral bypass, there was a strong correlation between the predicted ankle/brachial index and the actual post-bypass ankle/brachial index (r = 0.8735) (Fig. 4). Of the 49 ankle/brachial indices analyzed, only 2 (4%) did not increase to within 0.10 of the predicted index.

Patients receiving infrainguinal bypasses had a moderate correlation between the predicted ankle/brachial index and the actual post-bypass ankle/brachial index (r = 0.5961) (Fig. 5). The reason for this lower correlation was that 75% of the post-bypass ankle/brachial indices were greater than predicted. Of 134 ankle/brachial indices analyzed, only 9% did not increase to within 0.10 of that predicted.

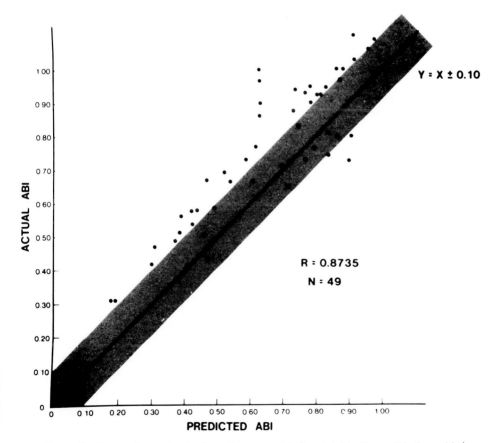

Figure 4 Comparison of actual postbypass ankle/brachial indices with the ankle/brachial indices predicted from preoperative pressure measurements for patients undergoing aortofemoral bypass.

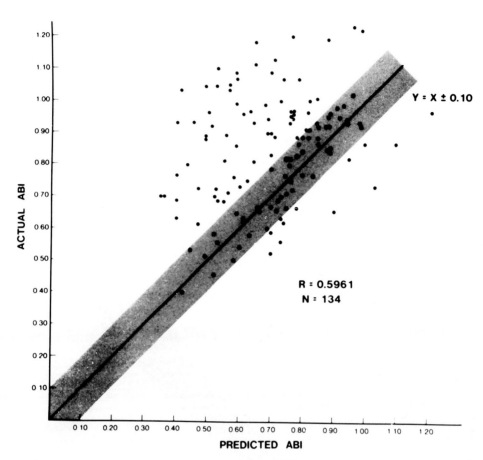

Figure 5   Actual post-bypass ankle/brachial indices compared with predicted indices for infrainguinal bypasses.

LIMITATIONS

One limitation encountered in predicting the ankle/brachial index to be expected post-bypass, is that ankle/brachial indices cannot be calculated if the pre-bypass proximal index is greater than 1.0. This usually does not pose a significant problem, however, since little change should be expected in the proximal pressure index post-bypass if it is already at the systemic level. It follows then that no significant change in ankle/brachial index should be expected post-bypass.

In addition, post-bypass ankle/brachial indices cannot be predicted in patients with no measureable blood pressure at the ankle preoperatively. Although previous authors have suggested that infrainguinal bypasses done with ankle/brachial indices of less than 0.20 will fail uniformly, our experience has been much more favorable.

Table 1 Patients with No Detectable Ankle Pressure
Preoperatively

Bypass	N^a	No. with ABI Postop[b]	Mean ABI
Aortofemoral	25	20 (80%)	0.75
Infrainguinal	13	12 (92%)	0.80

[a] N = Number with no detectable ankle blood pressure preoperatively.
[b] ABI = Ankle/brachial index.

Specifically, for patients undergoing aortofemoral bypass in this series, no detectable flow was recorded preoperatively in 25 pedal vessels (Table 1). Twenty of these vessels (80%) had a measureable pressure post-bypass, with a mean ankle/brachial index of 0.75.

For patients receiving infrainguinal bypass, in 13 pedal vessels with no detectable flow preoperatively, 12 (92%) had a measureable pressure post-bypass. The mean ankle/brachial index was 0.80. Thus, the expected post-bypass ankle/brachial index, as calculated from preoperative hemodynamic criteria, is a predictor of the minimum improvement to be expected. In the majority of cases, greater increases in ankle/brachial index will be realized. This is especially true in patients with no detectable pressure in the pedal vessels preoperatively.

The ability to predict the minimum increases in ankle/brachial indices make it possible to determine those patients who require bypass of only one proximal arterial segment to provide an adequate increase in ankle blood pressure. Since greater increases are often realized, one cannot decide only on the basis of ankle/brachial index, which patients require distal reconstruction in combination with more proximal bypass.

REFERENCES

1. Couch NP, Wheeler HB, Hyatt DF, et al: Factors influencing limb survival after femoropopliteal reconstruction. Arch Surg 95:163-169, 1967.
2. Stipa S, Wheelock FC: A comparison of femoral artery grafts in diabetic and nondiabetic patients. Am J Surg 121:223, 1971.
3. Reichle FA, Shuman CR, Tyson RR: Femorotibial bypass in the diabetic patient for salvage of the ischemic lower extremity. Am J Surg 129:603-605, 1975.
4. Dean RH, Yao JST, Stanton PE, Bergan JJ: Prognostic indicators in femoropopliteal reconstructions. Arch Surg 110:1287-1293, 1975.

5. Bouhoutsos J, Martin P: The influence of age on prognosis after arterial surgery for atherosclerosis of the lower limb. Surgery 74:637, 1973.

6. Bennion RS, Williams RA, Stabile BE, Fox MA, Owens ML, Wilson SE: Patency of autogenous saphenous vein versus polytetrafluoroethylene grafts in femoropopliteal bypass for advanced ischemia of the extremity. Surg Gynecol Obstet 160:239-242, 1985.

7. Miller VM: Femoropopliteal bypass graft patency: An analysis of 156 cases. Ann Surg 180:35, 1974.

8. DeWeese JA, Rob CG: Autogenous venous bypass grafts five years later. Ann Surg 174:346, 1974.

9. Koontz TS, Stansel HC: Factors influencing patency of the autogenous vein-femoropopliteal bypass graft: An analysis of 74 cases. Surgery 71:753, 1972.

10. Kaminski DL, Barner HB, Dorighiu JA, et al: Femoropopliteal bypass with reversed autogenous saphenous vein. Ann Surg 177:232, 1973.

11. Imparato AM, Kim GE, Madayag M, Haveson S: Angiographic criteria for successful tibial arterial reconstruction. Surgery 74:830-838, 1973.

12. O'Mara CS, Flinn WR, Neiman HL, Bergan JJ, Yao JST: Correlation of foot arterial anatomy with early tibial bypass patency. Surgery 89:743-752, 1981.

13. Ricco JB, Flinn WR, McDaniel MD, Yao JST, Bergan JJ: Objective analysis of factors contributing to failure of tibial bypass grafts. World J Surg 7:347-352, 1983.

14. Hiatt JG, Raviola C, Baker JD, Busuttil RW, Machleden HI, Moore WS: The limitations of predictability of success of femoral-popliteal bypass grafts. J Vasc Surg 1, 617-622, 1984.

15. Williams LR, Flanigan DP, Schuler JJ, O'Connor RJA, Castronuovo JJ: Prediction of improvement in ankle blood pressure following arterial bypass. J Surg Res 37:175-179, 1984.

16. Yao JST, Hobbs JT, Irvine WT: Ankle systolic pressure measurements in arterial disease affecting the lower extremities. Br J Surg 56:676-679, 1969.

17. O'Donnell TF, Lakey SJ, Kelly JJ, Ransil BJ, Millan VG, Korwin S, Callow AD: A prospective study of Doppler pressures and segmental plethysmography before and following aortofemoral bypass. Surgery 86:120-129, 1979.

18. Carson JD, Johnson WC, LoGerfo FW, Bush HL, Menzoian JO, Kumaki DJ, Nasbeth DC: Doppler ankle systolic blood pressure: Prognostic value in vein bypass grafts of the lower extremity. Arch Surg 113:932-935, 1978.

3

Tests for Selection of Patients for Suprainguinal versus Infrainguinal Bypass

D. PRESTON FLANIGAN
University of Illinois College of Medicine at Chicago
Chicago, Illinois

Many patients who require revascularization for lower extremity ischemia have arterial occlusive disease affecting only one of the three lower extremity arterial segments (aortoiliac, femoropopliteal, or tibial). In these patients, disease localization can be determined simply by history and physical examination. Arteriograms performed in these patients are usually just confirmatory and offer a "road map" to the surgeon in planning the details of the revascularization procedure. Other patients, usually those with worse ischemia, have disease affecting two or more arterial segments, and often neither the physical examination nor the arteriogram are adequate to assess the significance of the disease in each segment. Several non-invasive tests have been applied to this problem, but they have not been able to determine the need for suprainguinal versus infrainguinal revascularization in patients with combined aortoiliac and femoropopliteal disease.

Traditional teaching has been that in the presence of combined segment disease the more proximal segment should be bypassed as an initial step since an infrainguinal bypass below a diseased aortoiliac segment might thrombose because of inadequate inflow. Traditionally, the assessment of the adequacy of inflow has been made on the basis of femoral pulse palpation and arteriography, yet, using these methods, 10-15% of patients having aortofemoral bypass require subsequent downstream repair for relief of ischemia (1). Some of these repairs are required for disease progression whereas others are required because of lack of improvement following inflow revascularization.

More recently, minimally invasive techniques have been used to determine the need for suprainguinal versus infrainguinal revascularization (2-13). These techniques have employed intraarterial pressure measurements during rest and with

25

induction of vasodilatation. Although these latter methods are not perfect, they have allowed for significant improvement in the selection of the best revascularization procedure in patients with multisegment disease. Using these methods, early hemodynamic failure of a properly performed operation has been rare (3).

This chapter will delineate and discuss the various methods of selection of patients for suprainguinal versus infrainguinal bypass so that the reader will become well versed in the proper application and interpretation of the tests.

HISTORY AND PHYSICAL EXAMINATION

Patients with single-segment disease affecting the aortoiliac or femoropopliteal segment usually present with claudication rather than with more severe ischemic symptoms. Exceptions to this principle are acute occlusions and, occasionally, juxtarenal aortic occlusion. Patients with single segment tibial vessel disease often remain asymptomatic until rest symptoms develop, although with proximal tibial artery occlusions, claudication may be present. Patients with multisegment disease usually present with rest pain, ischemic ulceration, or gangrene.

Localization of single-segment disease by pulse palpation is usually not diffcult. One occasional exception is the patient with true vasculogenic claudication who has normal pulses to palpation. Such patients usually have a proximal infrarenal aortic stenosis that only becomes hemodynamically significant with exercise. De-Weese has termed this the disappearing pulse phenomenon, since pulses will no longer be papable following walking to the point of claudication (Fig. 1) (14). Recently, we have seen this same phenomenon in vigorous walkers who have no aortoiliac disease but who were found to have tight stenosis of the superficial femoral artery.

In patients with combined aortoiliac and femoropopliteal disease, selection of suprainguinal versus infrainguinal bypass traditionally is based on palpation of the common femoral pulse. Pulse palpation is a subjective test and, therefore, open to interpretation. Several authors have evaluated the accuracy of femoral pulse palpation in comparison to intraarterial pressure measurements with poor results (15-17). Sobinsky determined that the overall accuracy for the test was only 61%. In his study, a normal pulse to palpation correctly identified the absence of hemodynamically significant aortoiliac disease at rest 100% of the time. However, the positive predictive value of an abnormal pulse was only 29% (15). Johnston, on the other hand, found femoral pulse palpation neither sensitive nor specific (16). Thus, it would appear that although pulse palpation can be an important first step in the localization of lower extremity arterial occlusive disease it is not sufficiently accurate to determine the hemodynamic significance of aortoiliac disease in all cases and therefore is an inadequate test for the selection of suprainguinal versus infrainguinal bypass in patients with multisegment disease.

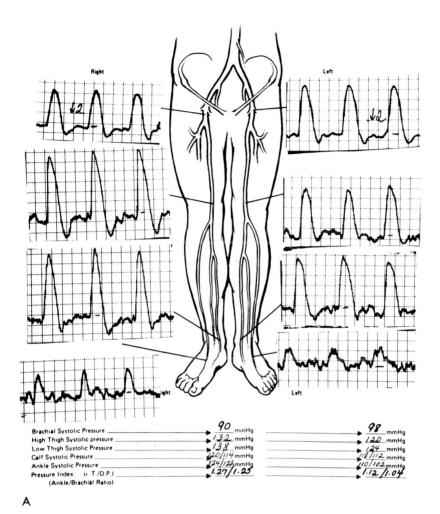

Brachial Systolic Pressure	90 mmHg	98 mmHg
High Thigh Systolic pressure	132 mmHg	120 mmHg
Low Thigh Systolic Pressure	138 mmHg	124 mmHg
Calf Systolic Pressure	120/114 mmHg	118/112 mmHg
Ankle Systolic Pressure	124/122 mmHg	110/102 mmHg
Pressure Index: (t.T./D.P.)	1.27/1.25	1.12/1.04
(Ankle/Brachial Ratio)		

A

Figure 1A Normal lower extremity Doppler examination except for an abnormal waveform at the left dorsalis pedis artery in a patient with claudication. All four foot pulses were palpable.

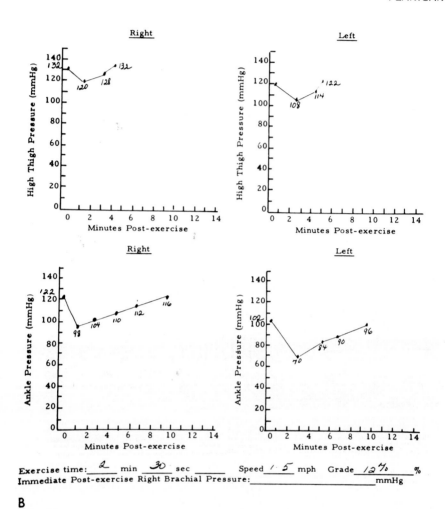

Figure 1B Exercise test showing severe reductions in lower extremity pressures with only 2.5 min of treadmill exercise.

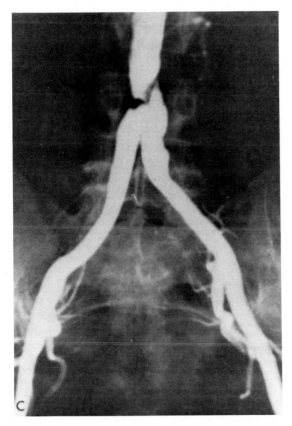

Figure 1C Aortogram in the same patient showing an aortic stenosis. This patient's symptoms were completely relieved by aortofemoral bypass.

ARTERIOGRAPHY

Arteriography generally has been used to verify physical findings and to help in planning the specifics of a revascularization procedure. This approach has been based on the belief that arteriography could determine the severity of the arterial occlusive process. In general, lesions causing greater than a 50% diameter stenosis are considered hemodynamically significant whereas those of a lesser degree were considered not to be of hemodynamic significance. There are two fallacies to this approach. The first fallacy is that the arteriogram can correctly quantitate the degree of stenosis. Moore and Hall have clearly shown that the arteriographic appearance of a stenotic plaque is dependent upon the plane in which it is viewed (Fig. 2) (11). Although multiple-plane arteriograms improve the accuracy of measurement, they are seldom obtained routinely. The second fallacy is that a 50% diameter

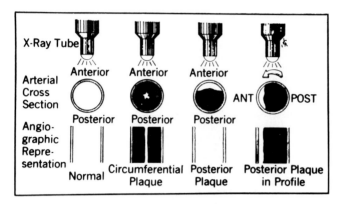

Figure 2 Diagram illustrating the variation in the arteriographic appearance of disease based upon the viewing plane. (From Moore WS, Ref. 11, with permission.)

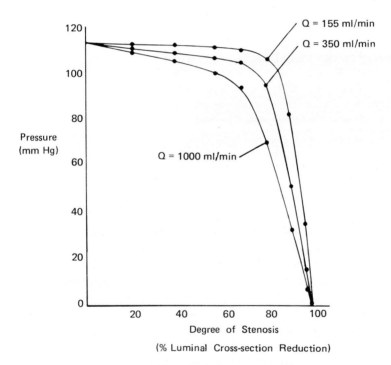

Figure 3 The effect of flow on pressure changes caused by different degrees of arterial stenosis. (From Flanigan DP et al., Annals of Surgery 186:663, 1977, with permission.)

stenosis is the cutoff for hemodynamic significance. Although it is generally true that stenoses greater than 50% diameter reduction (75% area reduction) cause reductions in flow and poststenotic pressure (critical stenoses) at rest in most arteries, such knowledge may not be pertinent in the assessment of human atherosclerotic disease for the determination of the proper bypass procedure because the degree at which a stenosis becomes critical is dependent upon the flow rate through the stenosis. Figure 3 demonstrates that at higher flow rates lesser stenoses can cause pressure effects. This fact is one of the reasons for the disappearing pulse phenomenon described above.

Clearly, arteriography is useful when it shows extremely severe stenoses but in single-plane "normal" studies or in studies showing borderline disease the hemodynamic significance of the disease cannot be assessed with certainty.

It is primarily because of the inaccuracy of the physical examination and arteriography that multiple noninvasive techniques were applied to the problem of assessing the hemodynamic significance of aortoiliac disease.

NONINVASIVE TECHNIQUES

In many patients with single-segment disease, segmental Doppler-derived pressures can both define the segment diseased and quantitate the severity of the disease. These techniques can easily and accurately assess aortoiliac disease when it is the only segment involved, but these measurements may also be affected by infrainguinal occlusive disease. As a result, more sophisticated noninvasive studies were developed. The major testing procedures in this category are common femoral artery Doppler analog waveform analysis, high-thigh Doppler-derived pressure measurements, and femoral pulsatility index.

The normal common femoral Doppler waveform is triphasic in nature, and increasingly severe disease causes pregressive deterioration of the waveform (Fig. 4). The changes in the waveform as they relate to the presence of aortoiliac disease have been analyzed extensively and found to be very sensitive indicators of disease (18). False-negative results are occasionally seen but, more importantly, false-positive results are commonly seen. Technical errors in sampling of Doppler information can result in a falsely abnormal waveform but not in a falsely normal waveform. Also, presence of scar tissue and a large amount of inguinal adipose tissue have been found to produce falsely abnormal waveforms. Primarily because of a high false-positive test rate, we have found the common femoral artery Doppler waveform to have an overall accuracy of only 80% in the detection of hemodynamically significant aortoiliac occlusive disease. Such an accuracy rate makes this technique insufficient as a selection criteria in the decision for suprainguinal versus infrainguinal bypass.

Measurement of the high-thigh Doppler-derived segmental pressure has been proposed as a method of evaluation of aortoiliac disease (19). An obvious problem

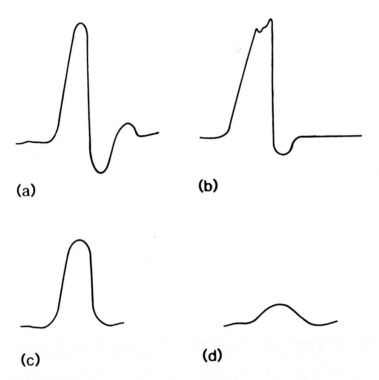

(a)   (b)

(c)   (d)

Figure 4 Doppler analog waveform changes associated with progressively tighter arterial stenoses. (a) Triphasic; (b) biphasic; (c) monophasic; (d) very flat ("damped"). (From Flanigan DP, in Roger M. Greenhalgh (ed): Diagnostic Techniques in Assessment Procedures in Vascular Surgery, Grune & Stratton, London, England, Fig. 25-1, pp. 286, with permission.)

with this approach is the distal location of the blood pressure cuff relative to the arterial segment being evaluated. Because of this problem the use of a narrow cuff has been suggested despite the fact that narrow thigh cuffs give falsely elevated pressures. To resolve this question, Flanigan et al. evaluated both wide (normal) and narrow-width thigh cuffs in the assessment of aortoiliac disease through comparisons to common femoral intraarterial pressure measurements (20). The accuracy for the detection of hemodynamically significant aortoiliac disease was poor for both normal (52%) and the narrow (73%) cuff techniques. False-positive tests were common with both techniques; the lowest false-negative rate was found using the normal size cuff (3%). The findings showed that superficial femoral artery disease accounted for nearly all false-positive tests and that the falsely elevated pressures obtained with the narrow cuff accounted for most of the false-negative tests. Thus, it appears that high thigh measurements are not sufficiently accurate to be used in the selection of suprainguinal versus infrainguinal bypass. Such measurements using a normal-width thigh cuff, however, are useful when normal to rule out hemodynamically significant aortoiliac disease at rest.

Femoral pulsatility index is the peak-to-peak Doppler waveform height divided by the mean frequency of the Doppler signal obtained from the common femoral artery. The advantage of this measurement is that it is independent of the Doppler probe angle. Flanigan et al. evaluated the femoral pulsatility index in both the canine laboratory and the clinical setting (21,22). In both experiments the femoral pulsatility index was compared to the intraarterially measured femoral/brachial pressure index. In the canine study, it was found that femoral pulsatility index was significantly affected by superficial femoral artery disease. This finding was verified in the clinical study in which femoral pulsatility index was only 66% accurate in the detection of hemodynamically significant aortoiliac disease. Although the femoral pulsatility index correlated with hemodynamic and morphologic changes in the aortoiliac segment, it was not found to be sufficient for operative decision-making purposes having false-positive and false-negative rates of 38% and 31%, respectively.

MINIMALLY INVASIVE TESTS

To date, a sufficiently accurate noninvasive technique to determine the hemodynamic significance of aortoiliac disease has not been found. The gold standard remains the measurement of intraarterial pressure at the level of the common femoral artery. Even this measurement is valid only at rest, however, and may not be applicable in patients with claudication who develop symptoms only during the vasodilatation caused by exercise. Vasodilatation in the lower extremities with exercise, and possibly following the performance of infrainguinal bypass grafting, causes an increase in flow through the aortoiliac segment and may cause a decrease in perfusion pressures distal to subcritical stenosis in the aortoiliac segment (Fig. 3). A subcritical stenosis is defined as one that does not cause a decrease in poststenotic pressure at rest but does so only with increased flow as seen with exercise or other inducements to vasodilatation. The identification of such lesions in the aortoiliac segment is of great importance in the assessment of patients with claudication and may also be important in patients requiring infrainguinal bypass. Thus, it is important to evaluate the aortoiliac segment both at rest and during vasodilatation.

Three methods of increasing lower extremity blood flow are available: exercise, reactive hyperemia, and pharmocologic means. Treadmill exercise is a poor method in the presence of intraarterial catheters. Reactive hyperemia is accurate but the painful nature of the procedure precludes many patients from study. Pharmocologic vasodilatation is applicable in nearly all patients and is the author's current method of choice. The use of papaverine hydrochloride for this purpose was first described by Sako in 1966 (23). This method was further evaluated by Quinn (8), Barber (4), Baron (9), and Archie (12).

Williams evaluated the technique in the canine model to assess the affect of superficial femoral artery occlusion on the test and found that results were unaffected by the status of the superficial femoral artery (24).

Previous investigators had performed the test in patients at the time of operation. This approach did not allow for a preoperative decision regarding the operation to be performed. Schwartz compared intraoperative measurements with measurements performed preoperatively in the vascular laboratory (25). This was done in 43 lower extremities and no statistically significant difference was found between results obtained from the two methods. Thus, in the author's practice, the test is now performed preoperatively in the vascular laboratory.

The test is performed by percutaneous puncture of the common femoral artery with a 19-gauge needle attached by arterial pressure tubing to a three-way stopcock (Fig. 5). The stopcock in turn is connected to a syringe containing 30 mg of papaverine hydrochloride diluted in saline solution to a total volume of 10 ml. Intraarterial pressure is measured by a calibrated pressure monitor and is recorded on a two-channel strip chart recorder. Common femoral artery blood velocity is measured simultaneously with a Doppler velocity meter also attached to the two-channel recorder. After measurement of common femoral and brachial artery base-

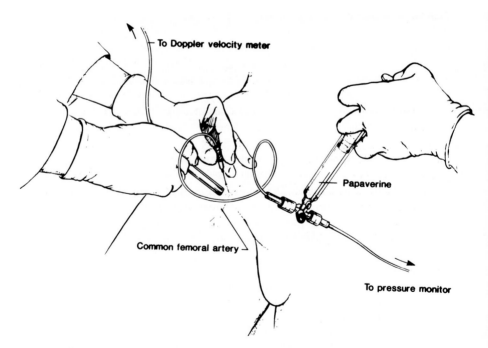

Figure 5   Illustration of the papaverine technique (see text). (From Flanigan DP, Ref. 3, with permission.)

line pressures, the papaverine is injected during simultaneous recording of pressure and velocity (Fig. 6). The percent decrease in the femoral brachial index (% △ FBI) is determined at the point of maximum vasodilatation.

Flanigan et al. performed the test in 41 lower extremities to determine a discriminate value for normal versus abnormal tests (2). This was done by comparing the results of the preoperative papaverine test with the postoperative clinical course of the patients. In patients operated upon for limb salvage, categorization into the clinical improvement group required healing of ischemic lesions or relief of rest pain in addition to an increase in the thigh/brachial pressure index of greater than or equal to 0.15 for aortofemoral, axillofemoral, and femorofemoral bypasses and to a postoperative value of greater than or equal to 0.9 for infrainguinal reconstructions. Categorization of claudicants into the clinically improved group required at least a 50% increase in treadmill exercise time regardless of the type of bypass performed. Additionally, claudicating limbs undergoing infrainguinal reconstruction required a postoperative thigh/brachial pressure index of greater than or equal to 0.9 to be considered improved. Postoperative assessment of the patients was made during the first three postoperative months. A discriminate value is needed for the interpretation of the papaverine test because normal patients have a mean decrease of femoral/brachial pressure index of 6% with papaverine injection. In relation to clinical course, receiver-operator characteristic analysis revealed a decrease in the

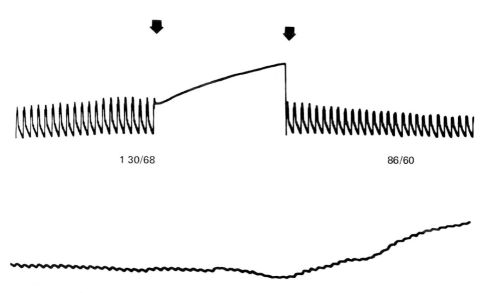

Figure 6 Strip chart recording of a positive papaverine test (see text). (From Flanigan DP, Ref. 3, with permission.)

femoral/brachial pressure index of greater than or equal to 15% following papaverine injection to be optimal in the detection of hemodynamically significant aortoiliac disease (2).

To test the validity of this discriminate value, 65 bypass procedures were chosen (suprainguinal vs. infrainguinal) on the basis of the papaverine test (3). These limbs were then compared to the first 41 lower extremities in which the decision for operation was based on arteriography. When the decision regarding the type of operation was based on arteriography, 80% of limbs experienced hemodynamic improvement. When the operation was chosen on the basis of papaverine testing, 98% of limbs improved (p < 0.01) (Fig. 7).

One additional test for the evaluation of the hemodynamic significance of lower extremity arterial disease is that of pedal ergometry. This test was first described by Moore and Hall but has had little utilization (11). The test is performed in the supine position. The feet rest on pedals, which the patient moves through dorsiflexion and plantar flexion of the feet against resistance (Fig. 8).

This apparatus was first assessed in the author's laboratory in comparison to treadmill testing in patients able to perform both tests (13). The treadmill test was considered the standard. There was strong correlation between maximum pressure drop (r = 0.8448) and recovery time to baseline (r = 0.8700) between the tests. Decision matrix analysis revealed that ergometer testing had a positive predictive value of 100%, a negative predictive value of 93%, and an overall accuracy of 96%.

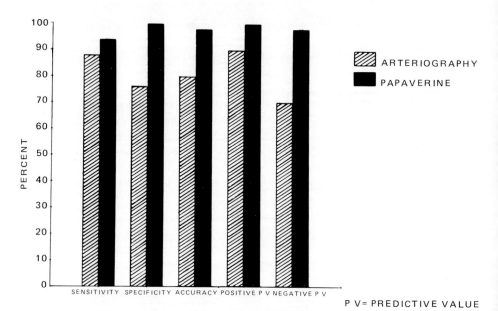

Figure 7 Clinical utility of arteriography versus papaverine testing in selection of proper revascularization procedures. (From Flanigan DP, Ref. 3, with permission.)

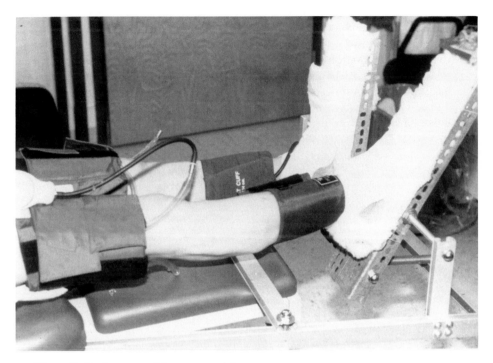

Figure 8   Patient exercising on a pedal ergometer.

In view of the above findings, it seemed appropriate to evaluate the use of pedal ergometer testing with intraarterial common femoral artery pressure measurements in the assessment of aortoiliac disease. This was performed in 35 extremities having both papaverine testing and pedal ergometer testing. The results were assessed in comparison to the clinical criteria described above. In this study, pedal ergometer testing was 100% accurate and papaverine testing was 97% accurate. The lower accuracy for the papaverine test was the result of two borderline results that were in error.

Both the papaverine test and the pedal ergometer test are sufficiently accurate to allow the surgeon to make a decision regarding suprainguinal versus infrainguinal bypass. In the author's experience, ergometer testing is somewhat limited because of patient cooperation whereas all patients have been able to have papaverine testing performed. As a result, the author's practice is to employ papaverine testing in all cases. When borderline results (% $\triangle$ FBI = 13-17%) are obtained, ergometer testing is added for confirmation.

In conclusion, the most accurate currently available tests for assisting in the decision for infrainguinal versus suprainguinal bypass are the papaverine and pedal ergometer tests. Although minimally invasive, these tests have led to no complication in several hundred applications. These tests are not performed routinely, rather, the need for testing is made following history and physical examination, routine noninvasive testing, and arteriography. In approximately two-thirds of patients, these evaluations are sufficient. The most common applications for minimally invasive tests are in patients with claudication, in patients with multisegment disease who do not have normal bi- or triplanar aortoiliac arteriography, and in the donor limb of patients being evaluated for femorofemoral bypass. Application of these tests in this manner should provide for uniform hemodynamic and symptomatic improvement in patients undergoing lower extremity revascularization procedures.

REFERENCES

1. Baird RJ, Feldman P, Miles JT, Madras PM, Gurry JF: Subsequent downstream repair after aorto-iliac and aorto-femoral bypass operations. Surgery 82:785, 1977.
2. Flanigan DP, Williams LR, Schwartz JA, Schuler JJ, Gray B: Hemodynamic evaluation of the aortoiliac system based on pharmacologic vasodilatation. Surgery 93:709, 1983.
3. Flanigan DP, Ryan TJ, Williams LR, Schwartz JA, Gray B, Schuler JJ: Aortofemoral or femoropopliteal revascularization? A prospective evaluation of the papaverine test. J Vasc Surg 1:215, 1984.
4. Barber GG, Fong H, McPhail NV, et al: Hemodynamic assessment of the aortoiliac segment: A prospective study. Can J Surg 23:542, 1980.
5. Brener BJ, Raines JK, Darling RC, et al: Measurement of systolic femoral artery pressure during reactive hyperemia: An estimate of aortoiliac disease. Cardiovasc Surg 49-50 (Suppl 2):259, 1974.
6. Brener BJ, Brief DK, Alpert J, et al: The usefulness of intra-arterial pressure measurements in occlusive arterial disease: Part I. Vasc Dis Ther 3:37, 1982.
7. Brewster DC, Waltman AC, O'Hara PJ, et al: Femoral artery pressure measurement during aortography. Cardiovasc Surg 60 (Suppl 1):120, 1979.
8. Quin RD, Evans DH, Bell PRF: Haemodynamic assessment of the aorto-iliac segment. J Cardiovasc Surg 16:586, 1975.
9. Baron HC, Schwartz M, Batri G: The papaverine test for blood flow potential of the profunda femoris artery. Surg Gynecol Obstet 153:873, 1981.
10. Udoff EJ, Barth KH, Harrington DP, et al: Hemodynamic significance of iliac artery stenosis: Pressure measurements during angiography. Radiology 132:289, 1979.
11. Moore WS, Hall AD: Unrecognized aortoiliac stenosis: A physiologic approach to the diagnosis. Arch Surg 103:633, 1971.
12. Archie JP Jr, Feldtman RW: Intraoperative assessment of the hemodynamic significance of iliac and profunda femora artery stenosis. Surgery 90:876, 1981.
13. Ryan TJ, Williams LR, Gray B, Schuler JJ, Flanigan DP: Supine exercise testing of the lower extremities using a pedal ergometer. Bruit 8:39, 1984.

14. DeWeese JA: Pedal pulses disappearing with exercise: A test for intermittent claudication. N Engl J Med 262:212, 1960.
15. Sobinsky KR, Borozan PG, Gray B, Schuler JJ, Flanigan DP: Is femoral pulse palpation accurate in assessing the hemodynamic significance of aortoiliac occlusive disease? Am J Surg 148:214, 1984.
16. Johnston KW, Demorais D, Colapinto RI: Difficulty in assessing the severity of aortoiliac disease by clinical and arteriographic methods. Angiology 32: 609, 1981.
17. Zupan TI, Gates K, Porter JM, Baur GM: Evaluation of common femoral artery hemodynamics. Bruit 7:45, 1983.
18. Nicolaides AN, et al: The value of Doppler blood velocity tracings in the detection of aortoiliac disease in patients with intermittent claudication. Surgery 80:774, 1976.
19. Heintz SE, et al: Value of arterial pressure measurement in the proximal and distal part of the thigh in arterial disease. Surg Gynecol Obstet 146:337, 1978.
20. Flanigan DP, Gray B, Schuler JJ, Schwartz JA, O'Connor RJA, Williams LR: Utility of wide and narrow blood pressure cuffs in the hemodynamic assessment of aortoiliac occlusive disease. Surgery 92:16, 1982.
21. Flanigan DP, Collins JT, Goodreau JJ, Burnham SJ, Yao JST: Femoral pulsatility index in the evaluation of aortoiliac occlusive disease. J Surg Res 31: 392, 1981.
22. Flanigan DP, Collins JT, Schwartz JA, O'Mara C, Flinn WR, Bergan JJ, Yao JST: Hemodynamic and arteriographic evaluation of femoral pulsatility index. J Surg Res 32:234, 1982.
23. Sako Y: Papaverine test in peripheral arterial disease. Surg Forum 17:141, 1966.
24. Williams LR, Flanigan DP: Detection of subcritical iliac artery stenoses with pharmacologic vasodilatation. Surg Forum 33:451, 1982.
25. Schwartz JA, Flanigan DP, Williams LR, Schuler JJ, Gray B: Preoperative hemodynamic evaluation of aortoiliac occlusive disease: Correlation with intraoperative measurements. Curr Surg 40:278, 1983.

4

Evaluation of Vasculogenic Impotence

JAMES J. SCHULER
University of Illinois College of Medicine at Chicago
Chicago, Illinois

Even though it is quite likely that sexual impotence had been recognized by mankind long before recorded history, the earliest references to impotence occur in the Old Testament (1), and the medical writings of Hippocrates and the ancient Hindus (2). Even as late as the 19th century such prominent medical authorities of the time as Herman Boerhaave and Benjamin Rush attributed impotence to masturbation and/or sexual promiscuity (2). In light of these presumed etiologies for impotence it is not surprising that up until the mid-20th century impotence was treated either by aphrodisiacs and/or witchcraft; and if not "treated," it was accepted as justifiable punishment for, or the consequences of, sexual excess.

It was not until 1948 in the reports of Kinsey (3) that much of the ignorance, myth, and folklore surrounding sexuality was replaced by the beginning of an objective approach toward sex and sexual dysfunction. The Kinsey Report not only set the stage for further research into human sexuality and sexual dysfunction but also initiated a change in societal attitudes toward sexuality that has allowed patients with sexual dysfunction to seek treatment without fear of being ignored, chastised, or labeled as sexually abnormal. As the population at large becomes better informed regarding the various causes of sexual dysfunction and learns that most of these causes are treatable, as the average age of the population in general increases, and as the geriatric population continues to experience an overall increase in its general level of health and quality of life, physicians are ever more frequently encountering patients who are unable to, and, in light of the success of present-day treatment modalities, should not be expected to accept sexual dysfunction as the normal sequela of various disease processes or the inevitable consequences of aging. With the various forms of psychological and sexual counseling developed by psychiatrists and psychologists; with the variety of new nerve-sparing operations being performed by the urologists, surgical oncologists, and vascular surgeons; with aortoiliac reconstructive procedures being performed in such a way as to preserve or restore pelvic perfusion; with specific hormonal replacement therapy available to endocrinologists; and with the newer penile prostheses being utilized by the urologists when the above methods fail or cannot be implemented; it is now possible in many instances to prevent iatrogenic impotence and in many others to restore erectile function. However, successful treatment is dependent upon an accurate pathophysiologic diagnosis. This chapter will deal with the various clinical and laboratory methods used to evaluate the etiology of impotence in general and vasculogenic impotence in particular.

Much of the misunderstanding surrounding sexual dysfunction in the past followed from a lack of a clear definition of impotence. Various types of sexual dysfunction such as retrograde ejaculation, premature ejaculation, loss of libido, sexual apathy, and others were all lumped together and referred to as "impotence." Impotence is defined as the inability to achieve or maintain a penile erection sufficient for vaginal intromission and the successful completion of sexual intercourse. Although there are suggestions that a female counterpart of vasculogenic impotence may occur in some women with aortoiliac occlusive disease (4) who experience a lack of vaginal lubrication and orgasmic failure, this report will deal solely with impotence in the male.

ANATOMY AND PHYSIOLOGY OF PENILE ERECTION

In the presence of a functioning endocrine system, normal penile erection is dependent upon an intact autonomic nerve system, adequate arterial inflow to the penis, and a competent venous outflow system from the penis. The arterial blood supply to the penis is derived from the paired internal pudendal arteries, which are the terminal branches of the internal iliac arteries. The internal pudendal arteries course along the pelvic floor and pass into the perineum between the pyriformis and coccygeus muscles through the lesser sciatic foramen. They traverse the perineum in an anteromedial direction, paralleling the lateral wall of the ischiorectal fossa, and enter the base of the penis where the bulbourethral branch originates and serves as the primary blood supply to the corpus spongiosum. Shortly after giving rise to the bulbourethral artery, the internal pudendal artery divides into its two terminal branches, the deep and dorsal penile arteries, the former of which are the main arterial blood supply to the corpora cavernosa, which are primarily responsible for erection.

Once blood enters the terminal branches of the penile arteries it can take one of two pathways: either into the cavernous spaces to produce erection or through arteriovenous shunts into the veins of the penis and back to the systemic venous circulation. Which of these two pathways the blood traverses is under neural control and, therefore, penile erection is dependent upon intact reflex arcs and the coordination of afferent signals in the thoracolumbar and sacral (S2-S4) erection centers as well as intact autonomic nerves to the penis. The entrances to the cavernous spaces contain valve-like structures called Ebners pads or polsters, which are composed of longitudinally oriented smooth muscle fibers under autonomic control. When the penis is flaccid, these pads are contracted causing them to protrude into the lumen of the openings into the cavernous spaces, thus, forming a series of alternating baffles which function as a valve and cause blood to be shunted into the arteriovenous fistulae rather than the cavernous spaces, thus, maintaining the flaccid state. During erection, these pads are relaxed and no longer form a series of baffles that function as a valve, thus, allowing blood to enter the cavernous spaces. As the cavernous spaces fill with blood, the corpora cavernosa enlarge and compress both the arteriovenous shunts and the circumflex veins of the penis between the tunica albuginea and Bucks fascia, thus, tending to restrict venous outflow and maintain the erect state (4-8). Although the structure and function of Ebners pads has recently been questioned (9), the majority of evidence supports their key role in achieving and maintaining erection. A recent report (10) indicates that at least part of the neural control of the Ebners pads may derive from a newly recognized class of nonadrenergic noncholinergic (peptidergic) nerves that are under the control of vasoactive intestinal peptide (VIP) and have been found in abundance in close association with the blood vessels and Edners pads of the penis.

CLASSIFICATION OF IMPOTENCE

Impotence occurs in two forms, primary and secondary. Primary impotence refers to a male who has never had a penile erection. This occurs in males who have anorchism, severe hypogonadism, or in males with chromosomal abnormalities such as Klinefelter's syndrome. Primary impotence may also be seen in individuals who have experienced severe psychiatric trauma in childhood that has left them with such a high degree of guilt, fear, or anxiety regarding sex that they never experience erections. Primary impotence is exceedingly rare, and is usually accurately diagnosed during adolescence or in the early postadolescent period.

Secondary impotence is much more common than primary impotence and refers to a male who has previously had normal erectile function and who subsequently loses the ability to achieve or maintain an erection. All instances of vasculogenic impotence are secondary. Secondary impotence is of two etiologic types: psychogenic and organic. Psychogenic impotence occurs in males with normal endocrine, metabolic, neurologic, and vascular function who because of guilt, fear, anxiety, depression, anger, or other psychological disturbances are impotent. Organic impotence occurs in males with abnormal function of one of the abovementioned physiologic systems. In the past, it was estimated that approximately 90% of all cases of secondary impotence were psychogenic in origin (11). Presently, with more accurate methods of defining the specific etiology of various types of impotence, it is estimated that approximately half of all patients with secondary impotence will be found to have some degree of organic dysfunction contributing to their impotence, and that the organic component of their impotence has caused whatever psychological problems may be present.

DIFFERENTIATION OF PSYCHOGENIC FROM ORGANIC IMPOTENCE

The first step in the evaluation of impotence is to obtain an accurate and complete sexual history aimed at differentiating psychogenic from organic impotence. As in most other disorders an accurate etiologic diagnosis can frequently be made on the basis of a thorough history alone.

Organic impotence is constant in that the degree of erectile dysfunction is the same with all sexual partners at all times and under all circumstances, whereas psychogenic impotence is usually inconstant in that the patient will experience normal erections under certain circumstances or with certain partners and at other times be impotent. Organic impotence is usually gradual in onset, increasing over 6 months to many years, and is usually first noticed as a gradual decrease in the degree of firmness of the penis or the gradual onset of the inability to maintain an erection until completion of intercourse; whereas psychogenic impotence is usually rapid in onset, complete but variable in that no degree of penile rigidity occurs under certain circumstances whereas normal erections occur at other times, and usually follows the onset of some degree of emotional stress such as the death of a loved one, guilt over divorce, separation, or an extramarital affair, loss of job or social standing, or recent serious illness. Nocturnal erections and erections present upon awakening in the morning are absent in those with organic impotence but present in those with psychogenic impotence. Normal sexual drive, desire, and libido, will be retained in patients with organic impotence whereas it will be variable (i.e., present and normal under certain circumstances and absent under other circumstances) in patients with psychogenic impotence.

Quite often the differentiation between psychogenic and organic impotence is clear cut. The hard-driving, goal-oriented, middle-aged executive who becomes impotent shortly after being passed over for a significant promotion; the "macho" man who becomes impotent shortly after learning of his wife's extramarital affair; and the previously healthy patient who experiences impotence shortly after fully recuperating from his myocardial infarction are all classic examples of psychogenic impotence. These patients will not benefit from a multitude of tests aimed at discovering an organic cause for their impotence but are more likely to be made worse or at least more refractory to successful psychological and sexual counselling since the various testing procedures will likely increase their level of fear or anxiety regarding their recovery of normal erectile function.

In contradistinction to the above examples are the patient who relates the gradual onset of less firm erections coincident with the gradual onset of intermittent claudication of the buttocks and thighs, which has progressed to complete impotence coincident with the worsening of his claudication; the diabetic patient who notes the gradual onset of partial impotence at the same time as he develops mild peripheral neuropathy and who progresses to complete impotence as he develops neurotrophic ulcers and signs of a neurogenic bladder; and the patient who finds himself impotent immediately following abdominal perineal resection for carcinoma of the rectum. These are all classic examples of organic impotence. No amount of counseling can be expected to restore potency in these patients. In between the two obvious extremes outlined above are a large number of patients in whom it is difficult or impossible to distinguish psychogenic from organic impotence and in whom components of both may be contributing to erectile dysfunction ("mixed" impotence). In these patients, more thorough evaluation aimed at discovering an organic etiology for impotence is definitely indicated since except for "classic" examples of psychogenic impotence it remains a diagnosis arrived at by exclusion.

TYPES OF ORGANIC IMPOTENCE

Organic impotence may be caused by congenital, mechanical, endocrinologic, metabolic, posttraumatic, postsurgical, neurologic, vascular, or pharmacologic factors. A list of the various known causes of organic impotence is outlined in Table 1. The vast majority of patients who are eventually found to be impotent on an organic basis are impotent secondary to pharmacologic, neurologic, or vascular causes.

A wide variety of pharmacologic agents have been shown to cause impotence. The major groups of drugs involved are the anticholinergic agents, ganglionic blocking agents, tricyclic antidepressants, monoamine oxidase inhibitors, and phenothiazine derivatives. A more complete listing of specific drugs known to cause impotence is outlined in Table 2.

After ruling out all of the other more easy to differentiate causes of organic impotence, the clinician is frequently faced with the problem of whether vascular occlusive disease, or neurologic dysfunction, or both, are contributing to organic impotence. This problem is especially pronounced because of the high incidence of impotence in patients with diabetes mellitus. The incidence of impotence in diabetics increases from approximately 25% in the 30-35-year age group to 75% in the 60-65-year age group (12). This incidence is approximately five times higher than the incidence of impotence in the general population studied by Kinsey and associates (3). It is well known that patients with diabetes frequently have an autonomic neuropathy as well as accelerated atherosclerosis. These two factors, in conjunction with the known predilection for diabetics to develop small-vessel as

Table 1 Organic Causes of Impotence

Congenital	Mechanical
Epispadias	Peyronie's disease
Hypospadias	Phymosis
Anorchism	Morbid obesity
Cryptorchidism	Carcinoma of penis
Klinefelter's Syndrome	Hydrocele
Chordee	Elephantiasis
Microphallus	
Postsurgical or posttraumatic	Inflammatory
Prostatectomy	Prostatitis
Abdominoperineal Resection	Seminal vesticulitis
Thoracolumbar Sympathectomy	Urethritis
Pelvic fracture	Cystitis
Genital irradiation	
Post priapism	
External sphincterotomy	
Endocrinologic	Neurologic
Diabetes mellitus	Spina bifida
Hyperthyroidism	Multiple sclerosis
Hypothyroidism	Spinal cord tumors or transection
Acromegaly	Tabes dorsalis
Addison's disease	Temporal lobe tumors
Adrenal neoplasms	Amyotrophic lateral sclerosis
Craniopharyngioma	Parkinsonism
Pituitary chromophobe adenoma	Subacute combined degeneration
Vascular	Miscellaneous
Arterial occlusive disease	Lead poisoning
Post priapism	Herbicide ingestion
Arteritis	Chronic renal failure
	Hepatic failure

well as large-vessel atherosclerosis, probably account for the increased incidence of impotence seen in the diabetic population. Because of this high incidence of impotence in the diabetic population where both neurologic dysfunction and arterial occlusive disease usually contribute to the impotence as well as a high percentage of mixed etiology impotence in the nondiabetic population (13), the complete evaluation of vasculogenic impotence quite frequently comes down to differentiating neurogenic from vasculogenic causes.

Table 2 Pharmacologic Agents Reported to Cause Impotence

Monoamine oxidose inhibitors	Tricyclic antidepressants
Tranylcypromine	Amitriptyline
Phenelzine sulfate	Nortriptyline
Pargyline	Protriptyline
Isocarboxazide	Desipramine
Iproniazid	Imipramine
Alpha-adrenergic blocking agents	Benzodiazepines
Phenoxybenzamine	Chlordiazepoxide
	Diazepam
	Oxazepam
Cholinergic blocking agents	Phenothiazines
Atropine	Chlorpromazine
Propantheline bromide	Fluphenazine
Methaneline bromide	Thioridazine
Trihexyphenidyl	
Scopolamine	
Benztropine	
Antihypertensive drugs	Miscellaneous
Clonidine	Ethyl alcohol
Alpha-methyldopa	Narcotics
Guanethidine	Marijuana
Propranolol	Methadone
Spironolactone	Barbiturates
Chlorthalidone	Cimetidine
Prazosin	Bromides
Reserpine	Clofibrate
Thiazides	Lithium carbonate
Hydralazine	Metoclopramide
Chlorthalidone	Probucol
	Hydroxyprogesterone
	Baclofen
	Perhexilene
	Diphenhydramine
	Hydroxyzine
	Haloperidol
	Ethionamide

THE PHYSICAL EXAMINATION IN THE
EVALUATION OF IMPOTENCE

The evaluation of vasculogenic impotence involves not only the obvious vascular examination but also a thorough genital and neurologic examination. Examination of the penis may reveal the fibrous plaques of Peyronies diesease or the diffuse fibrosis and edema that result from previous priapism. Palpation of the testicles will occasionally reveal soft atrophic testes and prompt further endocrinologic evaluation. Palpation of the prostate may reveal fibrosis and inflammation or a large prostatic mass and indicate that chronic prostatitis or carcinoma of the prostate invading the adjacent nerves is the cause of impotence.

The neurologic examination in the evaluation of impotence should be aimed at detecting autonomic neuropathy. Most patients with autonomic neuropathy have diabetes and associated peripheral neuropathy (14). The evaluation should include the assessment of motor strength, deep tendon reflexes, the Babinski reflex, and most importantly light touch, vibratory, and kinesthetic sense, which are usually impaired before the other more obvious signs of neuropathy are apparent. The function of the suprasacral and supraspinal nerve pathways are evaluated by asking the patient to voluntarily contract and relax the external anal sphincter. Absence of this ability implies that spinal cord nerve tracts or peripheral nerve dysfunction may be responsible for impotence. The integrity of the sacral spinal cord segment S2-S4, which is primarily responsible for the neurogenic control of blood supply and, thus, erection of the cavernosal bodies, is tested by eliciting the bulbocavernosus reflex. This reflex is tested by placing an examining finger in the anus to detect contraction of the bulbocavernosus muscle when the glans penis is squeezed. Absence of this reflex in an impotent patient indicates that a neurogenic cause is at least partially responsible for impotence.

The vascular aspect of the physical examination is aimed at assessing the adequacy of pelvic and, thus, penile blood flow. Absence of femoral pulses in conjunction with absence of an aortic pulse obviously precludes normal inflow to the internal iliac arteries and, thus, the penis. Leriche and Morel first described the syndrome of thrombotic obliteration of the abdominal aortic bifurcation in the English literature in 1948 (15). Because the symptoms of impotence and thigh and buttock claudication that characterize this syndrome fit so nicely with the easily detectable physical findings, many clinicians have drawn the erroneous conclusion that the presence of normal femoral pulses implies adequate pelvic and penile flow. This is not the case since the internal iliac arteries are frequently involved with atherosclerosis prior to the development of significant disease in the aorta, common iliac, or external iliac arteries (4, 16, 17). Likewise, the palpation of a normal dorsal penile artery pulse has been reported to be a fairly accurate method of ruling out vasculogenic impotence (18). This pulse is difficult to palpate and although we would agree that the presence of a palpable dorsal penile artery pulse probably rules out a vasculogenic cause of impotence, the absence of this pulse does not necessarily imply that the impotence is due to vascular occlusive disease since the abundant network of pelvic collateral flow will frequently provide for normal erectile function and yet, because the flow is via collateral channels, no penile pulses will be palpable.

THE LABORATORY EVALUATION OF IMPOTENCE

Laboratory studies other than the noninvasive assessment of penile flow, which will be discussed subsequently, play a limited role in the evaluation of impotence. These studies are needed only in ambiguous cases of impotence suspected to be of endocrine, psychogenic, or neurogenic origin since most of these can be accurately diagnosed on the basis of history and physical examination.

Thorough endocrinologic evaluation includes measurement of follicle-stimulating hormone (FSH), luteinizing hormone (LH), testosterone, prolactin, and occasionally thyroid function tests (19-24). Since these tests are both costly and time consuming and of "low yield," they are indicated only in those cases in which an endocrinologic cause of impotence is suspected on the basis of such physical evidence as soft atrophic testes, gynecomastia, or changes in other secondary sex characteristics. These tests are especially not indicated as part of the routine evaluation of impotence in diabetics since numerous authors have demonstrated that these patients, aside from their insulin deficiency, have normal hormonal function (19-24).

Nocturnal penile tumescence (NPT) has been of value in selected individuals to distinguish organic from psychogenic impotence (25-29). This test as described by Karacan et al. (26) is based upon the fact that normal males have fairly constant periods of penile erection during rapid eye movement (REM) periods of sleep. This test assumes that the relevant psychological factors causing psychogenic impotence will not be operable during sleep in psychogenically impotent men and therefore NPT will occur. However, this assumption has not been proven and therein lies the inaccuracy of the test (30,31). This test, likewise, assumes that, in men impotent on an organic basis, the organic factors will continue to be operable during sleep and NPT will not occur. Although the accuracy and clinical utility of this test is still being defined, it has become a popular method for evaluating the various causes of impotence and it is probable that the test is being overutilized. Nocturnal penile tumescence monitoring requires the patient to sleep for three nights in a specially designed room with a variety of monitoring instruments used to assess REM sleep periods and NPT, and is therefore costly. Because of this, in today's economic climate it would seem prudent to utilize other less costly methods of defining the etiology of impotence and reserve NPT for those truly ambiguous cases in whom the information gained will determine further evaluation and/or therapy.

In those patients suspected of being impotent on a neurologic basis but in whom the bulbocavernosus reflex is equivocal, two tests, the cystometrogram and bulbocavernosus reflex latency time, can be performed. Both of these tests are accurate, relatively easy to perform and interpret, and have a definite but limited role in the evaluation of impotence (13,14).

NONINVASIVE VASCULAR LABORATORY TESTING
IN THE EVALUATION OF VASCULOGENIC IMPOTENCE

Various noninvasive methods of measuring penile arterial flow have been developed and correlated with the presence or absence of impotence. Since both psychogenic and other organic factors may cause impotence, the presence of normal penile flow does not necessarily mean that a patient has normal erectile function; however, the detection of abnormal penile pressure indicates that impotence is caused, at least in part, by arterial occlusive disease.

Canning et al. in 1963 was the first to utilize noninvasive methods of assessing penile flow in the evaluation of vasculogenic impotence (32). An impedance plethysmographic technique with penile pulse volume waveform analysis was correlated with arteriographic evidence of pelvic arterial occlusive disease and impotence. Other noninvasive methods soon followed. The use of mercury strain gauge plethysmography was reported by Britt et al. in 1971 (33), oxyhemoglobin spectroscopy by Gaskell also in 1971 (34), and Doppler-derived waveform analysis by Malvar et al. in 1973 (35). These methods, as well as other noninvasive means of measuring penile flow (18,36,37), are no longer commonly employed. At present, there are three techniques: Doppler ultrasound, photoplethysmography, and pulse volume recordings, used to measure penile arterial pressure. All are safe, quick, inexpensive, and accurate.

Doppler ultrasonic measurement of penile systolic pressure is performed by applying a 2.5 × 9-cm pneumatic cuff around the base of the penis and using a 9-10-kHz Doppler ultrasound probe positioned over the dorsal penile or deep penile (cavernosal) arteries to detect the return of a flow signal as the cuff is deflated from suprasystolic pressures. The pressure at which flow returns is termed the penile systolic pressure and when divided by the simultaneously measured brachial systolic pressure yields a penile brachial index (PBI). Queral et al. (38), as well as Kempczinski (39) and others (16,40,41), have demonstrated that a PBI of less than 0.6 is diagnostic of vasculogenic impotence and a PBI of 0.6-0.75 to 0.6-0.8 is suggestive but not diagnostic of vasculogenic impotence, and a PBI of greater than 0.75-0.8 essentially rules out vascular occlusive disease as a cause of impotence.

Preoperative measurement of PBI is not only useful in ruling in or ruling out vascular occlusive disease, but Queral et al. (38) as well as the present authors (17, 40,41) have shown that PBI can be increased and erectile function restored to normal in patients with vasculogenic impotence when vascular reconstructive procedures for the treatment of aneurysmal or occlusive disease in the aortoiliofemoral area are modified so as to maintain or maximize pelvic and penile flow. Queral et al. (38) have likewise demonstrated that in vascular reconstructive procedures on the aortoiliac segment done in such a way as to diminish pelvic blood flow in previously potent patients the PBI will decrease and the majority of these patients will be rendered impotent on a vasculogenic basis.

Nath et al (42) have expanded the use of PBI to include an objective assessment of patients suspected of a "pelvic steal syndrome." This syndrome consists of an initially firm and normal erection that rapidly subsides following thigh and buttock muscle exercise during sexual intercourse. This is caused by a shunting of blood to the muscles of the thigh and buttocks and away from the penis via patent but stenotic internal iliac arteries serving as collateral blood supply to the legs. Assessment of the pelvic steal is performed by measuring PBI both at rest and immediately following vigorous buttock and thigh muscle exercise. A drop in PBI after exercise of 0.1 or more is considered significant and indicative of a possible pelvic steal. Nath et al. (42) report five patients with symptoms of pelvic steal and all five of these patients had a drop in PBI following leg exercise as well as pelvic arteriograms showing occlusive disease in a pattern that would be expected to cause pelvic steal. One of these patients experienced both a return of erectile function and postexercise PBI to normal following left iliac artery endarterectomy, which reversed his pelvic steal.

At present, it is our practice to obtain both a thorough sexual history as well as Doppler-derived penile systolic pressures on all patients who undergo segmental, lower extremity, Doppler pressure measurements as part of their preoperative evaluation prior to aortoiliofemoral reconstructive procedures. This is done for three reasons. First, the detection of a decreased PBI in an impotent patient with no other reasonable cause for impotence allows the surgeon to inform the radiologist that more thorough than usual aortoiliofemoral arteriography is required to tailor the planned operative procedure to maximize pelvic and penile flow. Second, if the PBI does not increase into the range compatible with relatively normal erectile function (≥ 0.6) following vascular reconstruction and the patient desires restoration of erectile function, the surgeon can refer the patient for evaluation for placement of a penile prosthesis rather than hold out the vain hope that the vascular reconstructive procedure will eventually restore erectile function. Third, the documentation of pre- and postoperative PBI may prove useful at a later date should medico-legal proceedings ensue concerning the alleged iatrogenic creation of impotence during the vascular reconstruction.

The second most commonly employed method for the noninvasive assessment of penile blood flow is the plethysmographic technique of pulse volume recordings (PVR). This method employs a digital plethysmographic cuff placed snugly around the base of the penis and inflated with an amount of air sufficient to attain mean arterial pressure. Penile PVR waveforms are recorded on a strip chart recorder at 25 mm/sec and either compared to simultaneously obtained index finger PVR recordings or interpreted separately. Both Depalma et al. (43) and Kempczinski (39) have demonstrated that PVR readings are accurate and reproducible in the measurement of penile flow.

The reported criteria for penile PVR recordings that distinguish normal from abnormal have varied (4, 44-46). DePalma (4, 45) has reported that a PVR amplitude of greater than 5 mm (range 6-30 mm), systolic upstroke, or time to maximum amplitude of less than 6 mm (range 4-6 mm), with the dicrotic notch either present or absent on the downslope of the curve all correlated with normal penile perfusion and erectile function. Rhodes et al. (46) have demonstrated that PVR amplitude varies considerably with penile cuff pressure being 14-8 mm at a cuff pressure of 60 mmHg; 25-12 mm at a cuff pressure of 80 mmHg; and 33-13 mm at a cuff pressure of 100 mmHg. They considered a PVR amplitude of <25 mm at all cuff pressures to indicate abnormal penile perfusion and showed a good correlation between abnormal PVR and both PBI and a history of impotence. From the above it can be seen that the interpretation of PVR recordings of penile perfusion pressure are considerably more subjective and variable than Doppler-derived penile systolic pressures. Because of this it is recommended that normal and abnormal values be established for each individual blood flow laboratory performing penile PVR.

DePalma et al. (43) and Merchant and DePalma (44) have shown that abnormal PVR recordings can be used to define patients impotent on the basis of vascular occlusive disease and that the return of penile PVR recordings into the normal range correlated well with return of erectile function following aortoiliofemoral vascular reconstruction.

Both Doppler-derived penile pressures and PVR assessment of penile flow have certain advantages and disadvantages. The Doppler technique has the following advantages: (a) it is more objective in that exact penile pressures are recorded; (b) it can separately measure pressure from both the right and left penile arteries as well as both the dorsal and deep penile arteries; and (c) penile pressure can be quite easily indexed to the brachial pressure. The Doppler technique has the following disadvantages: (a) because it can measure each penile artery pressure separately, results can occasionally be difficult to interpret such as when the PBI on one side is definitely normal (>0.8) and the PBI on the other side is abnormal (<0.6); (b) because the technique involves manipulation of the penis to find the optimal Doppler signals, it can produce embarassment and anxiety for both the patient and vascular technologist; and (c) it is more time consuming (15-20 min) than PVR recordings. The PVR method of assessing penile flow has the following advantages: (a) it measures the sum total of all arteries contributing to penile flow; (b) it is more acceptable to both patient and technologist; and (c) it is faster (5-10 min) than the Doppler technique. The PVR technique has the following disadvantages: (a) interpretation of results is more subjective than with the Doppler technique; (b) PVR amplitude is dependent on cuff pressure and, therefore, standardization of criteria for normal versus abnormal must be performed in each individual laboratory; and (c) because the PVR technique measures the sum total of penile flow, it cannot separately assess the contribution of each side of the pelvis to penile flow.

Recently two reports have evaluated photoplethysmography (PPG) in the evaluation of vasculogenic impotence (47,48). PPG consists of an infrared light-emitting diode and a photosensor. Changes in movement of erythrocytes (pulse) reflect the emitted light and when this signal is electronically processed it can be recorded on a strip chart recorder as a pulse waveform. The technique for measuring penile systolic pressures consists of placing a 2.5 X 9-cm cuff around the base of the penis with the PPG on the glans or lateral aspect of the penis distally and noting the pressure at which a pulse waveform reappears as the cuff is deflated from suprasystolic pressure. This pressure is recorded as penile systolic pressure. The accuracy of PPG as compared to PBI has been evaluated (47,48) and the two techniques have been shown to be equally accurate in measuring penile systolic pressure. However, the PPG possesses certain advantages in that in up to 16% of patients (48) no Doppler signal can be detected distal to the cuff whereas in all patients a PPG-derived penile systolic pressure can be recorded (47,48).

Additionally, the PPG assessment of penile pressure is quick (average 3.5 min) and, since it requires minimal penile manipulation, more acceptable to both patients and vascular technologists. However, the PPG shares with PVR recordings the disadvantage of not being able to assess selectively the contribution to total penile perfusion of each side of the pelvis separately. At present, it is our practice to use the PPG-derived penile systolic pressure as our standard noninvasive method of evaluating vasculogenic impotence and using Doppler-derived penile systolic pressure and PBI to assess the contribution of each side of the pelvis separately in those patients in whom a surgical procedure is planned that would affect perfusion from one side more than the other (i.e., unilateral internal iliac artery endarterectomy or femorofemoral bypass).

ARTERIOGRAPHY IN THE EVALUATION OF VASCULOGENIC IMPOTENCE

Selective catheterization and arteriography of the distal internal iliac artery to obtain internal pudendal and corpora cavernosa angiograms has been reported by various authors (49-52). This is usually not done for diagnostic purposes but rather as part of the preoperative evaluation of the distribution of arterial occlusive lesions in patients in whom a vascular bypass procedure from the femoral artery or inferior epigastric artery to the dorsal penile artery or directly to the cavernous spaces is planned. These "penile revascularization" procedures are presently available in only a few centers worldwide, require microsurgical technique, have a substantial complication rate consisting primarily of priapism, and overall less than a 50% success rate at 1-2-year follow-up (53-56). At present, although not considered experimental, these microsurgical penile revascularization procedures are still in their developmental stages and, thus, the indications for selective internal pudendal or cavernosal angiography are extremely limited.

In those patients in whom aortoiliac reconstruction is planned for the treatment of aneurysmal disease or arterial occlusive disease, slight modifications of the standard single-plane anteroposterior aortoiliofemoral arteriographic technique can be quite helpful in planning and performing the operative procedure in such a way as to maintain normal pelvic perfusion in those patients who are potent preoperatively and restore penile perfusion in those patients with vasculogenic impotence. We have found triplanar (anteroposterior, right, and left oblique) views of the pelvic and femoral areas quite useful in this regard (17,40,41). This more thorough arteriographic evaluation will occasionally demonstrate more severe degrees of proximal internal iliac artery stenosis than is revealed by an AP projection only, thus allowing for internal iliac endarterectomy, or bypass or reimplantation of the internal iliac artery to increase pelvic and penile perfusion (41,57). In those patients with arteriographic evidence of patent common and internal iliac arteries but occluded or severely stenotic external iliac arteries, the proximal aortic anastomosis should be done in an end-to-side fashion to preserve pelvic inflow. In those patients in whom aortobifemoral bypass is planned, thorough preoperative arteriography will occasionally reveal proximal common femoral artery disease thus allowing the surgeon to construct the distal anastomosis in such a way as to maximize retrograde flow up the external iliac arteries and into the internal iliac arteries. Likewise, oblique views of the femoral vessels will frequently reveal stenoses at the origin of the profunda femoris arteries which when bypassed will allow normal perfusion pressure into the rich collateral network of vessels between the profunda femoris and distal internal iliac system (40,44) and allow restoration of erectile function even in the presence of bilateral proximal internal iliac occlusion (17,40).

SUMMARY

On the basis of our experience and the abovementioned methods of evaluating vasculogenic impotence, we have devised and follow the clinical algorithm depicted in Figure 1. A thorough sexual history and physical examination in conjunction with a knowledge of the various causes of impotence will frequently be all that is needed prior to the institution of therapy or an appropriate and well-directed referral. In those patients in whom the etiology of impotence is still unclear following the sexual history and physical examination, appropriate application and interpretation of the evaluation procedures previously described will allow the clinician to arrive at an accurate etiologic diagnosis of impotence and treat it correctly.

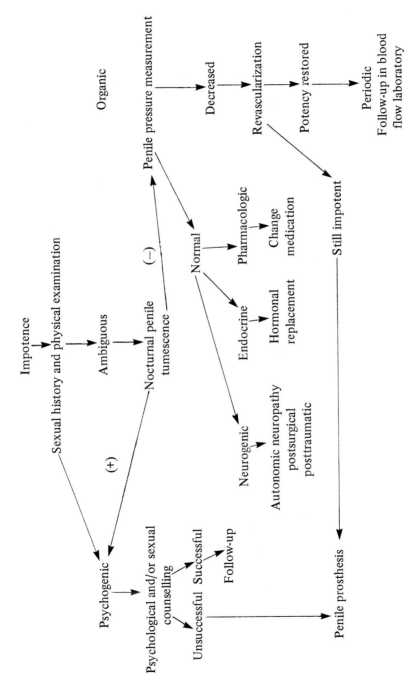

Figure 1 Clinical algorithm for the evaluation of secondary impotence.

REFERENCES

1. The Holy Bible: The Old Testament, Book of Genesis 20:13.
2. Gee WF: A history of surgical treatment of impotence. Urology 5:401, 1975.
3. Kinsey AC, Pomeroy WB, Marin CE: Sexual Behavior in the Human Male, WB Saunders Co, Philadelphia, p. 63, 1948.
4. DePalma RG, Kedia K, Persky L: Vascular operations for preservation of sexual function. In JJ Bergan and JST Yao (ed): Surgery of the Aorta and Its Body Branches, Grune and Stratton Inc., New York, p. 277, 1979.
5. Ruzbarsky V, Michal V: Morphologic changes in the arterial bed of the penis with aging: Relationship to the pathogenesis of impotence. Invest Urol 15: 194, 1977.
6. Fitzpatrick T: The corpus cavenosum intercommunicating venous drainage system. J Urol 113:494, 1975.
7. Fitzpatrick TJ, Cooper JF: A cavernosogram study on the valvular competence of the human deep dorsal vein. J Urol 113:497, 1975.
8. Fitzpatrick TJ: Venography of the deep dorsal venous and valvular systems. J Urol 111:518, 1974.
9. Benson GS, McConnell JA, Schmidt WA: Penile polsters: Functional structures or atherosclerotic changes? J Urol 125:800, 1981.
10. Polak JM, Gu J, Mina S, Bloom SR: Vipergic nerves in the penis. Lancet 2: 217, 1981.
11. Strauss EB: Impotence from the psychiatric standpoint. Br Med J 1:697, 1950.
12. Rubin A, Babbott D: Impotence and diabetes mellitus. J Am Med Assoc 168: 498, 1958.
13. Blaivas JG, O'Donnell TF, Gottlieb P, Labib KB: Comprehensive laboratory evaluation of impotent men. J Urol 124:201, 1980.
14. Ellenberg M: Impotence in diabetes: The neurologic factor. Ann Int Med 75: 213, 1971.
15. Leriche R, Morel A: The syndrome of thrombotic obliteration of the aortic bifurcation. Ann Surg 127:193, 1948.
16. Queral LA, Flinn WR, Bergan JJ, Yao JST: Sexual function and aortic surgery. In JJ Bergan and JST Yao (ed): Surgery of the Aorta and Its Body Branches, Grune and Stratton, Inc., New York, p. 263, 1979.
17. Flanigan DP, Schuler JJ, Keifer T, Schwartz JA, Lim LT: Elimination of iatrogenic impotence and improvement of sexual function after aortoiliac revascularization. Arch Surg 117:544, 1982.
18. Abelson D: Diagnostic value of the penile pulse and blood pressure: A Doppler study of impotence in diabetics. J Urol 113:636, 1975.
19. Chopp RT, Mendez R: Sexual function and hormonal abnormalities in uremic men on chronic dialysis and after renal transplantation. Fert Ster 29:661, 1978.
20. Wright AD, London DR, Holder G, Williams JW, Rudd BT: Luteinizing release hormone tests in impotent diabetic males. Diabetes 25:975, 1976.
21. Faerman I, Vilar O, Rivarola MA, Rosner JM, Jadzinsky MN, Fox D, Lloret AP, Bernstein-Hahn L, Saraceni D: Impotence and diabetes: Studies of androgenic function in diabetic impotent males. Diabetes 21:23, 1972.

22. Franks S, Jacobs HS, Martin N, Nabarro JDN: Hyperprolactinaemia and impotence. Clin Endocrinol 8:277, 1978.

23. Kolodny RC, Kahn CB, Goldstein HH, Barnett DM: Sexual dysfunction in diabetic men. Diabetes 23:306, 1974.

24. Benkert O, Horn K, Pickardt CR, Schmid D: Sexual impotence: Studies of the hypothalamic-pituitary-thyroid axis and the effect of oral thyrotropin-releasing factor. Arch Sexual Behav 5:275, 1976.

25. Karacan I, Hursch CJ, Williams RL: Some characteristics of nocturnal penile tumescence in elderly males. J Geron 27:39, 1972.

26. Karacan I, Hursch CJ, Williams RL, Thornby JI: Some characteristics of nocturnal penile tumescence in young adults. Arch Gen Psychiat 26:351, 1972.

27. Karacan I, Scott FB, Salis PJ, Attia SL, Ware JC, Altinel A, Williams RL: Nocturnal erections, differential diagnosis of impotence, and diabetes. Bio Psychiat 12:373, 1977.

28. Karacan I, Ware JC, Dervent B, Altinel A, Thornby JI, Williams RL, Kaya N, Scott FB: Impotence and blood pressure in the flaccid penis: Relationship to nocturnal penile tumescence. Sleep 1:125, 1978.

29. Karacan I, Williams RL, Thornby JI, Salis PJ: Sleep-related penile tumescence as a function of age. Am J Psychiat 132:932, 1975.

30. Wasserman MD, Pollack CP, Spielman AJ, Weitzman ED: Theoretical and technical problems in the measurement of nocturnal penile tumescence for the differential diagnosis of impotence. Psycho Med 42:575, 1980.

31. Marshall P, Morales A, Surridge D: Unreliability of nocturnal penile tumescence recording and MMPI profiles in assessment of impotence. Urology 17:136, 1981.

32. Canning JR, Bowers LM, Lloyd FA, Cottrell TLC: Genital vascular insufficiency and impotence. Surg Forum 14:298, 1963.

33. Britt DB, Kemmerer WT, Robison JR: Penile blood flow determination by mercury strain gauge plethysmography. Invest Urolol 8:673, 1971.

34. Gaskell P: The importance of penile blood pressure in cases of impotence. Can Med Assoc J 105:1047, 1971.

35. Malvar T, Baron T, Clark SS: Assessment of potency with the Doppler flowmeter. Urology 2:396, 1973.

36. Shirai M, Nakamura M, Ishii N, Mitsukawa S, Sawai Y: Determination of intrapenial blood volume using 99mTc-labeled autologous red blood cells. Tohoku J Exp Med 120:377, 1976.

37. Velcek D, Sniderman KW, Vaughan ED, Sos TA, Muecke ED: Penile flow index utilizing a Doppler pulse wave analysis to identify penile vascular insufficiency. J Urol 123:669, 1980.

38. Queral LA, Whitehouse WM, Flinn WR, Zarins CK, Bergan JJ, Yao JST: Pelvic hemodynamics after aortoiliac reconstruction. Surgery 86:799, 1979.

39. Kempczinski RF: Role of the vascular diagnostic laboratory in the evaluation of male impotence. Am J Surg 138:278, 1979.

40. Schuler JJ, Gray B, Flanigan DP, Williams LR: Increased penile perfusion and reversal of vasculogenic impotence following femoro-femoral bypass. Br J Surg 69 (Supplement):S6, 1982.

41. Flanigan DP, Sobinsky KR, Schuler JJ, Buchbinder D, Borozan PG, Meyer JP: Internal iliac artery revascularization in the treatment of vasculogenic impotence. Arch Surg 120:271, 1985.

42. Nath RL, Menzoian JO, Kaplan KH, McMillian TN, Siroky MB, Krane RJ: The multidisciplinary approach to vasculogenic impotence. Surgery 89:124, 1981.

43. DePalma RG: Impotence in vascular disease: Relationship to vascular surgery. Br J Surg 69 (Suppl.):S14, 1982.

44. Merchant RF, DePalma RG: Effects of femorofemoral grafts on postoperative sexual function: Correlation with penile pulse volume recordings. Surgery 90: 962, 1981.

45. DePalma RG, Kedia K, Persky L: Surgical options in the correction of vasculogenic impotence. Vasc Surg 14:92, 1980.

46. Rhodes BA, Grossman DS, Gupta SK, Weiser RK, Veith FJ, Samson RH: Improved technique for diagnosis of vasculogenic impotence. Bruit 8:171, 1984.

47. Lane RJ, Appleberg M, Williams W: A comparison of two techniques for the detection of the vasculogenic component of impotence. Surg Gynecol Obstet 155:230, 1982.

48. LaRosa, MP, Buchbinder D, Gray B, Zasadzinski J, Schuler JJ, Woelfel GF, Flanigan DP: Penile arterial study by photoplethysmography. Bruit 8:225, 1984.

49. Ginestie' J-F: Pudendal angiography. In AW Zorgniotti and G Rossi (eds): Vasculogenic Impotence: Proceedings of the first international conference on corpus cavernosum revascularization, Charles C. Thomas, Springfield, Illinois, p. 125, 1978.

50. Padula G: Problems of pudendal angiography. In AW Zorgniotti and G Rossi (eds): Vasculogenic Impotence: Proceedings of the first international conference on corpus cavernosum revascularization, Charles C. Thomas, Springfield, Illinois, p. 143, 1978.

51. Juhan CM, Huguet JF, Clerissi JA, Courjaret P: Classification of internal pudendal artery lesions in one hundred cases. In AW Zorgniotti and G Rossi (eds): Vasculogenic Impotence: Proceedings of the first international conference on corpus cavernosum revascularization. Charles C. Thomas, Springfield, Illinois, p. 153, 1978.

52. Michal V, Pospichal J, Blazkova' J: Arteriography of the internal pudendal arteries and passive erection. In AW Zorgniotti and G Rossi (eds): Vasculogenic Impotence: Proceedings of the first international conference on corpus cavernosum revascularization. Charles C. Thomas, Springfield, Illinois, p. 169, 1978.

53. LeVeen HH, Diaz C: Treatment by corpus cavernosum revascularization. In AW Zorgniotti and G Rossi (eds): Vasculogenic Impotence: Proceedings of the first international conference on corpus cavernosum revascularization. Charles C. Thomas, Springfield, Illinois, p. 217, 1978.

54. Ginestie' J: Results of the revascularization of the corpus cavernosum. In AW Zorgniotti and G Rossi (eds): Vasculogenic Impotence: Proceedings of the first international conference on corpus cavernosum revascularization. Charles C. Thomas, Springfield, Illinois, p. 235, 1978.

55. Casey WX, Kaufman JJ: Revascularization of the penis for erectile disability: Results in nine patients. In AW Zorgniotti and G Rossi (eds): Vasculogenic Impotence: Proceedings of the first international conference on corpus cavernosum revascularization. Charles C. Thomas, Springfield, Illinois, p. 257, 1978.
56. Houttuin E, Hawatmeh IS, Gregory JG, Hedgebeth CB, Blair OM: Femoro-cavernosal shunt by autogenous saphenous vein graft. In AW Zorgniotti and G Rossi (eds): Vasculogenic Impotence: Proceedings of the first international conference on corpus cavernosum revascularization. Charles C. Thomas, Springfield, Illinois, p. 273, 1978.
57. Cronenwett JL, Gooch JB, Garrett HE: Internal iliac artery revascularization during aortofemoral bypass. Arch Surg 117:838, 1982.

5

Methods of Preoperative Selection of Amputation Level

JOSEPH R. DURHAM*
University of Arizona
  Health Sciences Center
Tucson, Arizona

GARY G. ANDERSON
Veterans Administration
  Medical Center
Tucson, Arizona

JAMES M. MALONE
Tucson Veterans Administration
  Medical Center and
University of Arizona
  Health Sciences Center
Tucson, Arizona

There are between 50,000 and 60,000 new lower extremity amputations performed in the United States each year (1-3). Lower extremity amputation comprises approximately 2% of all operations performed each year in the Veteran Administration Hospital system, and the total economic impact approaches $6 billion per year (3). Two-thirds to 80% of all lower extremity amputations are required for peripheral vascular insufficiency and/or complications of diabetes mellitus. For those patients with diabetes mellitus, it is estimated that the risk of loss of the second leg in the ensuing 5 years after amputation of the first leg ranges from 15% to 33% (3-7%/year) (4); however, one-third to one-half of amputees with diabetes mellitus will die of complications from cardiorespiratory diseases or diabetes prior to undergoing amputation of their second extremity.

Accurate amputation level selection is of critical importance not only for morbidity and mortality, but also for eventual prosthetic rehabilitation. If too proximal an amputation, such as midthigh amputation, is performed, the patient

Supported in part by Veterans Administration R E R&D Research Grant Project #146.

Present affiliation: University of Illinois College of Medicine at Chicago, Chicago, Illinois may be deprived of the opportunity for subsequent ambulation and rehabilitation, even though the amputation might heal without difficulty. On the other hand, if too distal an amputation site is selected and the blood supply is inadequate for amputation healing, then further surgery will be required to achieve healing of an amputation at a higher level. This latter approach often results in increased morbidity and mortality and, in addition, may ultimately result in rehabilitation failure. The overall objective of preoperative amputation level selection is to determine the most distal amputation site that will heal. The general requirements for amputation level selection are as follows: (a) The proposed amputation must remove all necrotic, painful, or infected tissue; (b) the amputation stump must be able to be fitted with a functional and easily applied prosthesis; and (c) the blood supply at the level of proposed amputation must be sufficient to allow primary skin healing.

In prior decades, the majority of patients requiring lower limb amputation underwent above-knee amputation to assure amputation healing. With time, however, the inherent advantages of below-knee amputation have become increasingly apparent. In general, a unilateral below-knee amputee requires a 10-40% increase in energy expenditure for ambulation compared with the energy required for walking with an intact extremity (4). By contrast, a unilateral above-knee amputee, using a prosthesis with either a locked or free knee, requires approximately a 50-70% increase in energy expenditure (4). In comparison, crutch walking without a lower extremity prosthesis utilizes approximately a 60% increase in energy expenditure, while wheelchair use necessitates only a 9% increase in energy expenditure (4). Young patients will often walk quite well with an above-knee amputation; however, elderly patients, especially those with significant coronary artery disease and/or chronic obstructive pulmonary disease, may be physically unable to provide the additional energy expenditure required for ambulation on an above-knee prosthesis. In addition, conversion of a failed below-knee amputation to an above-knee amputation often converts a patient from independent ambulation to nonambulatory status.

The decision for an amputation level that will remove necrotic, painful, or infected tissue, as well as planning an amputation stump that can be fitted with a prosthesis is usually not a difficult problem. In contrast, however, the decision regarding the adequacy of blood supply at a proposed amputation level has been one of the most perplexing problems facing the amputation surgeon. Early workers in the field of amputation surgery solved the problem of level selection by performing above-knee amputations in almost all patients. The earliest attempts at objective amputation level selection utilized the presence of pulses in the affected extremity, skin temperature, correlation of arteriographic findings, skin edge bleeding at the time of surgery, and "clinical judgment." It is now generally well documented that none of these indirect selection techniques has a consistent enough correlation with amputation healing to provide a sound basis for clinical decision-making. However, one physical finding that has some predictive value is the presence of dependent rubor. Skin that develops dependent rubor is clearly ischemic and, therefore, skin with dependent rubor, like gangrenous tissue, is an absolute contraindication to amputation at that level. However, the absence of dependent rubor does not necessarily guarantee healing ability. Although Lim and co-workers demonstrated in the 1960s (5) that 83% of patients requiring lower extremity amputation would heal a below-knee amputation, empiric below-knee amputation potentially deprives some patients of a more distal lower extremity amputation, such as a foot or forefoot amputation. In addition, objective identification of the 20-30% of patients in whom a below-knee amputation is doomed to failure would be advantageous so that either a more proximal amputation, such as a knee disarticulation or an above-knee amputation, could be performed primarily or vascular reconstructive procedures could be considered in an effort to salvage a below-knee amputation.

The need for more sensitive and objective methods of preoperative amputation level selection has led to the development of numerous noninvasive diagnostic techniques. The following sections of this chapter will evaluate and discuss each of the currently used amputation level selection techniques. In addition, major levels of lower extremity amputation including the toe, the foot and forefoot, and below knee and above knee will be reviewed and the relative successes of amputation level selection techniques for each amputation level will be reviewed.

TECHNIQUES OF AMPUTATION LEVEL SELECTION

Clinical Judgment/Empiric Amputation Level Selection

Unfortunately, "clinical judgment" probably continues to be the most widely practiced method for amputation level selection. However, there is increasing objective data that clearly documents the pitfalls of empiric judgment. In a recent study by Robbs and Ray (6), the morbidity, mortality and rates of healing of lower limb amputations in 214 patients were analyzed restrospectively. Of 67 primary above-knee amputations, 6 (8.9%) had to be revised to a higher level. Thirty-seven of 147 below-knee amputations (25%) also had to be revised to a higher level. Most importantly the mortality from below-knee amputation increased almost threefold, from 1.5% to 4.1%, when amputation revision was required. The authors concluded "that flap viability could not be predicted by the extent of ischemic lesion in relation to the ankle joint, the popliteal pulse status, or lower limb angiography" (6). Unfortunately, however, these authors also concluded that, despite the increased mortality from amputation revision, a policy of primary empiric below-knee amputation was justified. Silverman et al. (7), in a recent study on fiberoptic fluorometry, noted that only 26 of 39 amputations healed (67%) when empiric criteria were used for amputation level selection, and that for amputations for below the ankle, the failure rate was 60%. In comparing the results between fiberoptic fluorometry and empiric amputation level selection, those authors concluded that "this study confirms the importance of skin perfusion in the selection of amputation level in the dysvascular extremity" (7,8). However, another recent study by Cederberg et al. (9) suggests that clinical findings are a sound basis for amputation level selection. In addition, their study demonstrated no significant relationship between Doppler-derived systolic calf pressure or calf/arm pressure index and the rate of primary healing of below-knee amputations in either diabetic or nondiabetic patients (9). In their study, 61 of 67 below-knee amputations, which were chosen on clinical judgment alone, healed primarily and only 23 of those limbs had calf systolic blood pressures >70 mmHg.

Summary calculations of the above studies suggest that empiric lower extremity amputation level selection resulted in successful primary healing in only 258 of 320 lower extremities (80%). This healing rate is not much different than that published by Lim et al. (5) in 1967 (83%). This data is in marked contrast to published reports which suggest that the healing rates for objective amputation level selection techniques range from 84 to 100% for below-knee amputation, and 86 to 100% for for toe and forefoot amputations (4).

Doppler Systolic Blood Pressure Measurements

The techniques for toe, ankle, calf, and popliteal Doppler systolic blood pressure determinations have been previously well described and will not be covered in the text of this chapter (4). The advantages of Doppler-derived blood pressures are that they are easy to obtain, inexpensive, noninvasive, and have good ability to predict amputation healing. However, the major problem with Doppler segmental pressures for amputation level selection is their relative inability to predict which amputations will not heal (negative predictive value). In an effort to increase the accuracy of Doppler ankle systolic pressures, several authors have suggested the adjunctive use of pulse volume recordings (PVR). Although Raines et al. (10) reported 100% successful healing of 27 below-knee amputations using a combination of ankle and calf blood pressures with PVR, Gibbons et al. (11) were unable to duplicate those results and concluded, in fact, that "there are no consistent criteria which are more accurate and reliable than clinical judgment and no ankle pressure above which primary healing was guaranteed." The success rates for amputation level selection using Doppler-derived pressures have varied with both the amputation level and the absolute pressure chosen as a selection point. Lepantalo et al. (12) reported 100% healing in 31 below-knee amputations where the calf systolic pressures were ⩾68 mmHg and the distal thigh systolic pressures were ⩾100 mmHg. In that study, when calf blood pressures were <35 mmHg and distal thigh pressures were <60 mmHg, all amputations failed to heal. The authors also noted that diabetes mellitus had no effect on the rate of amputation healing. Those data coincide nicely with a report by Nicholas et al. (13) wherein 33 of 34 (97%) below-knee amputations healed when the calf systolic blood pressure was ⩾70 mmHg. In the latter study, 39 of 43 below-knee amputations (91%) healed if the ankle systolic blood pressure was ⩾30 mmHg; however, the false-negative rates for the calf and ankle systolic blood pressure measurements were 32% and 40%, respectively. Nicholas et al. (13) concluded that Doppler systolic blood pressures can predict successful amputation healing but its use cannot reliably predict amputations that will fail to heal.

Although Doppler systolic pressures are reasonably accurate for below-knee amputation level selection, they have not fared quite so well for foot or forefoot amputations. Boeckstyns and Jensen recently reported primary healing in only 17 of 63 foot and forefoot amputations when the systolic ankle blood pressure was >40 mmHg (14). They also noted that there was no apparent correlation between diabetes mellitus and amputation healing. Holstein (15) suggested that digital systolic blood pressures might be more useful than ankle systolic blood pressures for distal forefoot and toe amputations. He noted a 78% success rate (51/65) for toe and forefoot amputation healing when the digital systolic blood pressure was ≥30 mmHg but only a 72% success rate (47/65) when the ankle systolic blood pressure was ≥100 mmHg. Holstein also noted that diabetes did not seem to have an effect on the success of digit and transmetatarsal amputations. The problems with the Doppler-derived pressures for amputations below the ankle were nicely summarized by Mehta et al. (16) who noted that "for forefoot amputation a high Doppler ankle blood pressure did not guarantee successful healing and a low ankle pressure did not contraindicate primary healing."

In summary then, Doppler systolic blood pressures have been used for amputation level selection at the toe, forefoot, foot, and below-knee level with varying success rates. Amputation healing can be accurately predicted when the systolic pressure is above a predetermined number, however, Doppler systolic pressures do not appear to have accuracy in predicting those patients who will fail to heal primarily their lower extremity amputation.

Fluorescein Dye Measurements

Although more invasive than Doppler systolic pressure measurements, assessment of skin blood flow based on skin fluorescence with a Wood's ultraviolet lamp after the intravenous injection of the fluorescein dye (Funduscen, Cooper Vision, San Germain, Puerto Rico) has demonstrated promise as an amputation level selection technique. Preliminary data reported by McFarland et al. (17) suggested an accuracy rate of 80% for skin fluorescence compared with only 47% for Doppler popliteal systolic blood pressure (≥50 mmHg) for prediction of healing of below-knee amputations. In addition, McFarland et al. (17) noted that when skin fluorescence and Doppler systolic pressures did not agree on the level of amputation, fluorescein always predicted a more distal level. The commercial availability of a new fiberoptic fluorometer (Diversotronics, Broomall, Pennsylvania), which is able to provide objective numerical readings (without a Wood's lamp), should further enhance the use of the fluorescein technique. Silverman et al. (7) recently reported their data on fiberoptic fluorometry for amputation level selection at the below-ankle, below-knee, and above-knee levels in dysvascular limbs. Overall, fiberoptic fluorometry successfully predicted amputation healing in 36 of 39 lower extremities (92%). Success ranges were as follows: 18/20 below ankle (90%), 12/12 below knee, and 6/7 above knee (80%). Discriminate analysis demonstrated an optimum reference point between healing and nonhealing amputations and a dye fluorescence index (DFI) of 44 had a 93% accuracy for amputation level selection. Validation of the preliminary data reported by Silverman et al. (7) is, of course, required, but fiberoptic fluorometry appears to have considerable potential for amputation level selection, especially since it appears to have a high accuracy rate at all levels of major lower extremity amputation.

Laser Doppler Velocimetry

Laser Doppler velocimetry is a technique that uses the Doppler principle much as the ultrasonic Doppler does, but it uses light rather than sound. Laser Doppler velocimetry has been compared to Xenon-133 skin blood flow measurements and blood flow measurements using microspheres and electromagnetic flow probes. These comparative studies have shown a linear relationship among techniques, but with a fair amount of variance (18-21). In addition, these studies have suggested that there is difficulty in calibrating laser Doppler velocimetry techniques against other more direct blood flow measurements. Holloway et al. (20,21) have suggested that the accuracy of laser Doppler velocimetry may be enhanced by local skin heating. Resting laser Doppler blood flow measurements in patients with ischemic vascular disease have much the same range as measurements in patients without vascular disease; however, when the skin under the laser probe was heated to 44°C for 10 min, patients with peripheral vascular disease demonstrated markedly diminished hyperemic responses as compared to normal patients (20,21). Holloway and Burgess (21) recently reported their experience with laser Doppler velocimetry in 20 lower extremity amputations at the foot, forefoot, below- and above-knee levels and the accuracy rates were: foot/forefoot 2/6 (33%); below knee 8/8 (100%); and above knee 6/6 (100%). To date, researchers using laser Doppler velocimetry have not reported actual numerical levels or patterned responses to heating which can be used as objective criteria for the successful prediction of amputation healing. The preliminary data reported by Holloway and colleagues (18-21) have clearly suggested that there is too much overlap and too low a predictability for unheated laser Doppler velocimetry to be an acceptable technique; however, the use of local skin heating may enhance the accuracy of the laser Doppler and make it a more valuable test for amputation level selection. The promising work reported so far remains to be validated in further studies.

Photoelectric Skin Perfusion Pressure (PSPP)

Skin perfusion pressure (SPP) measured by isotope washout techniques has consistently proved a reliable method of amputation level selection for below- and above-knee amputations (15,22-26). However, isotope-derived skin perfusion pressures determinations are time consuming, invasive, and require sophisticated nuclear medicine and computing equipment. Photoelectric measurement of skin perfusion pressure may offer a less invasive and simpler method of determining skin blood flow than isotope techniques. The technique for PSPP has been described in detail by Stockel et al. (27); briefly, the equipment consists of a photodetector that is placed against the patient's skin and connected to a plethysmograph (Medimatic, Denmark). External counter pressure over the photodetector is applied with a blood pressure cuff. Pressure on the photodetector is raised to suprasystolic level and then reduced in a constant slow speed. When capillary inflow begins, the plethysmographic tracing changes direction and the skin perfusion pressure (minimal external pressure to prevent reddening after blanching of the skin) is read as the external counter pressure (in mmHg) at that point. Apparently there have been difficulties interpreting tracings in patients with low lower-extremity systolic blood pressures, so a standardized reading technique has been developed whereby the systolic pressure is measured directly by a strain gauge technique at the same level of the leg at which the photoelectric tracing is being performed (27). Oveson and Stockel (28) recently reported that 34 of 40 below-knee amputations healed when the photoelectric SPP was $\geqslant 21$ mmHg; however, some healing failures occurred at pressures $\leqslant 60$ mmHg. In that same study 19/19 above-knee amputations healed primarily when the PSPP was $\geqslant 21$ mmHg. The authors concluded that the standardized photoelectric technique can, in many cases, replace isotope washout techniques as a routine method for lower extremity amputation level selection; however, the isotope technique should be the method of choice when technically satisfactory photoelectric tracings cannot be measured, or in cases where systolic pressures cannot be accurately obtained (28). The exact role for photoelectric skin perfusion pressures for amputation level selection will have to await comparative studies with fiberoptic fluorometry, transcutaneous oxygen, and isotope skin blood flow studies by other investigators.

Isotope Measurement of Skin Perfusion Pressure (SPP)

Holstein (15,22) and Holstein et al. (23-26) have published numerous studies on isotope-derived skin perfusion pressures. In general, skin perfusion pressures derived from isotope clearance studies have correlated well with isotope skin blood flow measurements reported by Moore, Malone, and colleagues (4).

Estimation of local tissue perfusion pressure by isotope washout was originally described by Nilsen et al. (29) and Holstein (26) using Xenon-133 in muscle and skin. For the measurement of skin perfusion pressure, [133]I antipyrine was found by Holstein et al. (24) to be more reliable than Xenon-133, since [133]I antipyrine is not trapped in the subcutaneous fat. Munck and Anderson (30) observed that ^{131}I antipyrine was unstable, splitting off iodine, but Munck, Anderson, and Binder (31) found no basis for favoring labeled antipyrine over sodium or iodide for assessment of subcutaneous tissue circulation. In a more recent publication Holstein et al. (26) found so significant difference among (NA) [131]I, ^{131}I antipyrine, and Tc^{99m}-pertechnetate for measurement of SPP.

Holstein modified the radioisotope clearance method originally described for measurement of muscle perfusion for use in the skin (15). Skin perfusion pressure was measured as the external counterpressure necessary to stop the clearance of intradermal of ^{133}I antipyrine. In Holstein's preliminary study of 29 amputations, failure of healing occurred if the skin perfusion pressure at the proposed amputation level was <20 mmHg; however, if the skin perfusion pressure was >40 mmHg 80% of the amputations healed successfully. In a subsequent study, Holstein et al. (25) presented isotope SPP data on 67 lower extremity amputations: if SPP was <20 mmHg, a 25% healing rate was noted; a 67% healing rate occurred when the SPP was between 20 and 30 mmHg; and for SPP >30 mmHg the healing rate was 90%. In a recent review of isotope skin perfusion pressure measurements, Holstein et al. compared ^{131}I antipyrine, Na (^{131}I), and pertechnetate (Tc^{99m}) and reported that isotopically derived skin perfusion pressure was significantly correlated with skin blood flow, systolic blood pressure, angiographic findings, and transcutaneous oxygen measurements (26). Although these reports by Holstein (15,22) and Holstein et al. (23-26) suggest that there is a correlation between isotopically derived skin perfusion pressure and successful amputation healing, it is also clear that SPP does not provide a sharp demarcation point above which all amputations heal and below which no amputations heal.

Skin Temperature

Although empiric amputation level selection techniques, including clinical assessment of skin temperature, do not provide a rational basis for amputation level selection, recent data have been published which suggests that new techniques for skin temperature measurement may provide valid data for objective amputation level selection. Frank Golbranson recently presented data demonstrating that skin temperature measurement had a high degree of accuracy (90%) for selecting below-knee versus above-knee amputation levels (32). In addition, a recent study by Spence and Walker (33) documented a clear correlation between three different temperature isotherms (1.8°C separation), and isotopically derived skin blood flow (p < 0.001). In the latter study color thermograms (0.6°C separation) were mapped into 10 sets of isotherms on the lower extremities of dysvascular patients all of whom underwent lower extremity amputations. These isotherms were compared to skin blood flow data calculated from the cutaneous isotope washout of 4-^{125}I-iodoantipyrine and a statistical correlation between skin blood flow at three isotherm levels (with 1.8°C separation) was noted. Thermographic mapping may have considerable promise for objective amputation level selection, especially since thermographic examinations can be easily performed and the test provides a contoured isothermic map of the lower limb, which might be useful for surgical flap design.

Transcutaneous Oxygen Measurements (TcPO$_2$)

Promising work with a modified Clark-type heated oxygen electrode has been reported by several groups. Franzeck et al. (34) reported that the mean transcutaneous

PO_2 ($TcPO_2$) valves of patients who primarily healed their lower extremity amputation compared with those who failed to heal were 36.5 ± 17.5 mmHg and <0.3 mmHg, respectively. However, three of nine patients with $TcPO_2$ measurements <10 mmHg healed primarily, suggesting that the ability of $TcPO_2$ to predict failure to heal may be somewhat less accurate than its ability to predict successful healing. Burgess et al. (35) found that 15/15 below-knee amputations healed if the $TcPO_2$ was >40 mmHg, 17/19 healed if the $TcPO_2$ was >0 but <40 mmHg and 0/3 amputations healed if the $TcPO_2$ = 0 mmHg. Katsamouris et al. (36) more recently found that 17/17 lower extremity amputations healed primarily if the $TcPO_2$ was >38 mmHg or if the $TcPO_2$ index (chest wall control site) was >0.59. In addition, this latter group followed $TcPO_2$ measurements during the healing stages after amputation and found a lower $TcPO_2$ on the posterior flap as compared with the skin immediately anterior to the suture line, the direct opposite of the usual preoperative findings. They felt that this change in $TcPO_2$ was compatible with the partial debulking/devascularization of the posterior flap and/or angulation of the flap associated with surgery. Such observations only serve to reemphasize the necessity for gentle, meticulous surgical technique with careful skin coaptation, to obtain primary healing. Ratliff et al. (37) recently reported their experience in the Royal South Hants Hospital in South Hampton, United Kingdom. Eighteen below-knee amputations healed if the $TcPO_2$ was >35 mmHg whereas 10/15 failed to heal if the $TcPO_2$ was <35 mmHg. In addition, the $TcPO_2$ data for above knee amputations suggested that there was a wide difference between the mean $TcPO_2$ valves for those patients that healed primarily ($TcPO_2$ = 53 mmHg) and those that failed ($TcPO_2$ = 20 mmHg). In summary, all of these studies suggest that transcutaneous oxygen measurements can successfully predict amputations healing with a high degree of accuracy; however, the ability of $TcPO_2$ to predict failure to heal is promising, but not yet well defined. In addition, as pointed by Ratliff et al. (37), failure of amputation healing is often due to postoperative factors and is multifactorial in origin, so that a preoperative test of whatever nature cannot be expected always to predict the outcome with complete reliability.

Several recent articles have attempted to explain the discrepancy between $TcPO_2$ and actual skin blood flow measurements at low $TcPO_2$ valves (<10 mmHg). Such data may, in fact, provide a partial explanation of why patients heal amputations with low $TcPO_2$ measurements. Matsen et al. (38) reported that there is a nonlinear relationship between $TcPO_2$ and local cutaneous blood flow. In that study $TcPO_2$ readings of 0 mmHg were obtained in the presence of significant local cutaneous blood flow (AV gradients = 13-34 mmHg). $TcPO_2$ measurements are dependent upon the ratio of arterial-venous gradients and vascular resistance. Heating ($44°C$) minimizes local vascular resistance and tends to make $TcPO_2$ measurements more parallel with local cutaneous blood flow. Although it could be expected that ischemic limbs would have a low vascular resistance, the use of a heated $TcPO_2$ electrode seems warranted. Spence et al. (39) suggested that the $TcPO_2$ values are not directly related to tissue PO_2 and may not represent local oxygen availability since oxygen extraction and utilization is significantly altered in ischemic tissues. However, they concluded that $TcPO_2$ might be closely related to actual arterial perfusion pressure, especially in ischemic areas, since the autoregulation mechanisms are presumably abolished in the face of significant ischemia.

Other investigators have attempted to find ways of enhancing the accuracy of $TcPO_2$ measurements by methods other than local skin heating. Spence et al. (39) demonstrated an increase in $TcPO_2$ measurements of over 300% in patients breathing oxygen for 4 min. That data was obtained with a microelectrode with a 15-μm platinum-tip wire, which most probably measured actual cellular oxygen partial pressure rather than $TcPO_2$. Spence et al. (39) concluded that "the oxygen breathing response of local tissue," as measured by $TcPO_2$, with the patient breathing oxygen, may be as important or more important than the $TcPO_2$ measurement with the patient breathing room air. A somewhat similar approach to enhance the accuracy of $TcPO_2$ measurements was reported by Mustapha et al. (40). That study evaluated changes in $TcPO_2$ after breathing oxygen, through a 2-liter mask or following the intravenous infusion of Naftidrofuryl (a drug that has been shown to increase oxydative cellular metabolism). Their data suggest that a $TcPO_2 \geqslant 40$ mmHg indicates adequate perfusion for healing, whereas a recording of $\leqslant 30$ mmHg is inadequate. In addition, they demonstrated a significant increase in $TcPO_2$ after oxygen breathing (42 mmHg to 56 mmHg) or naftidrofuryl infusion (42 mmHg to 52 mmHg) and an even more striking increase was noted after drug infusion and oxygen together (42 mmHg to 64 mmHg) (40). However, it is unclear from their preliminary report whether such data have direct clinical application for prospective amputation level selection. Yet a different approach was taken by Ito et al. (41), who suggested mapping oxygen isobars on the lower limb based upon circumferential $TcPO_2$ measurements. The potential advantage of the oxygen isobar technique is that surgical flaps could be modified to match the $TcPO_2$ isobars. In their study of foot, below-knee, and above-knee amputations, Ito et al. (41) reported that 28/31 amputations healed if the $TcPO_2$ was $\geqslant 30$ mmHg. In a report evaluating the use of transcutaneous oxygen measurements for peripheral vascular disease, Kram et al. (42) suggested that transcutaneous oxygen recovery halftime (TORT) provided increased discrimination for objective evaluation of room air $TcPO_2$ measurements. Perhaps, more importantly, their data also suggested that TORT measurements had a clear-cut relationship for quantitatively evaluating residual disease *after* operative reconstructive surgery. Finally, Harward et al. (43) recently published an elegant analysis on $TcPO_2$ measurements for amputation level selection. That study evaluated the accuracy of $TcPO_2$ measurement while patients were breathing room air and again while breating oxygen. Amputation levels evaluated included the toe, foot and forefoot, below knee and above knee (with midcalf measurements). At all amputation levels, the oxygen breathing allowed increased accuracy for amputation level selection. Harward et al. (43) reported that a $TcPO_2 \geqslant 10$ mmHg when breathing room air or > 10 mmHg increase after oxygen breathing provided accurate prediction for amputation healing or failing. For the below-knee amputation level, the sensitivity of their test criteria was 95%, specificity was 100%, the accuracy was 95%, the positive predictive value was 100%, and the negative predictive value was 50%. Not surprisingly, the accuracy of the test was higher for above-knee amputations and lower for toe and transmetatarsal amputations.

We have just begun a comparison study at the Tucson VA Medical Center evaluating $TcPO_2$, transcutaneous PCO_2 ($TcPCO_2$), and Xenon-133 skin blood flow measurements for lower extremity amputation level selection. To date 17 major lower extremity amputations have been evaluated: 3 foot, 9 below knee; and 5 above knee. Fifteen/seventeen amputations with $TcPO_2$ values $\geqslant 20$ mmHg healed primarily. One failure had a $TcPO_2 = 37$ mmHg but the failure was due to infection rather than ischemia. The other failure had a $TcPO_2 = 13$ mmHg and the failure was due to ischemic necrosis. The mean $TcPO_2$ for amputations that successfully healed was 35 mmHg (N = 15), whereas it was 20 mmHg (N = 2) for those that failed. We have previously used 2.6 ml/100 g tissue/min as the optimum point for amputation level selection with Xenon-133 skin blood flow. The two amputations that failed in this preliminary study had xenon values of 3.0 and 1.6 ml/100 g tissue/min. The xenon of 3.0 ml/100 g tissue/min corresponded to a $TcPO_2$ of 13 mmHg, whereas the xenon of 1.6 ml/100 g tissue/min corresponded to a $TcPO_2$ of 37 mmHg. The former amputation failed due to ischemic necrosis, whereas the latter amputation failed due to infection. The relative merits of $TcPO_2$ as compared with Xenon-133 skin blood flow for prospective amputation level selection is unclear from our preliminary data. More patients and further analysis will be required before any definitive conclusions can be reached.

Transcutaneous Carbon Dioxide Measurements ($TcPCO_2$)

As mentioned in the section on $TcPO_2$ measurements, our group has been evaluating $TcPO_2$, $TcPCO_2$, and Xenon-133 skin blood flow for prospective amputation levels selection. We have been utilizing a Nova Matrix^{TM} system, which incorporates a combined transcutaneous PO_2/PCO_2 electrode. The exact correlation between $TcPCO_2$, skin blood flow, and amputation healing is, of course, unknown at the present time. In addition, whether or not $TcPCO_2$ behaves in a nonlinear fashion with respect to blood flow, such as was previously discussed for $TcPO_2$, is unclear. The combined electrode uses a heated element, and all measurements were made at 44°C after allowing time for membrane equilibration. $TcPCO_2$ measurements ranged from 21.5 to 43 mmHg. Primary amputation healing was seen in 16/17 patients with $TcPCO_2 < 40$ mmHg. There were two amputation failures in our initial 17 patients and one failure was due to ischemic necrosis ($TcPCO_2 = 43$ mmHg) and one failure was due to infection ($TcPCO_2 = 21.5$ mmHg). The exact accuracy of $TcPCO_2$ measurements for amputation level selection and their correlation with $TcPO_2$ and Xenon-133 skin blood flow measurements remain to be further evaluated.

Xenon-133 Skin Blood Flow Measurements

The authors' greatest experience for prospective amputation level selection is with the use of Xenon-133 skin blood flow techniques (4,44). Xenon-133 skin blood flow is determined in the Nuclear Medicine Department using an intradermal injection of Xenon-133 gas dissolved in saline and the rate of isotope clearance is measured with a gamma camera interfaced to a minicomputer (4,44). Dual point testing (1 cm separation) is performed in order to eliminate injection error. The monoexponential washout rate of the intradermal Xenon-133 during the first 6 min after injection is entered into the Schmidt-Kety equation and blood flow is calculated in milliliters/minute per 100 g of tissue. The reproducibility of the method in normal subjects and repeat measurements in study subjects are satisfactory. Room/environment temperature control during measurement is extremely important since skin blood flow changes with environmental temperature in a nonlinear "sigmoid" manner (45). It has been our practice to offer a below-knee amputation to any patient when the Xenon-133 skin blood flow is between 2.0 and 2.6 ml/min per 100 g of tissue, in spite of the fact that the objective reference point for successful prediction of amputation healing is 2.6 ml/min per 100 g of tissue. Previous reports from our center have suggested that the rates of primary healing for major lower extremity amputation based upon Xenon-133 skin blood flow measurements are as follows: toe, 83%; transmetatarsal, 89%; Symes, 92%; below knee, 97%; above knee, 100%. As mentioned in previous sections, we are in the process of comparing Xenon-133 skin blood flow data with $TcPO_2$ and $TcPCO_2$ measurements. In our initial 17 patients, one amputation failure (due to infection) was correctly predicted by Xenon-133 skin blood flow of 1.6 ml/min per 100 g of tissue; however, one failure due to ischemic necrosis had a below-knee Xenon-133 skin blood flow of 3.0 ml/100 g tissue per minute, a value of which should have predicted successful healing.

One of the major difficulties with the application of Xenon-133 skin blood flow techniques for amputation level selection has been the reproducibility of results by other investigators. Holloway and Burgess (19) were unable to document a clear-cut end point above which all amputations healed. On the other hand, Silberstein et al. (46) recently reported that 38/39 patients (11 Ak, 18 BK/TMA, and 9 no amputation) healed when Xenon-133 skin blood flow was >2.4 ml/min per 100 g of tissue, and that when flow was less than 2.4 ml/min per 100 g of tissue only 4/7 patients healed. Prior analysis of failure to heal in our patients with satisfactory Xenon-133 skin blood flow levels suggested three main reasons for failure: (a) computing error, which occured early in our experience and is no longer a problem; (b) infection and/or errors in surgical judgment, with performance of a primary amputation through areas of cellulitis; and (c) late stump trauma after primary skin healing, but in which cases there was ischemic muscle underlying the healed skin.

Intradermal Xenon-133 skin blood flow techniques and radioisotope skin perfusion pressure studies yield approximately the same results with the same selection end points for prospective amputation level selection (4). Common problems with intradermal radioisotope injections for measurements of skin blood flow or skin perfusion pressure are that the tests are invasive, they require sophisticated computing equipment and computer software, and they must be performed in a very precise manner by trained technicians. For just these reasons a prior publication on the epicutaneous application of Xenon-133 by Kostuik et al. (47) deserves discussion. In a blind study of 17 below-knee amputations, two failures occurred with a skin blood flow <0.5 ml/min per 100 g of tissue. Fourteen/fifteen amputations healed primarily when the skin blood flow was >0.9 ml/min per 100 g of tissue. It has suggested that the difference between the results of Kostuik et al. (47) and those of Moore, Malone, and colleagues (3, 4, 44) are possibly due to differences between epicutaneous versus intradermal radioisotope clearance. The technique of epicutaneous Xenon-133 administration obviates the need for intradermal injection; however, sophisticated computing equipment is still required for calculation of skin blood flow. Be that as it may, Kostuik et al. (47) have suggested that a minimum skin blood flow of 1.5 ml/min per 100 g of tissue should serve as a criterium for prospective below-knee amputation level selection.

OVERVIEW OF PROSPECTIVE LOWER EXTREMITY AMPUTATION LEVEL SELECTION

Toe Amputation

A review of the current published results for amputation level selection at the digit level are shown in Table 1. The accuracy rate ranges from a low 78% (Doppler digital systolic pressure) to a high of 100% (photoplethysmography), and the overall average was 86% (140/163). The accuracy rate of Doppler systolic pressure measurements for amputations at this level, especially in diabetic patients, will be significantly altered by the presence of calcified vessels. $TcPO_2$ measurements may be abnormally low due to AV shunting. Xenon-133 skin blood flow measurements may be falsely elevated due to measurement in areas of cellulitis or hyperemia. The available data suggest that the best technique for selection of digital amputation is photothysmographic digit or forefoot systolic blood pressure measurements and that Doppler ankle systolic pressure measurements are a reasonable second choice.

Table 1 Toe Amputation

Selection Criteria	Reference #	Healing Extremities (%)
Doppler *toe* systolic pressure $\geqslant 30$ mmHg	22	47/60 (78)
Doppler *ankle* systolic pressure $\geqslant 35$ mmHg	50	44/46 (96)
Photoplethysmographic digit or TMA systolic pressure $\geqslant 20$ mmHg	51	20/20 (100)
$TcPO_2$ $\geqslant 10$ mmHg *or* $\geqslant 10$ mmHg increase on 100% oxygen	43	24/31 (77)
Xenon-133 skin blood flow >2.6 ml/100 g tissue/min	44	5/6 (83)
Totals		140/163 (86)

Foot and Forefoot Amputation

An overview of published data for amputation level selection at the foot and fore-foot level is shown in Table 2. The accuracy rate for prospective amputation level selection below the ankle ranges from a low of 33% (Doppler ankle systolic pressure $\geqslant 40$ mmHg or laser Doppler velocimetry) to a high of 100% ($TcPO_2$ and $TcPCO_2$). The accuracy rate of ankle Doppler systolic blood pressures is clearly related to the absolute pressure used for prediction of amputation healing. The accuracy rate for $\geqslant 40$ mmHg is only 33%, whereas the accuracy rate for $\geqslant 70$ mmHg is 75%. Both fiberoptic fluorometry and $TcPO_2$ and $TcPCO_2$ appear to have excellent potential for prediction of amputation healing at this level. Xenon-133 skin blood flow measurements have a rather high predictive accuracy; how-ever, the test is somewhat more invasive than other techniques and, as previously noted, requires special nuclear medicine and computing capabilities. The published data suggests that the most accurate techniques are fiberoptic fluorometry and $TcPO_2$ or $TcPCO_2$ measurements. If available, Xenon-133 skin blood flow measure-ments also have excellent accuracy rates. Doppler ankle systolic pressure measure-ments would certainly serve as a standby technique if nothing else is available. The overall ability for noninvasive tests to predict correctly healing of foot and fore-foot amputations was only 67% (163/244); however, deletion of the poor results reported with laser Doppler velocimetry and Doppler ankle systolic pressure <70 mmHg results in an overall accuracy rate of 81% (127/157).

Table 2 Foot and Forefoot Amputation

Selection Criteria	Reference #	Healing Extremities (%)	
Doppler *ankle* systolic pressure			
⩾40 mmHg	14	20/60	(33)
⩾50 mmHg	22	14/21	(66)
⩾70 mmHg	13,52	70/93	(75)
Doppler *toe* systolic pressure			
⩾30 mmHg	22	4/5	(80)
Fiberoptic fluorometry DFI (Dye Fluoresence index: >44)	7	18/20	(90)
Laser doppler velocimetry	21	2/6	(33)
$TcPO_2$			
⩾10 mmHg *or* ⩾10 mmHg increase on 100% oxygen	43	6/8	(75)
⩾28 mmHg	a	3/3	(100)
$TcPCO_2$			
⩽40 mmHg	a	3/3	(100)
Xenon-133 skin blood flow			
⩾2.6 ml/100 g tissue per min	a	23/25	(92)
Totals		163/244	(67)

a = Current text.

Below-Knee Amputation

An overview of the current status for prospective amputation level selection in over 600 below-knee amputations is shown in Table 3. Accuracy rates range from a low of 71% ($TcPO_2 < 10 > 40$ mmHg) to a high of 100% (many tests); however, deletion of the poor results with low $TcPO_2$ values suggests accuracy rates from 80% to 100% are easily attainable. In that light, it is important to emphasize that empiric below-knee selection can achieve success rates of 80% (5-7,9). With the exceptions of non-fiber optic fluoroscein dye techniques and low $TcPO_2$ values, all other techniques for prospective below-knee amputation level selection result in a 5-20% improvement in amputation healing compared with empiric below-knee selection (Table 3). There are a variety of tests that provide accurate prospective amputation level selection at the below-knee level, and the choice of a specific technique

Table 3 Below-Knee Amputation

Selection Criteria	Reference #	Healing Extremities (%)	
Doppler *ankle* systolic pressure			
⩾30 mmHg	10,13	66/70	(94)
Doppler calf systolic pressure			
⩾50 mmHg	53	36/36	(100)
⩾68 mmHg	12,13,54	96/97	(99)
Empiric BK	5,6,9	209/260	(80)
Fluorescein dye	17	24/30	(80)
Fiberoptic flurometry			
(Dye Fluoresence Index: DFI > 44)	7	12/12	(100)
Laser Doppler velocimetry	21	8/8	(100)
Pertechnetate 99m (skin			
perfusion press: SPP)	23	24/26	(92)
Photoelectric skin perfusion			
press (PSPP) ⩾20 mmHg	27,28	60/71	(85)
TcPCO$_2$			
⩽40 mmHg	a	7/8	(88)
TcPO$_2$			
= 0 mmHg	35	0/3	(00)
⩾10 mmHg *or* ⩾10 mmHg			
increase on 100% oxygen	34,43	76/80	(95)
⩾10 ⩽40 mmHg	a	5/7	(71)
⩾35 mmHg	35-37,a	51/51	(100)
TcPO$_2$ index >0.59	36	17/17	(100)
Xenon-133 skin blood flow			
epicutaneous			
⩾0.90 ml/100 g tissue per min	47,55	14/15	(93)
Intradermal ⩾2.4 ml/100 g tissue			
per min	19,44,a,46	83/89	(93)
Totals (excludes empiric BK and TcPO$_2$ = 0)		579/617	(94)

a = Current text.

will depend upon equipment and facilities available to the amputation surgeon. Doppler ankle or calf systolic blood pressure measurements certainly provide a simple and accurate baseline against which other tests can be compared. Fiberoptic fluorometry, laser Doppler velocimetry, $TcPO_2$, $TcPCO_2$, photoelectric skin perfusion pressure, and Xenon-133 skin blood flow measurements all provide diagnostic techniques that have good to excellent accuracy for below-knee prospective amputation level selection. Overall, excluding empiric below-knee selection and low $TcPO_2$ values, prospective below-knee level selection tests have an accuracy rate of 94% (574/610). It is important to emphasize that this overall rate of 94% is a 14% improvement over empiric below-knee selection and that the increased salvage of this many knee joints (86 = 14% X 617) has significant impact on patient rehabilitation.

Above-Knee Amputation

Since it is assumed by most surgeons that above-knee amputations will heal without difficulty, it is interesting that many investigators have chosen to evaluate prospective amputation selection techniques at the above-knee level. Recognizing

Table 4 Above-Knee Amputation

Selection Criteria	Reference #	Healing Extremities (%)	
Fiberoptic flurometry DFI > 44	7	6/7	(86)
Laser Doppler velocimetry	21	6/6	(100)
Photoelectric skin perfusion pressure (PSPP)			
≥21 mmHg	28	19/19	(100)
$TcPCO_2$			
≤38 mmHg	a	5/5	(100)
$TcPO_2$			
≥10 mmHg *or* ≥10 mmHg			
increase on 100% oxygen	43	15/23	(65)
≥23 mmHg	a	2/2	(100)
≥35 mmHg	37,[a]	21/24	(88)
Xenon-133 skin blood flow			
≥2.4 ml/100 g tissue/min	44,[a],46	20/20	(100)
Totals		94/106	(89)

[a] = Current text.

that most above-knee amputations are performed in dysvascular amputees and that primary amputation at this level is rather uncommon for simple complications of diabetes mellitus, it is perhaps not surprising that there is a failure rate for primary healing of above-knee amputations. The reported data for prospective amputation level selection at the above-knee level are shown in Table 4. The overall accuracy was 98/108 or 89%. It should not, however, be extrapolated from this data that one expects an 11% failure rate for above-knee amputation, since the primary function of these studies was to evaluate prospective selection criteria. Nevertheless, it has been our experience that there is approximately a 2% failure rate when above-knee amputations are performed in dysvascular amputees. The accuracy rates for amputation level selection for above-knee amputation range from a low of 65% (calf $TcPO_2$) to a high of 100% (most tests). Although one might argue that aggressive attempts at prospective amputation level selection may not be indicated at the above-knee level, since the failure rate is so low, prior sections of this chapter have pointed out that amputation revision for failure results in increased patient morbidity and mortality, and, therefore, prospective amputation level selection for above-knee amputation is clearly indicated. In addition, if objective level selection techniques suggest that a below-knee amputation is not possible and that only an above-knee amputation will heal, then that patient should be reevaluated for lower extremity vascular reconstruction in an effort to lower the amputation level from an above-knee to a below-knee level.

ANCILLARY FACTORS OF IMPORTANCE

It has been our experience, as well as that of others, that diabetes mellitus has no significant impact on success rates for primary healing after major lower extremity amputation (1,3,4,18,44).

The role for hemodilution as an adjunct for amputation healing is unclear. Bailey et al. (48) have suggested that preoperative hemoglobin level may be important in diabetic patients undergoing lower extremity amputation. In that series, 18 amputations performed in patients with preoperative hemoglobin levels <12 g healed primarily whereas 30 amputations performed in patients with the hemoglobin level >13 g failed to heal. However, Kacy et al. (2) noted that below-knee healing was improved by low hemoglobin levels in patients with diabetes mellitus and cellulitis, but not in patients with diabetes mellitus without cellulitis. That same study by Kacy et al. (2) also noted that the absence of femoral pulses uniformly predicted a nonhealing below-knee amputation in patients with cellulitis, whereas in patients without cellulitis healing occurred 85% of the time. In addition Kacy et al. (2) found that cellulitis of the foot did not significantly affect healing of below-knee amputation in patients with diabetes mellitus (82.5% with cellulitis vs. 87.5% without cellulitis), but did affect healing in nondiabetic patients with (66.7%) and without (81.8%) cellulitis (p ≤ 0.05). The exact value of hemodilution, especially in patients with small vessel disease, marginally viable skin, or borderline skin blood flow, is unclear; however, Gatti et al. (8) have suggested that isovolemic hemodilution might be a valuable technique for the salvage of marginally ischemic tissues.

Finally, a recent publication by Dickhuat et al. (49) describing the effects of nutritional status for predicting wound healing after amputation, reported a significant correlation between serum albumin ($\geq$3.5 g/dl) and lymphocyte count ($>$1500 m^3). That study examined the influence of nutritional status on morbidity in 23 diabetic patients who underwent a Symes amputation. Six of seven patients with proper nutritional criteria healed at the Symes level; in contrast only two of 11 patients who healed and did not meet the same nutritional criteria. It is important to note that all 23 patients in that study met Wagner's criteria for a Symes level amputation (49).

SUMMARY

Multiple semiinvasive, noninvasive, and invasive techniques are available for prospective amputation level selection for major and minor lower extremity amputations. Depending upon the technique chosen and the amputation level studied, success rates for these techniques vary from acceptable to excellent. The benchmark for amputation level selection techniques must be 80% primary healing at the below-knee level, since that statistical end point can be achieved by empiric below-knee selection with disregard to findings on physical examination or objective selection criteria. The failure to achieve primary healing after lower extremity amputation results in significantly increased patient morbidity, mortality, and rehabilitation failures. In the authors' opinion, major lower extremity amputation should not be done without preoperative objective amputation level selection. Objective healing criteria can serve to advise the amputation surgeon of the likelihood of primary healing at the chosen level of amputation or the requirement for preamputation vascular reconstruction to achieve healing at the level chosen for amputation.

REFERENCES

1. Huston CC, Bivins BA, Ernst CB, Griffen WO Jr: Morbid implications of above-knee amputations. Report of a series and review of the literature. Arch Surg 115:165-167, 1980.
2. Kacy SS, Wolma FJ, Flye MW: Factors affecting the results of below knee amputation in patients with and without diabetes. Surg Gyn Obstet 155:513-518, 1982.
3. Malone JM, Moore WS, Goldstone J, Malone SJ: Therapeutic and economic impact of a modern amputation program. Ann Surg 189:798-802, 1979.

4. Malone JM, Goldstone J: Lower extremity amputation. In Moore WS (ed): Vascular Surgery: A Comprehensive Review, Grune & Stratton, New York, pp. 909-974, 1984.

5. Lim RC Sr, Blaisdell FW, Hall AD, Moore WS, Thomas AN: Below knee amputation for ischemic gangrene. Surg Gyn Obstet 125:493-501, 1967.

6. Robbs JV, Ray R: Clinical predictors of below-knee stump healing following amputation for ischemia. South African J Surg, 20(4):305-310, 1982.

7. Silverman DG, Rubin SM, Reilly CA, Brousseau DA, Norton KJ, Wolf GL: Fluorometric prediction of successful amputation level in the ischemic limb. J Rehab Res Dev 22:29-34, 1985.

8. Gatti JE, LaRossa D, Neff SR, Silverman DS: Altered skin flap survival and fluorescin kinetics with hemodilution. Surgery 92:200-205, 1982.

9. Cederberg PA, Pritchard DJ, Joyce JW: Doppler-determined segmental pressures and wound-healing in amputations for vascular disease. J Bone Joint Surg 65(3):363-365, 1983.

10. Raines JK, Darling RC, Buth J, Brewster DC, Austen WG: Vascular laboratory criteria for the management of peripheral vascular disease of the lower extremities. Surgery 79:21-29, 1976.

11. Gibbons GW, Wheelock FC Jr, Siembieda C, Hoar CS Jr, Rowbotham JL, Persson AB: Noninvasive prediction of amputation level in diabetic patients. Arch Surg 114:1253-1257, 1979.

12. Lepantalo MJA, Haajanen J, Linfors O, Paavolainen P, Sheinin: Predictive value of preoperative segmental blood pressure measurements in below-knee amputations. Acta Chir Scand 148:581-584, 1982.

13. Nicholas GG, Myers JL, Demuth WE: The role of vascular laboratory criteria in the selection of patients for lower extremity amputation. Am Surg 195:469-473, 1982.

14. Boeckstyns MEH, Jensen CM: Amputation of the forefoot: Predictive value of signs and clinical physiological tests. Acta Orthop Scand 55:224-226, 1984.

15. Holstein P: Distal blood pressure as a guide in choice of amputation level. Scand J Clin Lab Invest 31 (Suppl 128):245-248, 1973.

16. Mehta K, Hobson RW II, Jamil Z, Hart L, O'Donnell JA: Fallibility of doppler ankle pressure in predicting healing of transmetatarsal amputation. J Surg Res 28:466-470, 1980.

17. McFarland DC, Lawrence PF: Skin fluorescence. A method to predict amputation site healing. J Surg Res 32:421-415, 1982.

18. Holloway GA Jr: Cutaneous blood flow responses to infection trauma measured by laser doppler velocimetry. J Invest Dermatol 74:1-4, 1980.

19. Holloway GA Jr, Burgess EM: Cutaneous blood flow and its relation to healing of below-knee amputation. Surg Gynecol Obstet 146:750-756, 1978.

20. Holloway GA Jr, Watkins BW: Laser doppler measurement of cutaneous blood flow. J Invest Dermatol 69:300-309, 1977.

21. Holloway GA Jr, Burgess EM: Preliminary experiences with laser Doppler velocimetry for the determination of amputation levels. Prosthetics and Orthotics International 7:63-66, 1983.

22. Holstein P: The distal blood pressure predicts healing of amputations on the feet. Acta Orthop Scand 55:227-233, 1984.

23. Holstein P, Lassen NA: Assessment of safe level of amputation by measurement of skin blood pressure. In Rutherford RB (ed): Vascular Surgery, WB Saunders Co., pp. 105-111, 1977.

24. Holstein P, Lund P, Larsen B, Schomacker T: Skin perfusion pressure measured as the external pressure required to stop isotope washout. Methodological considerations and normal values on the legs. Scand J Clin Lab Invest 30:649-659, 1977.

25. Holstein P, Sager P, Lassen NA: Wound healing in below knee amputations in relation to skin perfusion pressure. Acta Orthop Scand 40:49-58, 1979.

26. Holstein P, Trap-Jensen J, Bagger H, Larsen B: Skin perfusion pressure measured by isotope washout in legs with arterial occlusive disease. Clin. Physiol 3:313-324, 1983.

27. Stockel M, Ovesen J, Brochner-Mortensen J, Emneus H: Standardized photoelectric technique as routine method for selection of amputation level. Acta Orthop Scand 53:875-878, 1982.

28. Ovesen J, Stockel M: Measurement of skin perfusion pressure by photoelectric technique—an aid to amputation level selection in arteriosclerotic disease. Prosthetics and Orthotics International 8:39-42, 1984.

29. Nilsen R, Dahn I, Lassen NA, Wastling GA: On the estimation of local effective perfusion pressure in patients with obliterative arterial disease by means of external compression over an Xenon-133 Depot. Scand J Clin Lab Invest 99 (Suppl):29-32, 1967.

30. Munck O, Anderson AM: Decomposition of iodine labelled antipyrine. Scand J Lab Invest 19:256-259, 1967.

31. Munck O, Anderson AM, Binder C: Clearance 4-iodo-antipyrine-125-I after subcutaneous injection in various regions. Scand J Lab Invest 99 (Suppl):39-45, 1967.

32. Golbranson F: Amputation level determination. Presented at the annual meeting of the American Academy of Orthotists & Prostehtists, San Diego, CA, Jan 1983.

33. Spence VA, Walker WF: The relationship between temperature isotherms and skin blood flow in the ischemic limb. J Surg Res 36:278-281, 1984.

34. Franzeck UK, Talke P, Bernstein EF, Golbranson FL, Fone KA: Transcutaneous PO_2 measurement in health on peripheral arterial occlusive disease. Surgery 91:156-163, 1982.

35. Burgess EM, Matsen FA, Wyss CR, Simmons CW: Segmental transcutaneous measurements of PO2 in patients requiring below the knee amputation for peripheral vascular insufficiency. J Bone Joint Surg 64A:378-382, 1982.

36. Katsamouris A, Brewster DC, Megerman J, Cina C, Darling RC, Abbott WW: Transcutaneous oxygen tension in selection of amputation level. Am J Surg 147:510-516, 1984.

37. Ratliff DA, Clyne CAC, Chant ADB, Webster JHH: Prediction of amputation would healing: the role of transcutaneous pO_2 assessment. Br J Surg. 71:219-222, 1984.

38. Matsen FA, Wyss CR, Robertson CL, Oberg PA, Holloway GA: The relationship of transcutaneous PO_2 and laser doppler measurements in a human model of local arterial insufficiency. Surg Gyn Obstet 159:418-422, 1984.

39. Spence VA, McCollum PT, Walker WF, Murdoch G: Assessment of tissue viability in relation to the selection of amputation level. Prosthetic and Orthotics International 8:67-75, 1984.

40. Mustapha NM, Jain SK, Dudley P, Redhead RG: The effect of oxygen inhalation and intravenous naftidrofuryl on the transcutaneous partial oxygen pressure in ischemic lower limbs. Prostetics and Orthotics International 8:135-138, 1984.

41. Ito K, Ohgi S, Mori T, Urbanyi B, Schlosser V: Determination of amputation level in ischemic legs by means of transcutaneous oxygen pressure measurement. Int Surg 69:59-61, 1984.

42. Kram HB, Appel PL, White RA, Shoemaker WC: Assessment of peripheral vascular disease by postocclusive transcutaneous oxygen recovery time. J Vasc Surg 1:628-634, 1984.

43. Harward TRS, Volny J, Golbranson F, Bernstein EF, Fronek A: Oxygen inhalation-induced transcutaneous PO_2 changes as a predictor of amputation level. J Vasc Surg 2:220-227, 1985.

44. Malone JM, Leal JM, Moore WS, Henry RE, Daly MJ, Patton DD, Childers SJ: The "Gold Standard" for amputation level selection: Xenon-133 clearance. J Surg Res 30:449-455, 1961.

45. Daly MJ, Henry RE: Quantitative measurement of skin perfusion with Xenon-133. J Nucl Med 21:156-160, 1980.

46. Silberstein EB, Thomas S, Cline J, Kempczinski R, Gottesman: Predictive value of intracutaneous Xenon clearance for healing of amputation and cutaneous ulcer sites. Radiology 147:227-229, 1983.

47. Kostuik JP, Wood D, Hornby R, Feingold S, Mathews V: Measurement of skin blood flow in peripheral vascular disease by the epicutaneous application on Xenon-133. J Bone Joint Surg 58:833-837, 1946.

48. Bailey MJ, Johnston CLW, Yates CJP, Somerville PG, Dormandy JA: Preoperative Haemaglobin as predictor of outcome of diabetic amputations. Lancet 28:168-170, 1979.

49. Dickhaur SC, Delee JC, Page CP: Nutritional status: Importance in predicting wound healing after amputation. J Bone Joint Surg 66-A:71-75, 1984.

50. Verta MJ, Gross WS, Van Bellan B, Yao JST, Bergan JJ: Forefoot perfusion pressure and minor amputation surgery. Surgery 80:729-734, 1976.

51. Schwartz JA, Schuler JJ, O'Connor RJA, Flanigan DP: Predictive value of distal perfusion pressure in the healing of amputation of the digits and the forefoot. Surg Gyn Obstet 154:865-869, 1982.

52. Baker WH, Barnes RW: Minor forefoot amputation in patients with low ankle pressure. Am J Surg 133:331-332, 1977.

53. Yao JST, Bergan JJ: Application of ultrasound to arterial and venous diagnosis. Surg Clin North Am 54(1):23-38, 1974.

54. Barnes RW, Shanik GD, Slaymaker EE: An index of healing in below-knee amputation: Leg blood pressure by Doppler ultrasound. Surgery 79:13-20, 1976.

55. Cheng EY: Lower extremity amputation level: Selection using noninvasive hemodynamic methods of evaluation. Arch Phys Med Rehabil 63:475-479, 1982.

6

Noninvasive Evaluation of Chronic Venous Insufficiency

LARRY R. WILLIAMS
University of South Florida
Tampa, Florida

Veterans Administration Medical Center
Bay Pines, Florida

The evolution of modern diagnostic techniques has made a significant impact on the noninvasive evaluation of venous disease. Accurate hemodynamic assessment has resulted in more complete understanding of this common but complex pathophysiologic process.

Lower extremity venous insufficiency is estimated to affect 3-5% of the population (1). Although not ordinarily life threatening, the disease is debilitating and painful and is a source of substantial economic losses in terms of patient productivity and dependency on others. In the past, many patients were destined to protracted courses, due to the unavailability of or poor understanding of appropriate diagnostic and therapeutic measures. Now innovative operative treatments for venous insufficiency are more readily available. Therefore, accurate noninvasive means of objective evaluation of the hemodynamics of venous disease and operative results has become mandatory.

CLINICAL FEATURES

The patient with chronic deep venous insufficiency does not usually present a difficult diagnostic problem. Symptoms include aching, swelling, tiredness, and heaviness of the leg. Long-standing edema with cutaneous pigmentation and thickened skin attest to the chronicity of the condition. Skin breakdown and ulceration result in frequent infection and severe pain.

Superficial venous varicosities are obvious upon inspection of the patient in the upright position. Serpentine, dilated varicosities cause local pain, are unsightly, and are prone to bleeding with minimal trauma.

PATHOPHYSIOLOGY

The clinical presentation of lower extremity venous insufficiency is a direct result of the relatively basic pathophysiologic process of ambulatory venous hypertension. Etiologies for this elevation in venous pressure to be considered include valvular incompetence on a familial or occupational basis, or valvular destruction due to previous deep venous thrombosis with recanalization. In some cases chronic venous occlusion may be the source of the ambulatory venous hypertension.

Three separate disease states can be identified. Primary varicose veins pertain to valvular dysfunction limited to the superficial venous system. Secondary varicose veins are associated with underlying deep venous obstruction or valvular incompetence. Postphlebitic syndrome is a result of deep and perforator venous incompetence. Regardless of the etiology or classification, it is the elevated ambulatory venous pressure as well as valvular incompetence that provide the basis for objective measurement.

PATIENT EVALUATION

Physical assessment of the patient with chronic venous insufficiency requires careful documentation of the status of the extremity. This should include measurement of circumferences, description of ulcerations and skin changes, and cultures of any open wounds. The venous compression test, or Trendelenburg test, is sometimes useful in the bedside evaluation of abnormal venous hemodynamics (Fig. 1). This test attempts to document the rapid filling of lower extremity superficial veins by gravity with and without tourniquet compression of the superficial saphenous system. In this way, patients with superficial venous insufficiency supposedly can be differentiated from patients with deep venous insufficiency.

The Trendelenburg test has many drawbacks. In most patients with chronic venous insufficiency, it is difficult to evaluate filling of the superficial veins of the lower extremity due to longstanding skin changes and pigmentation. In addition, obese patients very seldom have easily delineated superficial veins. The accurate differentiation of deep system insufficiency from combined valvular insufficiency and isolated perforator incompetence is not possible by physical assessment in most instances.

INVASIVE PRESSURE MEASUREMENTS

The "gold standard" for documenting abnormal hemodynamics in patients with suspected venous insufficiency is by direct pressure measurements (2-4). By placing

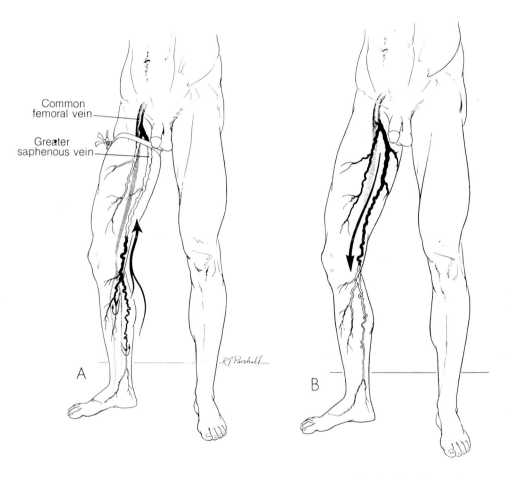

Common femoral vein

Greater saphenous vein

A

B

Figure 1 Trendelenburg test. (A) A constricting tourniquet is placed at the groin while supine with the leg elevated. Upon standing, superficial calf veins normally fill slowly (>20 sec) from distal to proximal. (B) Rapid filling of superficial veins upon removal of the tourniquet indicates saphenofemoral valvular incompetence. (From Flanigan and Williams, Ref. 23, with permission.)

a needle in a superficial vein of the foot, intraluminal pressure can be measured either with a mercury or water column or via a pressure transducer.

Resting pedal venous pressures in the normal erect individual average between 60 and 100 mmHg (Fig. 2). The resting pressure is roughly equal to the hydrostatic pressure of a column of blood extending from the level of the catheter to the middle of the right atrium.

Patients with deep or superficial venous insufficiency, regardless of etiology, have resting venous pressures that do not differ from normal individuals. With walking or vigorous calf muscle contraction, however, venous pressure responses vary

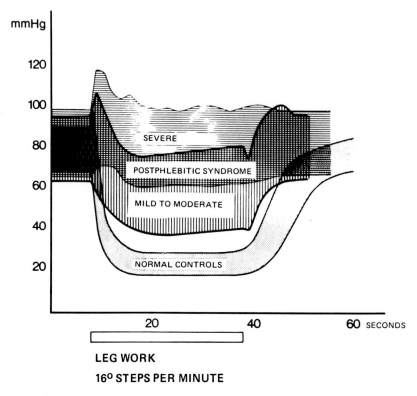

Figure 2   Venous pressure during and after exercise in patients with varying de-grees of venous insufficiency as compared with normals. (From Nachbur, Ref. 4, with permission.)

with different pathologic processes (Fig. 2). The normal response is a marked de-crease in pedal venous pressure. This is due to the effective pumping of blood from the superficial to the deep system and proximally out of the calf.

Nachbur (4) has documented that this venous emptying process occurs in a phasic manner. As the deep veins empty, pressure in the superficial veins is higher than deep venous pressure, therefore, blood flows from superficial to deep. During muscle contraction, deep venous pressure increases and valves in the perforating veins prevent flow from deep to superficial. With cessation of exercise there is a gradual return of venous pressure to normal levels. Normal refilling is slow, with the majority of the volume replacement coming from the arterial circulation via the capillary beds.

In patients with venous insufficiency, the reduction in venous pressure with calf muscle exercise is not as dramatic as in normal individuals. Pedal venous pressure may fall to only 40 mmHg, depending on the severity of reflux. Most striking, however, is the rapid refilling of the lower extremity from proximal veins, with correspondingly rapid return to baseline pressure.

Patients with severe postphlebitic syndrome demonstrate little or no fall in pedal venous pressure during exercise (5). Pressure rapidly returns to baseline when exercise is stopped. During prolonged exercise, as occurs with walking, venous pressure may initially fall, however, it does not stay reduced, and it frequently exceeds the baseline value.

The presence of proximal venous obstruction, either due to venous thrombosis or external compression, likewise results in ambulatory venous hypertension. The calf muscle pump works against venous outflow obstruction and pedal venous pressure rises. Slow recovery down to baseline following exercise occurs as pressures equalize.

Although highly accurate, the measurement of venous pressures by cannulation of a lower extremity vein is invasive. It is not well tolerated by the patient and is cumbersome for the physician. In most instances, venous pressure measurements have been supplanted by a variety of noninvasive techniques for the evaluation of patients with chronic venous insufficiency.

NONINVASIVE ASSESSMENT

Noninvasive diagnosis of altered lower extremity venous hemodynamics is based on the premise that changes in leg volume and skin blood content are a direct reflection of the underlying pressure. Several different types of plethysmography are available for this purpose. Foot volumetry has, likewise, been employed. In addition to volume assessments, directional Doppler ultrasound and B-mode imaging have been utilized to document valvular function.

PLETHYSMOGRAPHY

Plethysmography, very simply, is the measurement of increases or decreases in volume (6). When applied to lower extremity venous hemodynamics, a variety of plethysmographic techniques have been used. Water and air plethysmographs determine the displacement of blood volume from the leg within a chamber. Both are rather cumbersome and, therefore, are seldom used in clinical practice. The two most commonly utilized plethysmographic techniques for assessment of chronic venous insufficiency are strain gauge plethysmography and photoplethysmography.

Strain Gauge Plethysmography

Strain gauge plethysmography uses the change in leg circumference to calculate changes in volume flow. The strain gauge consists of a mercury-filled, silicone rubber tube with a measuring circuit that detects changes in length. Leg volume changes can be calculated on the basis of the changes in calf circumference and are expressed as milliliters per 100 ml of tissue per minute (ml/100 ml per min).

Holm et al. (7) measured the time required for calf volume to return to normal following exercise as a means of estimating venous insufficiency. With the patient in the erect position, blood is emptied from the leg by having the patient raise themselves on their toes three to five times. Recovery time to baseline in normal limbs averaged 22 ± 7 sec. In patients with venous insufficiency, recovery times were much shorter, averaging 7 ± 3 sec. Primary varicose veins could be distinguished from secondary varicose veins by compressing the saphenous vein in the thigh and repeating the test. In patients with primary varicose veins, venous recovery time was nearly normalized (18 ± 8 sec) whereas in patients with secondary varicose veins, recovery times remained much shorter (7 ± 2 sec).

Strain gauge venous recovery times can also be performed with the patient seated with the legs dangling. Barnes et al. (8) have determined that measurement of the recovery half time (time required for the calf to regain half the volume expelled during exercise) allows more precise interpretation. He has found that the normal recovery half time is 3.4 ± 1.4 sec whereas in patients with venous insufficiency the average value is 1.3 ± 1.0 sec.

Another modification of the strain gauge evaluation of venous insufficiency is the measurement of maximum venous reflux flow (MVRF) (9) (Fig. 3). With the leg resting horizontally, arterial inflow and venous outflow are prevented by inflating a 300 mmHg cuff at the thigh. Rapid inflation of a more distal 50 mmHg cuff causes blood to reflux down the leg. With venous insufficiency, a large degree of reflux is determined as a rapid increase in calf volume (mean = 13 ± 7 ml/100 ml per min). In normal individuals MVRF is less than 6 ml/100 ml per min.

Photoplethysmography

The photoelectric plethysmographic (PPG) measures the reflection of infrared light from subcutaneous red cells as an estimate of blood content in the microcirculation. Abramowitz et al. (10) have shown that venous recovery times determined with the PPG correlate very well with intraluminal pedal pressure measurements. This correlation holds true for normal individuals as well as patients with postphlebitic syndrome.

The test is performed by applying the PPG transducer to the skin on the medial aspect of the lower leg (Fig. 4). The patient is seated with legs dangling. Vigorous foot dorsiflexion causes emptying of blood from subcutaneous tissues of the legs. Upon relaxation, skin blood content gradually returns to baseline. In normal individuals recovery times average 47.8 ± 21.6 sec, and recovery half times average 9.7 ± 4.3 sec (9).

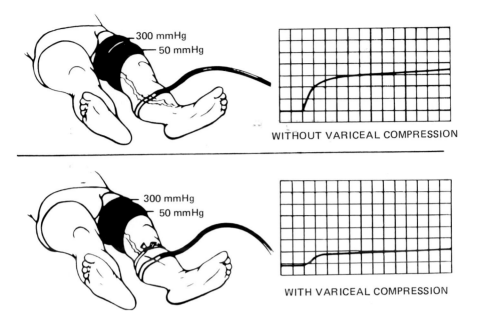

300 mmHg
50 mmHg

WITHOUT VARICEAL COMPRESSION

300 mmHg
50 mmHg

WITH VARICEAL COMPRESSION

Figure 3 Technique of measuring maximum venous reflux flow (MVRF) before and after tourniquet compression of superficial varices. (From Barnes, Ref. 8, with permission.

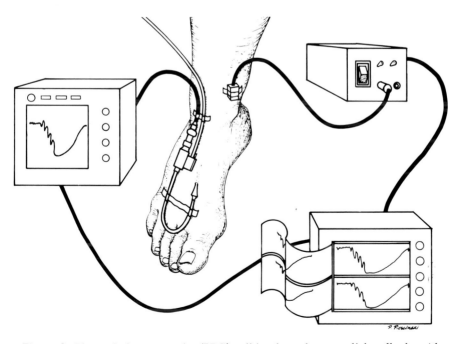

Figure 4 Photoplethysmography (PPG) cell in place above medial malleolus. Also demonstrated is simultaneous intravenous pressure measurement.

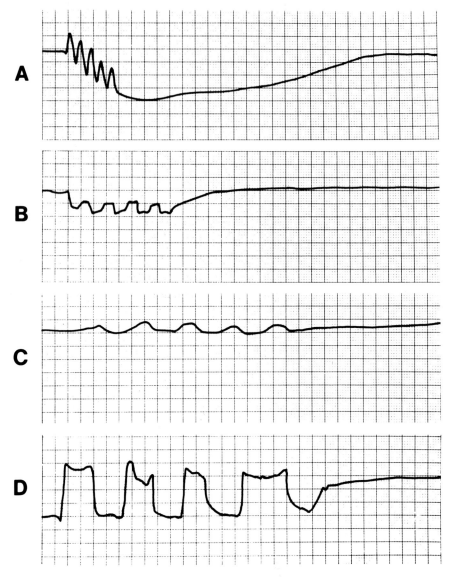

Figure 5 Photoplethysmography recordings during and after exercise demonstrating normal (A), decompressive (B), static (C) and congestive (D) patterns. (From Barnes, Ref. 11, with permission.)

In patients with venous insufficiency, recovery times are less than 20 sec and recovery half times average 3.7 ± 2.0 sec. Recovery half-time is elevated to 5.5 ± 2.8 sec in patients with primary varicose veins by the application of a tourniquet to compress the superficial venous system.

In addition to the venous recovery time, Barnes and Yao (11) have noted patterns of PPG recordings that may provide a clue to the underlying venous pathophysiology (Fig. 5). In patients with mild stasis dermatitis without ulceration, a decompressive pattern is commonly observed. Skin blood content decreases with calf exercise, however, the recovery time is extremely short (10 sec). In the majority of patients with severe postphlebitic syndrome, a static pattern (no significant change in skin blood content) or congestive pattern (increase in skin blood content) is seen with exercise. Although these patterns are difficult to quantitate, their notation in conjunction with recovery times provides useful information.

Norris et al. (12) have devised a system for gaining additional quantitative information for the PPG examination in venous insufficiency. By calibrating the full-scale deflection of the PPG output to correspond with the pressure difference from supine to erect position, an estimation of ambulatory venous pressure can be made. Norris et al. found a high degree of correlation between the PPG measurements and actual intraluminal pedal venous pressures (r = 0.97) with this technique.

FOOT VOLUMETRY

Although not commonly employed in the United States, foot volumetry has been pioneered by Norgren and Thelesius (13-15) in Europe. Quite simply, relative foot volumes are determined by the displacement of water in an open container (Fig. 6). Output from a damped photoelectric float-sensor is continuously recorded at rest and after knee bends to determine the foot volume expelled and the rate at which refilling occurs.

Thelesius (16) has determined that the ratio of refilling time to expelled volume provides the most sensitive determinant for the diagnosis of venous insufficiency. Differentiation of primary from secondary varicose veins can be made by application of an occluding tourniquet to the lower leg.

DOPPLER ULTRASOUND

Directional Doppler ultrasound has been found to be useful in several aspects of the evaluation of patients with venous disease. Although not a quantitative analysis, Doppler ultrasound has proven quite accurate in the detection of deep vein thrombosis and chronic venous occlusion (17-19).

In the evaluation of venous insufficiency, subjective assessment of the direction of blood flow in any particular vein can easily be determined with a pencil-

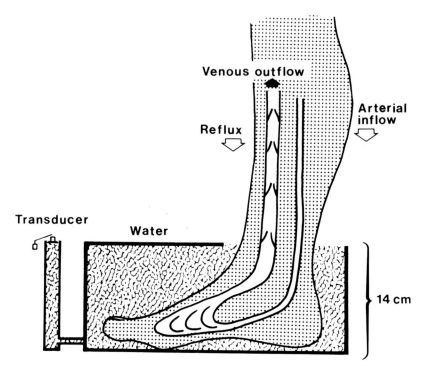

Figure 6   Foot volumetry apparatus. (From Thelesius, Ref. 16, with permission.)

probe directional Doppler (19). In normal individuals, reflux distal to competent venous valves does not occur when the leg is compressed proximally. In patients with incompetent valves in the vein being examined, proximal compression above the Doppler will result in reversal of flow within the vein. This flow reversal may also be detected during coughing or the Valsalva maneuver. In this way competence of the valves can be evaluated at any level on the saphenofemoral, popliteal, and deep venous system.

In addition, midthigh and calf perforating veins can be assessed for competent valves (17) (Fig. 7). The proximal deep and superficial venous systems are occluded with a 60 mmHg cuff and the distal superficial system is occluded with a tourniquet. Doppler evaluation is performed at 1-cm intervals on one side of the tourniquet while compressing the calf on the other side. Incompetent communicating veins will be easily detected by Doppler ultrasound.

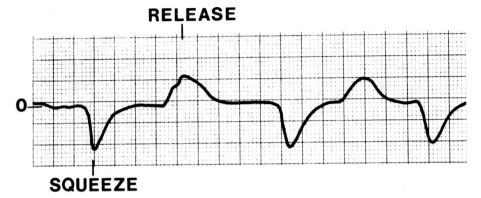

Figure 7 Detection of calf perforator vein incompetence (bidirectional flow) by Doppler ultrasound. (From Yao, JST, Ref. 28, with permission.)

B-MODE IMAGING

Real-time B-mode ultrasound imaging has become an innovative addition to the noninvasive evaluation of lower extremity venous disease. It is often used in conjunction with pulsed-wave Doppler analysis, which allows selective measurement of blood flow at a specific distance from the probe. Cranley et al. (20,21) have had a tremendous amount of experience with this modality and report that the superficial and deep veins of the entire lower extremity can be assessed in detail in over 90% of cases.

Sandager et al. (22) have described the normal thin, bicuspid, highly reflective valve cusp in clear detail (Fig. 8). This can be easily distinguished from the thickened, motionless diseased valve. Valve function can be readily assessed at any level in the leg in the majority of patients. Key observations include location and number of valves in each vein segment; valve movement in response to respiration, valsalva, and leg compression; direction of venous blood flow; and the presence of thrombus, manifest by filling defects or inability to coat the vein walls by compression with the probe.

Drawbacks of B-mode imaging include the inability to assess accurately venous structures above the inguinal ligament and the fact that findings are often subtle. Considerable experience is necessary both on the part of the examiner and the physician interpreting the results.

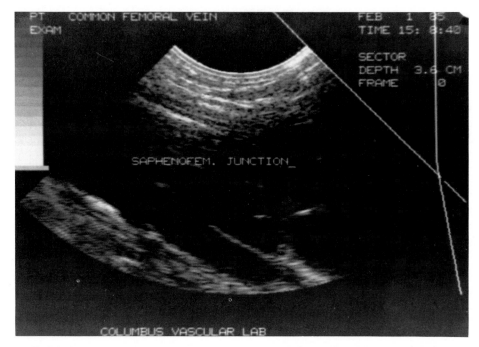

Figure 8 B-mode ultrasound image of a normal lower extremity venous valve. (Courtesy of WR Flinn, MD and G Sandager, RN, RVT.)

OPERATIVE SELECTION

The selection of patients for operation for chronic venous insufficiency is based on the presence of severe symptoms that have not responded to aggressive nonoperative management. Complete evaluation requires thorough history and physical examination, noninvasive hemodynamic assessment, and anatomic investigation with B-mode imaging and/or ascending and descending venography.

The major roles of noninvasive hemodynamic assessment are documentation of the elevated ambulatory venous pressure and definition of the relative contribution of the superficial, deep and perforator venous systems. The algorithms shown in Figure 9 are examples of how photoplethysmography in conjunction with segmental tourniquets is useful (23). Orderly examination of lower extremity hemodynamics in this fashion pinpoints the pathologic venous segment. Similar algorithms for venous pressures, strain gauge plethysmography, and foot volumetry can be devised (13,18). Appropriate operative procedures can then be planned to attack the system most responsible for the abnormal hemodynamics.

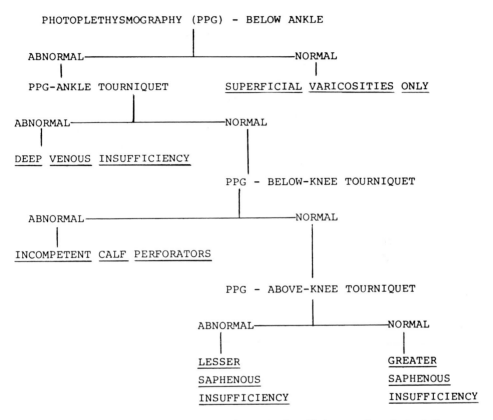

Figure 9 Algorithm for localization of valvular insufficiency using photoplethysmography and sequential tourniquets. (From Flanigan and Williams, Ref. 23, with permission.)

B-mode imaging of specific vein segments may prove to be particularly useful in selecting patients for new operative approaches. Femoral vein valve repair, valve transpositions, and free segment valve transplant are procedures in which specific venous segments are involved. Currently, most decisions regarding operation are based on ascending and descending venography. B-mode imaging should provide important information to help guide operative decisions. Further investigation is necessary with this innovative diagnostic tool to define its role clearly in operative selection.

POSTOPERATIVE ASSESSMENT

Noninvasive documentation of lower extremity venous hemodynamics is particularly useful in the evaluation of patients following operative intervention. The tests are well tolerated by the patient and essentially without risk, thus, assessment of postoperative results can be performed in the early postoperative period and at selected intervals.

Since noninvasive evaluation has only relatively recently been accepted, many surgeons continue to evaluate operative results with venous pressure studies and venography in conjunction with noninvasive tests (24-26). Johnson et al. evaluated the results of femoral venous valve surgery and found photoplethysmographic recovery time to correlate well with direct pressure measurements both pre- and postoperatively (24). However, they found that isolated repair of femoral venous valve segments very often did not totally correct abnormal limb hemodynamics. Therefore, careful follow-up with objective assessment helped to identify those patients in whom further operations were necessary.

We have, likewise, documented the utility of photoplethysmography in assessing results of venous surgery (27). Eight patients underwent venous reconstruction (venous bypass, vein segment transplant, or vein valve transposition). Photoplethysmographic recovery times correlated well with venous pressure readings (r = 0.8179). Successful correction of abnormal limb hemodynamics was documented in seven patients. One patient, whose photoplethysmographic recovery time was still abnormal postoperatively, was found to have a thrombosed venous reconstruction that was not suspected on clinical grounds.

The role of B-mode imaging has yet to be defined. It should, however, prove to be quite useful in the assessment of a variety of venous reconstructive procedures both in terms of thrombosis and venous valve function.

REFERENCES

1. Coon WW, Willis PW III, Kellis JB: Venous thromboembolism and other venous diseases in the Tecumsa Health Study. Circulation 48:839, 1973.
2. Warren R, White EA, Belcher CD: Venous pressures in the saphenous system in normal, varicose and postphlebitic extremities. Surgery 26:435-445, 1949.
3. DeCamp PT: Ambulatory venous pressure determinations in postphlebitic and related syndromes. Surgery 29:44, 1951.
4. Nachbur B: Assessment of venous disorders by venous pressure measurements. In Hobbs JT (ed): The Treatment of Venous Disorders, Lippincott, Philadelphia, pp. 75-85, 1977.
5. Walker AJ, Longland CJ: Venous pressure measurement in the foot in exercise as an aid to investigation of venous disease in the leg. Clin Sci 9:101-114, 1950.
6. Yao JST, Flinn W: Plethysmography. In Kempezinski R, Yao JST (ed): Practical Noninvasive Vascular Diagnosis, Yearbook Medical Publishers, Inc., Chicago, pp. 49-62, 1982.
7. Holm JSE: A simple plethysmographic method for differentiating primary from secondary varicose veins. Surg Gynecol Obstet. 143:609-611, 1976.

8. Barnes RW, Collincott PE, Mozersky DJ: Noninvasive quantitation of venous reflux in the postphlebitic syndrome. Surg Gynecol Obstet 136:769, 1973.

9. Barnes RW, Ross EA, Strandness DE Jr: Differentiation of primary from secondary varicose veins by Doppler ultrasound and strain gauge plethysmography. Surg Gynecol Obstet 141:207, 1975.

10. Abramowitz HB, Queral LA, Flinn WR, Nora PF, Peterson LK, Bergan JJ, Yao JST: The use of photoplethysmography in the assessment of venous insufficiency: A comparison to venous pressure measurements. Surgery 86: 434-441, 1979.

11. Barnes RW, Yao JST: Photoplethysmography in chronic venous insufficiency. In Bernstein EF (ed): Noninvasive Diagnostic Technique in Vascular Disease, CV Mosby Co, St. Louis, Missouri, pp. 514-521, 1982.

12. Norris CS, Bergan A, Barnes CW: Quantitative photoplethysmography in chronic venous insufficiency: A new method of noninvasive estimation of ambulatory venous pressure. Surgery 94:758-764, 1983.

13. Norgren L: Functional evaluation of chronic venous insufficiency by foot volumetry. Acta Chir Scand (Suppl) 444:9-48, 1974.

14. Norgren L, Thelesius O: Pressure-volume characteristics of foot veins in normal cases and patients with venous insufficiency. Blood Vessels 12:1-12, 1975.

15. Gjores JE, Thelesius O: Compression treatment in venous insufficiency evaluated with foot volumetry. VASA 6:364-368, 1977.

16. Thelesius O: Foot volumetry. In Bernstein E (ed): Noninvasive Diagnostic Techniques in Vascular Disease, CV Mosby Co, St. Louis, Missouri, pp. 508-513, 1982.

17. Yao JST, Blackburn D: Doppler venous survey. In Kempezinski R, Yao JST (ed): Practical Noninvasive Vascular Diagnosis, Yearbook Medical Publishers, Inc, Chicago, pp. 263-275, 1982.

18. Barnes RW: Doppler ultrasonic diagnosis of venous disease. In Bernstein E (ed): Noninvasive Diagnostic Techniques in Vascular Disease, CV Mosby Co, St. Louis, Missouri, pp. 452-458, 1982.

19. Folse R, Alexander RH: Directional flow detection for localizing venous valvular incompetency. Surgery 67:114, 1970.

20. Flanagan LD, Sullivan ED, Cranley JJ: Venous imaging of the extremities using real-time B-mode ultrasound. In Bergan JJ, Yao JST (ed): Surgery of the Veins, Grune & Stratton, New York, pp. 89-98, 1985.

21. Sullivan ED, Peter DJ, Cranley JJ: Real-time B-mode venous ultrasound. J Vasc Surg 1:465-473, 1984.

22. Sandager G, Williams LR, McCarthy WJ, Flinn WR, Yao JST: Assessment of venous valve function by duplex scan. Bruit (in press).

23. Flanigan DP, Williams LR: Venous insufficiency of the lower extremities: New methods of diagnosis and therapy. In Nyhus LM (ed): Surgery Annual, Appleton Century Crofts, Norwalk, Connecticut, 14:359-380, 1982.

24. Johnson ND, Queral LA, Flinn WR, Yao JST, Bergan JJ: Late objective assessment of venous valve surgery. Arch Surg 116:1461-1466, 1981.

25. Harris J, Halliday P, DeDomenico M, Kidd J, Burnett A, May J: Non-invasive assessment of venous cross-over grafts for thrombotic iliac venous occlusion. Bruit 8:209-212, 1984.
26. Bergan JJ, Flinn WR, Yao JST: Venous reconstructive surgery. Surg Clin NA 62:399-410, 1982.
27. Williams LR, Flanigan DP: Evaluation of venous insufficiency and results of venous surgery by photoplethysmography. Unpublished communication, 1984.
28. Yao JST, Bergan JJ: Application of ultrasound to arterial and venous diagnosis. Surg Clin NA 54:23-38, 1974.

7

Preoperative Noninvasive Cerebrovascular Testing

D. PRESTON FLANIGAN
University of Illinois College of Medicine at Chicago
Chicago, Illinois

Noninvasive studies are an extension of the physical examination and, if accurate, are especially valuable in areas of the body giving poor access to physical examination. Unlike the arteries of the lower extremity, which are easily palpable in several locations, the internal carotid artery is not directly accessible to accurate palpation and neither are its distal branches. Another factor that would tend to increase the value of accurate noninvasive testing is the lack of specificity of the history and physical findings in a given disease state. In patients with lower extremity arterial occlusive disease, the history and physical examination are most often sufficient to establish the diagnosis whereas cerebrovascular symptoms and physical findings are often less specific. This lesser specificity dictates the need for objective diagnostic studies to establish the correct diagnosis in patients with suspected cerebrovascular disease.

Nonspecificity of symptoms leads to a higher incidence of negative diagnostic studies, thus, it is particularly important that the diagnostic test be safe. Contrast arteriography has been the gold standard for cerebrovascular diagnosis but is not without risk. Stroke rates as high as 5% have been reported with arteriography (1). Additional risks include catheter complications and reactions to contrast media. Risk-free, noninvasive, tests would obviously be preferable provided their accuracy were acceptable.

TYPES OF NONINVASIVE
CEREBROVASCULAR TESTS

Noninvasive cerebrovascular tests have been categorized into direct and indirect tests. Direct tests evaluate the extracranial carotid artery by taking measurements directly over the area of the artery, whereas indirect tests attempt to assess extracranial carotid artery disease by assessing the effects of the disease on the more distal internal carotid artery circulation.

Indirect Tests

All indirect tests are based on the fact that the ophthalmic artery is the first branch of the internal carotid artery and that its branches and end organ, the ocular globe, are accessible for measurement. Ophthalmodymamometry was probably the first attempt to assess indirectly disease at the carotid birfurcation with noninvasive testing. Very low accuracy was obtained with the technique, however, such that it is seldom used for this purpose currently (2).

The fact that the supraorbital and infraorbital arteries, which are branches of the ophthalmic artery, anastomose through collateral beds with the superficial temporal and facial arteries led to the development of the periorbital Doppler examination for the evaluation of extracranial cerebrovascular occlusive disease. Flow in these orbital arteries is normally from an intracranial to an extracranial direction. When the orbital arteries are serving as collateral vessels secondary to severe stenosis or occlusion of the ipsilateral internal carotid artery, the flow is reversed. Additionally, compression of the superficial temporal or facial arteries should normally lead to an increase in amplitude of the orbital artery signal (Fig. 1). Attenuation of this signal with compression maneuvers indicates internal carotid artery occlusive disease. Numerous reports have demonstrated variable accuracy with the test in the detection of severe stenoses (Table 1) (3-11). Because the test has not been shown to be accurate with lesser stenoses, its application has been limited, however (12).

Ocular pulsations should occur simultaneously in each eye. The belief that carotid artery disease might delay pulse arrival is the basis for oculoplethysmography. In this test, suction cups are placed on the ocular globes. These cups are attached to volume plethysmographs, which are connected to a strip chart recorder. Plethysmographs also may be attached to an ear lobe to monitor the pulse arrival by way of the external carotid artery circulation. In the normal patient, the pulse upstroke should begin simultaneously in both eyes and ears. Delays in upstroke indicate carotid occlusive disease (Fig. 2). When the test was described by Kartchner and McRae, it was combined with carotid phonoangiography (Fig. 3) (13). The accuracy of this test in the detection of severe stenosis has been reported in a wide range (Table 2) (8,10,13-17). Like the Doppler periorbital examination,

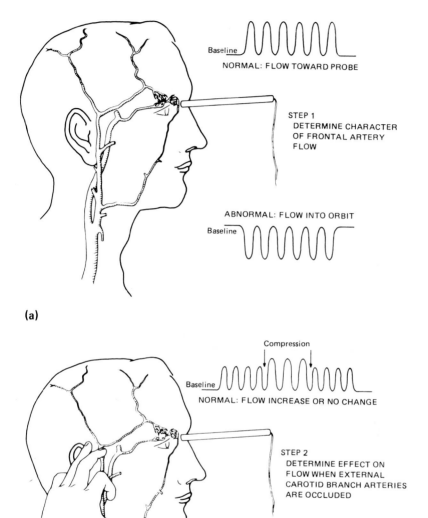

Baseline
NORMAL: FLOW TOWARD PROBE

STEP 1
DETERMINE CHARACTER
OF FRONTAL ARTERY
FLOW

ABNORMAL: FLOW INTO ORBIT
Baseline

(a)

Compression
Baseline
NORMAL: FLOW INCREASE OR NO CHANGE

STEP 2
DETERMINE EFFECT ON
FLOW WHEN EXTERNAL
CAROTID BRANCH ARTERIES
ARE OCCLUDED

Compression
Baseline
ABNORMAL: FLOW DECREASE

(b)

Figure 1 Periorbital Doppler examination without (a) and with (b) collateral compression. (From McDonald PT, Ref. 10, with permission.)

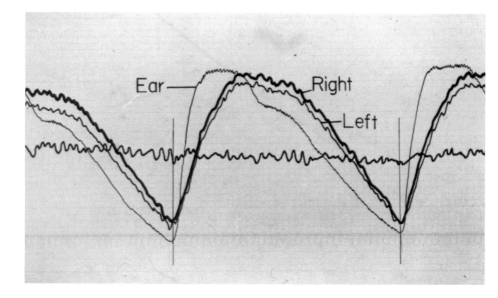

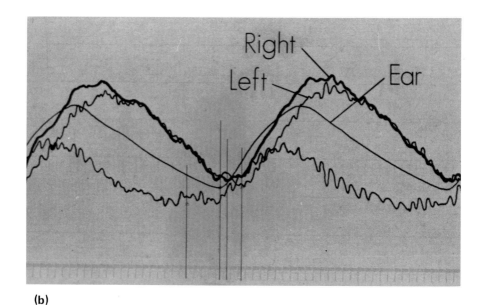

(b)

Figure 2   (a) Normal oculoplethysmogram.   (b) Left carotid stenosis tracing.

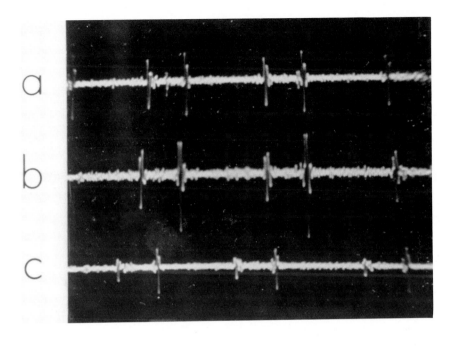

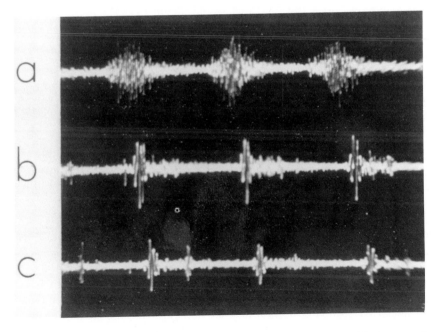

Figure 3 *Above*: Normal carotid phonoangiogram. *Below*: carotid phonoangiogram showing a bifurcation bruit.

Table 1 Reported Accuracy of Periorbital Doppler

Author (Ref.)	Accuracy (%)	Angiographic Standard (%)[a]
Lynch (4)	89	50
Bone (3)	93	50
Gross (8)	59	75
Malone (5)	92	50
Machleder (6)	54	60
McDonald (10)	74	60
Barnes (7)	95	50
Towne (11)	65	60

[a]Diameter stenosis.

Table 2 Reported Accuracy of Oculoplethysmography

Author (Ref.)	Accuracy (%)	Angiographic Standard (%)[a]
Bone (17)	92	>50
Gross (8)	90	Variable
McDonald (10)	86	>60
Keagy (15)	84	>60
Blackshear (16)	50	Variable
Satiani (14)	86	Variable
Kartchner (13)	90	>40

[a]Diameter stenosis.

this test also loses accuracy in the detection of lesser stenoses. Additionally, this test is limited somewhat in patients with bilateral disease.

Lesions that produce critical stenoses cause a decrease in pressure distal to the stenosis. Generally, these are thought to be lesions compromising 75% or more of the cross-sectional lumen of the artery. Gee, in an attempt to capitalize on these pressure changes caused by critical stenoses, developed a technique called oculo-pneumoplethysmography (18). This technique also employs suction cups that are attached to plethysmographs and a strip chart recorder. The cups are also attached to a vacuum source allowing high suction (300-500 mmHg) to be placed on the ocular globes resulting in circulatory arrest in the globe that is detectable by the plethysmographs. As the suction is reduced, pulsatile circulation returns to the globes and the pressure at which this occurs can be recorded (Fig. 4). The differences in ocular pressures between the two eyes as well as the pulse amplitude and the relationship to systemic blood pressure can then be assessed. A pressure difference of $\geqslant 5$ mmHg between the two eyes is indicative of significant unilateral stenosis. Bilateral stenoses can be diagnosed using comparisons to brachial pressure using a discriminate function nomogram. Results of this test (Table 3) (4,8,19-21) are also quite variable. Also, as with the previously mentioned indirect tests, the test is not accurate in the detection of lesser stenoses.

Although the indirect tests were just a beginning, they were useful in the detection of severe disease and were applied widely as screening procedures. The indirect tests, particularily oculopneumoplethysmography, remain as good evaluators of the hemodynamic effects of carotid stenoses. However, symptoms secondary to carotid artery disease are, to a large part, due to embolism rather than the hemodynamic effects of severe stenoses. Emboli, of course, can arise from plaques that

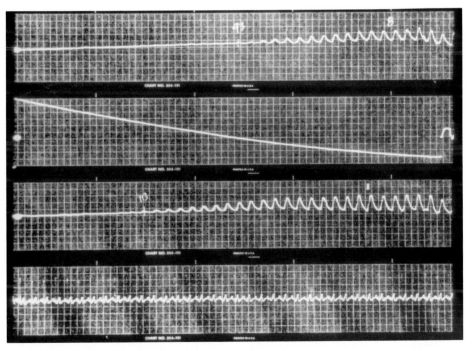

Figure 4 Oculopneumoplethysmographic tracing showing unilateral carotid artery disease.

Table 3 Reported Accuracy of Oculopneumoplethysmography

Author (Ref.)	Accuracy (%)	Angiographic Standard (%)[a]
Lynch (4)	94	>50
Gross (8)	31	Variable
McDonald (19)	97	>60
Schwartz (21)	62	>50
McDonald (20)	97	>50

[a]Diameter stenosis.

are not hemodynamically significant. Thus, the ability to detect these lesser stenoses is necessary in the proper evaluation of patients suspected of having extracranial cerebrovascular disease. Such assessment currently requires highly sensitive, direct measurements at the carotid bifurcation.

Direct Tests

Direct tests evaluate the cervical carotid artery directly rather than by the evaluation of effects on the distal circulation.

One of the first attempts to evaluate the carotid bifurcation directly was with the use of direct Doppler recordings from the common, internal, and external carotid arteries. If a pulsed Doppler is used in conjunction with a memory oscilloscope, an image of the arterial lumen can be constructed (pulsed Doppler arteriograph). As can be seen from Figure 5, these images are somewhat crude, but as shown by Barnes, there is agreement within 25% of the stenosis measured by this method when compared with arteriography 71% of the time. Barnes further showed that this accuracy could be enhanced by the addition of carotid sound spectrum analysis (98% agreement within 25% of the angiographically determined stenosis) (22). Although this is a useful diagnostic method, particularily when combined with sound spectrum analysis, it is limited by both calcification in the arterial wall, which appears as a stenosis by blocking ultrasound penetration, and from lack of resolution.

Doppler sound analysis consists of both the evaluation of the analog Doppler tracing and of spectral analysis of the Doppler signal using fast Fourier transform analysis. Each part of the carotid artery has a specific analog Doppler tracing. The tracing from the external carotid artery is similar to that in the extremities and contains forward and reverse components due to the peripheral resistance created by its distal perfusion bed. Intracerebral vascular resistance is low, however, giving the internal carotid artery a tracing that not only has an absent reversed (below

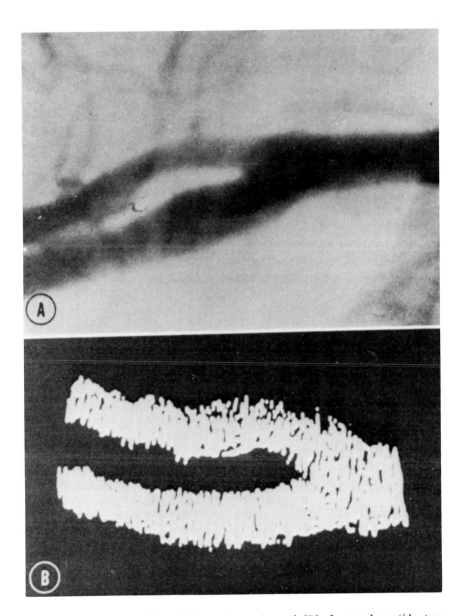

Figure 5 Arteriogram (A) and ultrasonic arteriograph (B) of normal carotid artery. (From Barnes RW, Ref. 22, with permission.)

baseline) component but one that indicates continued forward flow throughout systole and diastole by never returning to baseline during the entire cardiac cycle. Tracings from the common carotid artery are a hybrid of the internal and external carotid tracing in that the tracing returns to but not below baseline during diastole. These characteristics of the waveforms are helpful in the blind identification of each artery. Changes in the waveforms that reflect disease are similar to these seen in peripheral arterial disease and, as such, are not of high diagnostic accuracy.

Sound spectrum analysis of Doppler waveforms, however, has been shown to be a fairly accurate predictor of disease. The main criterion used by this method to quantitate disease is the peak systolic frequency. Barnes has shown this method to be 98% sensitive for stenoses greater than 50% but only 71% sensitive for those stenoses less than 50% (23). Use of this procedure alone is of limited accuracy in the evaluation of all degrees of stenosis, but the accuracy is greatly enhanced when combined with imaging procedures as mentioned above with pulsed Doppler arteriography. Even this combination is somewhat limited, however, because of the limitations of both methods as regards resolution and the evaluation of minimal and moderate degrees of disease. Diagnostic techniques that are for the evaluation of a disease which is largely embolic in nature should be accurate for all degrees of stenosis.

The development of real-time, B-mode ultrasonic imaging of the carotid bifurcation has enabled the accurate evaluation of all degrees of carotid stenosis (24). These instruments have the ability to achieve submillimeter resolution of the carotid artery, thus, enabling the evaluation of minimal disease. B-mode imaging has some limitations, especially in the evaluation of severe stenosis versus occlusion and in the evaluation of hypoechoic plaques. The addition of pulsed Doppler sound spectrum analysis to the system (duplex scanning) complements imaging by providing additional diagnostic information (Fig. 6). Accuracy obtained with duplex scanning has been high. Dagle (25) has reported negative and positive predictive values of greater than 94% for all degrees of stenosis. Occluded vessels gave a negative predictive value of 99% and a positive predictive value of 71%. Difficulty with the diagnosis of total occlusion was also experienced by Comerota in a multicenter study as well (26). Advances in Doppler technology are already starting to improve the accuracy in the diagnosis of total occlusion by duplex scanning.

The accuracy of duplex instrumentation for all degrees of stenosis begs the question of whether noninvasive studies could begin to replace invasive arteriography in the evaluation of cerebrovascular disease. There is little disagreement that duplex scanning is now the standard to which other noninvasive tests must compare. Accurate assessment of extracranial cerebrovascular disease and its progression or regression is now possible using duplex scanning. The use of the technique in patients for whom nonsurgical therapy is intended is appropriate and widely employed. It has not yet been determined if the technique is sufficiently

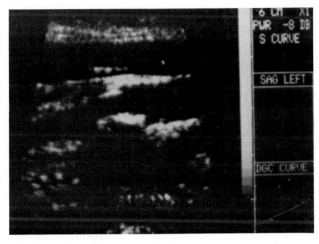

(a)

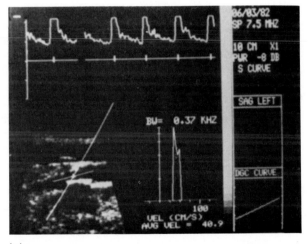

(b)

Figure 6 (a) B-mode ultrasound scan of the carotid artery demonstrating a bifurcation plaque. (b) Duplex scanning adds sound spectrum analysis localized to the diseased area. (From Daigle RJ, Ref. 25, with permission.)

accurate to be the sole evaluator of cerebrovascular disease in patients for whom surgical therapy is being considered.

In an attempt to begin to analyze this question, Flanigan et al. analyzed 157 carotid artery segments studied both by duplex scanning and contrast arteriography (27). The analysis was specifically done to assess the role of carotid duplex scanning in the surgical decision-making process. All studies, along with history and physical data, were analyzed in a blind study by two vascular surgeons, one who operates on only symptomatic patients and the other who operates on both symptomatic and selected asymptomatic (stenosis greater than 50% diameter reduction and/or "significant" ulceration) patients. The data were analyzed to determine if there was agreement regarding decision for carotid endarterectomy based on scan findings compared with decisions based on arteriographic findings. There was agreement between the two studies regarding the need for carotid surgery in 91% and 89% of arteries studied according to the two surgeons, respectively.

Data were also analyzed in this study to assess the four most commonly employed factors in surgical decision-making: (a) presence or absence of disease; (b) ulceration; (c) stenosis greater than 50% diameter reduction; and (d) total occlusion. The accuracy for duplex scanning in the assessment of these factors in comparison to arteriography was 81%, 90%, 83%, and 99%, respectively.

This information allowed the creation of a clinical algorithm for the management of patients being evaluated for cerebrovascular disease (Fig. 7). In this algorithm both symptomatic and asymptomatic patients undergo duplex scanning as their initial testing procedure. Patients with focal carotid territory symptoms with scans demonstrating appropriate disease go to surgery without additional diagnostic studies. This approach is supported by the fact that operated patients with abnormal scans but with normal arteriograms had disease documented at operation. One possible drawback to this approach is that additional intracranial and/or intrathoracic cerebraovascular disease might not be diagnosed. In this case it is our policy

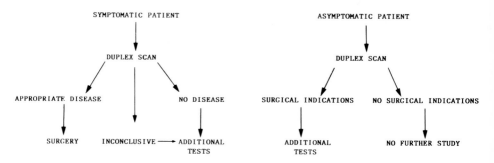

Figure 7 Algorithm for management of patients with suspected cerebrovascular disease. (From Flanigan DP, Ref. 27, with permission.)

to perform carotid endarterectomy as the initial procedure, since Borozan et al. have previously shown that symptomatic patients with multifocal disease are most often relieved of symptoms following carotid endarterectomy (28). If patients are not relieved of symptoms following this approach, reevaluation is still possible, however, we have not found this necessary.

Patients having focal carotid territory symptoms in this algorithm who have normal duplex scans should undergo further diagnostic evaluation. This follows since there were 6% and 8% of scans for surgeons A and B, respectively, not demonstrating disease that was visualized arteriographically. All patients who were actually operated upon had their arteriographic findings confirmed at operation. This method is also supported by the finding of an accuracy of only 81% in the category of presence or absence of disease when comparing duplex scans with arteriograms. Patients with vertebrobasilar symptoms pose a different situation. Noninvasive carotid testing in this group is focused on the hemodynamic significance of carotid lesions. This determination could be done with only an 83% accuracy in the above-mentioned study. Thus, when the degree of stenosis in the carotid artery is inconclusive following duplex scanning in patients with nonfocal symptoms, additional studies are warranted. It is in this situation that indirect noninvasive testing may be useful. Asymptomatic patients with duplex scans showing disease severity suggesting the need for surgery should probably undergo confirmatory studies, since the accuracy for determining a hemodynamically significant stenosis was only 83%. Asymptomatic patients with normal duplex scans or scans demonstrating insufficient disease severity for surgical indications should not undergo further studies, since in this group acts of omission are not likely to be serious errors. Obviously patients with inconclusive scans would require additional diagnostic testing for proper diagnosis if clinically indicated.

Application of the algorithm to the same patient cohort would have resulted in a 31% utilization of arteriography and an error rate of 0.6%. An evaluation of the algorithm is currently underway using angiographic control to determine its reliability prospectively. Until such validation is obtained, arteriography remains an integral part in the evaluation of patients with cerebrovascular disease.

CONCLUSION

The noninvasive diagnosis of extracranial cerebrovascular disease has undergone rapid evolution in the last decade. Initial techniques of indirect evaluation have progressed to a stage where the accuracy of noninvasive testing now rivals contrast arteriography. Noninvasive testing has already replaced arteriography in the initial evaluation of asymptomatic patients and patients with nonlocalizing symptoms and early evidence suggests that duplex scanning might be able to replace arteriography in selected patients being evaluated for carotid endarterectomy.

REFERENCES

1. Steiner TJ, McIvor J, Perkin GD, Greenhalgh RM, Rose FC: Morbidity of arch and carotid angiography: Perspective survey. In R Greenhalgh, FC Rose (eds): Progress in Stroke, Pittman Books, Ltd., London, p. 136, 1983.
2. Galin M, Baras I, Best M, et al: Methods of suction ophthalmodynamometry. Ann Ophthalmol 1:439, 1970.
3. Bone GE, Slaymaker EE, Barnes RW: Noninvasive assessment of collateral blood flow of the cerebral hemisphere by Doppler ultrasound. Surg Gynecol Obstet 145:873, 1977.
4. Lynch TG, Wright CB, Miller EV: Oculopneumoplethysmography, Doppler examination, and supraorbital photoplethysmography: A comparison of hemodynamic techniques in assessing cerebrovascular occlusive disease. Ann Surg 194:731, 1981.
5. Malone JM, Bean B, Laguna J, Hamilton R, Labadie E, Moore WS: Diagnosis of carotid artery stenosis: Comparison of oculoplethysmography and Doppler supraorbital examination. Ann Surg 191:347, 1980.
6. Macleder HI, Barker WF: Noninvasive methods for evaluation of extracranial cerebrovascular disease: A comparison. Arch Surg 112:944, 1977.
7. Barnes RW, Garrett WV, Slaymaker EE, Reinertson JE: Doppler ultrasound and supraorbital photoplethysmography for noninvasive screening of carotid occlusive disease. Am J Surg 134:183, 1977.
8. Gross WS, Verta MJ, van Bellen B, Bergan JJ, Yao JST: Comparison of noninvasive diagnostic techniques in carotid artery occlusive disease. Surgery 82: 271, 1977.
9. LeGerfo FW, Mason FR: Directional Doppler studies of supraorbital artery flow in internal carotid stenosis and occlusion. Surgery 76:723, 1974.
10. McDonald PT, Rich NM, Collins GA, Andersen CA, Kozloff L: Doppler cerebrovascular examination, oculoplethysmography, and ocular pneumoplethysmography: Use in detection of carotid disease: A prospective clinical study. Arch Surg 113:1341, 1978.
11. Towne JP, Salles-Cunha S, Bernhard VM: Periorbital ultrasound findings: Hemodynamics in patients with cerebral vascular disease. Arch Surg 114:158, 1979.
12. Bone GE, Barnes RW: Limitations of the Doppler cerebrovascular examination in hemispheric cerebral ischemia. Surgery 79:577, 1976.
13. Kartchner MM, McRae LP, Crain V, Whitaker B: Oculoplethysmography: An adjunct to arteriography in the diagnosis of extracranial carotid occlusive disease. Am J Surg 132:728, 1976.
14. Satiani B, Cooperman M, Clark M, Evans WE: An assessment of carotid phonoangiography and oculoplethysmography in the detection of carotid artery stenosis. Am J Surg 136:618, 1978.
15. Keagy BA, Pharr WF, Thomas DD, Bowes DE: Oculoplethysmography/carotid phonoangiography: Its value as a screening test in patients with suspected carotid artery stenosis. Arch Surg 115:119, 1980.

16. Blackshear WM Jr, Thiele BL, Harley JD, Chikos PM, Strandness DE Jr: A prospective evaluation of oculoplethysmography and carotid phonoangiography. Surg Gynecol Obstet 148:201, 1979.
17. Bone GE, Dickinson D, Pomajzl MJ: A prospective evaluation of indirect methods for detecting carotid atherosclerosis. Surg Gynecol Obstet 152:587, 1981.
18. Gee W, Smith CA, Hinson CE, et al: Ocular pneumoplethysmography in carotid artery disease. Med Instrum 8:244, 1974.
19. McDonald KM, Gee W, Kaupp HA, Bast RG: Screening for significant carotid stenosis by ocular pneumoplethysmography. Am J Surg 137:244, 1979.
20. McDonald PT, Rich NM, Collins GJ, Kozlof L, Andersen CA: Ocular pneumoplethysmography: Detection of carotid occlusive disease. Ann Surg 189:44, 1979.
21. Schwartz JA, Flanigan DP, Schuler JJ, Ryan TJ, Castronouvo JJ: Indirect assessment of carotid occlusive disease by ocular pneumoplethysmography 500 mmHg vacuum pressure measurements and ocular pulse timing. Stroke 15:521, 1984.
22. Barnes RW, Bone GE, Reinertson J, Slaymaker EE, Hokanson DE, Strandness DE Jr: Noninvasive ultrasonic carotid angiography: Prospective validation by contrast arteriography. Surgery 80:328, 1976.
23. Barnes RW, Rittgers SE, Putney WW: Real-time Doppler spectrum analysis: Predictive value in defining operable carotid artery disease. Arch Surg 117:52, 1982.
24. Blackshear WM Jr, Phillips DJ, Thiele BL, Hirsch JH, Chikos PN, Marinelli MR, Ward KJ, Strandness DE Jr: Detection of carotid occlusive disease by ultrasonic imaging and pulsed Doppler spectrum analysis. Surgery 86:698, 1979.
25. Daigle RJ, Gardner M, Smazal SF, Dreisbach JN: Accuracy of duplex ultrasound scanning in the evaluation of carotid artery disease. Bruit 17:17, 1983.
26. Comerota AJ, Cranley JJ, Katz M, Cook SE, Sippel PJ, Hayden WG, Fogarty TJ, Tyson RR: Real-time B-mode carotid imaging: A three-year multicenter experience. J Vasc Surg 1:84, 1984.
27. Flanigan DP, Schuler JJ, Vogel M, Borozan PG, Gray B, Sobinsky KR: The role of carotid duplex scanning in surgical decision making. J Vasc Surg 2:15, 1985.
28. Borozan PG, Schuler JJ, LaRosa MP, Ware MS, Flanigan DP: The natural history of isolated carotid siphon stenosis. J Vasc Surg 1:744, 1984.

8

Selection of Patients
for Renal Revascularization

JAMES C. STANLEY,
THOMAS W. WAKEFIELD
University of Michigan Medical School
Ann Arbor, Michigan

LINDA M. GRAHAM
University of Michigan
Medical School and
Ann Arbor Veterans
Administration
Medical Center
Ann Arbor, Michigan

Preoperative assessment of candidates for renal revascularization is directed at two specific populations: (a) patients with renal artery occlusive disease, manifest by renin-mediated hypertension or ischemic deterioration of renal function; (b) patients with renal artery aneurysms, which carry the potential for either life-endangering or kidney-threatening rupture, as well as secondary hypertension from thromboembolization of aneurysmal contents or compromised blood flow through distorted adjacent arteries. Selection criteria for operation are different for these two patient populations and warrant individual discussion.

RENAL ARTERY OCCLUSIVE DISEASE

Renal artery stenotic lesions are the most common cause of surgically correctable hypertension. The prevalence of renovascular hypertension among all patients with moderate or severe diastolic hypertension is approximately 5%, and the frequency is clearly greater among pediatric patients, women less than 50 years of age, and patients of both sexes with de novo development of hypertension beyond the age of 50 years.

Clinical manifestations of renovascular hypertension are as varied as the heterogeneic group of occlusive diseases producing the stenoses, and will result in many errors if used alone as the basis for pursuing diagnostic studies (1). Nevertheless, patients with renovascular hypertension, compared with essential hypertensives, are more likely to have: (a) a negative family history of hypertension, (b) hypertension of shorter duration, (c) accelerated hypertension with grade III or IV retino-pathy, and (d) abdominal or flank bruits. Unfortunately, renovascular hypertension can affect both sexes at any age and its severity may range from mild to severe, with medical control usually possible if diligently pursued. Thus, additional data regard-ing the kidney's role is needed to establish a diagnosis of renovascular hyperten-sion.

Laboratory tests contributing to a working diagnosis of renovascular hyperten-sion may be divided into three categories: (a) functional studies related to dimin-ished blood flow and urine production that are accompanied by changes in renal mass or clearances of various substances from the blood stream, (b) anatomic imag-ing of the renal artery, and (c) tests documenting activation of the renin-angioten-sin system with accompanying increased vasopressor activity (2). No single test serves as a totally reliable basis to confirm the diagnosis of renovascular hyperten-sion. Indeed, the only infallible evidence of renovascular hypertension is the nor-malization of blood pressure after successful renal revascularization or nephrec-tomy. However, a thorough understanding of contemporary diagnostic and prog-nostic investigations for patients suspected of renovascular hypertension becomes critical in clinical practice.

Hypertensive Urography

Rapid sequence excretory urography is suggestive of renal ischemia in the presence of: (a) unilateral delays in caliceal appearance of contrast medium, (b) differences in renal length, with the right kidney being 1.5 cm smaller than the left or the left being 2.0 cm smaller than the right, or (c) hyperconcentration of contrast media on delayed films. In addition, ureteral notching due to indentations by tortuous collateral vessels is an important, although inconsistent, finding of advanced renal artery occlusive disease.

Bilateral functionally important disease in approximately 15% of cases, and existence of occasional patients having segmental disease not interfering with the involved kidney's total excretory function, limits the overall sensitivity of uro-graphy to 85% at best. The Cooperative Study on Renovascular Hypertension re-ported abnormal urograms in 78% of patients with renal artery stenoses greater than 50% (3,4). This was in contrast to abnormal urograms in only 11% of patients with essential hypertension. Most patients in the Cooperative Study with renovas-cular hypertension had unilateral atherosclerotic lesions, a disease most likely to place the entire affected renal mass at risk for ischemia. In the University of Michi-gan experience, the 72% frequency of abnormal urograms among patients with atherosclerotic disease was similar to that of the Cooperative Study (5). However, abnormal studies in the Michigan experience were encountered in only 24% of pediatric and 47% of adult fibrodysplastic renovascular hypertensives (Table 1).

Despite an occasional report documenting high specificity of urograms among renovascular hypertensives and an unusually low incidence of abnormal studies in

Table 1 Hypertensive Urography in Renovascular Hypertension Cured by Surgery[a]

	Abnormal Urogram (%)	Normal Urogram (%)
Pediatric disease	24	76
Adult fibrodysplastic disease	47	53
Arterosclerotic disease	72	28

[a]Data from University of Michigan Experience; see original publication for definition of patient populations (5).

essential hypertensives (6), it would appear that rapid sequence excretory urography is unjustified for routine screening of patients suspected of renovascular hypertension (7).

Split Renal Function Tests

Individual kidney *p*-aminohippurate (PAH) and inulin clearances may be used to assess diminished renal blood flow. However, because of the high incidence of abnormal tests in patients with nonrenovascular disease, they have limited diagnostic applicability. Two particular studies have been used most frequently in evaluating renal ischemia: (a) the Howard test, documenting greater sodium and creatinine

Table 2 Split Renal Function Studies in Essential Hypertension and Renovascular Hypertension Cured by Surgery[a]

	Positive Studies	
	Essential Hypertension (%)	Renovascular Hypertension (%)
Classic criteria	2	50
Half-classic criteria	2	72
Lateralizing criteria	10	92

[a]Data from Vanderbilt Experience (9). Definition of criteria: (1) classic—40% reduction in urine volume, 50% increase in creatinine concentration, 100% increase in PAH concentration; (2) half-classic—20% reduction in urine volume, 25% increase in creatinine concentration, 50% increase in PAH concentration; (3) lateralizing—consistent lateralization in each of three collection periods with decrease in urine volume and increase in creatinine and PAH concentrations.

concentrations in reduced volumes of urine from the ischemic kidney, and (b) the Stamey test, which documents greater concentrations of PAH from the ischemic kidney following a urea-induced duiresis. The Vanderbilt group reported increased sensitivity of split renal function studies with a liberalization of the criteria for an abnormal test (8,9) (Table 2). In their experience, applying classic criteria, very few patients with essential hypertension had abnormal studies but only half of those with renovascular hypertension had abnormal studies. Use of less rigid diagnostic criteria resulted in greater test sensitivity, but was accompanied by appreciable numbers of abnormal studies in patients without renovascular disease. Thus, even though the sensitivity of split renal function tests may be improved by liberalizing the definition of abnormal studies, unacceptably high false-positive rates continue to limit their use as predictors of renovascular hypertension.

Isotope Renography

Radionuclides provide a noninvasive means of assessing kidney function in suspected cases of renovascular hypertension (10-12). Isotope renography may be used by direct imaging of the kidney, or with analysis of the renal washout curves of various tracers, the most common being ^{131}I orthoiodohippurate. Compounds such as this are cleared in a manner reflecting both renal blood flow and excretory function, similar to that of PAH in split renal function studies.

Unfortunately, false-positive radionuclide studies are common in essential hypertension, with certain states of abnormal hydration, or in situations where increased renal resistance causes flow abnormalities. Data reported from the Cooperative Study revealed a 75% specificity and 76% sensitivity in patients suspected of renovascular hypertension (13) (Table 3). Renal perfusion-excretion ratios may enhance the usefulness of radionuclide screening for renal ischemia. In this regard,

Table 3   Renography in Essential Hypertension and Renovascular Disease[a]

	Abnormal Renogram (%)
Essential hypertension	25
Renovascular disease, degree of stenosis	
Less than 50%	44
50-80%	69
Greater than 80%	77
100%	94

[a]Data from Cooperative Study on Renovascular Hypertension (13). Renograms were abnormal in 76% of all renovascular cases having stenoses greater than 50%.

^{99m}technetium DMSA and ^{99m}technetium DPTA renography has increased the accuracy of measuring differential excretory function. Transit time assessment with this technique appears to be an important advancement in diagnostic isotopic renography, although these studies are perhaps best used in longitudinal documentation of total and individual renal plasma flow.

Conventional Arteriography

Anatomic definition of the renal vasculature is accomplished best by aortography and selective renal arteriography. The morphologic character of renal artery stenotic disease has important prognostic implications. In addition, the presence of collateral

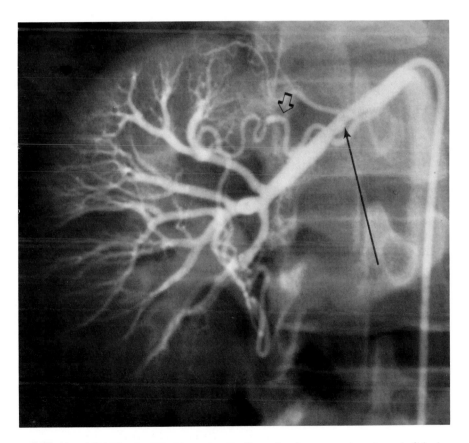

Figure 1 Selective renal arteriogram revealing a benign-appearing stenosis (black arrow) associated with a large collateral vessel circumventing the lesion (open arrow) that documents its hemodynamic significance. (Reproduced with permission, from Stanley, Graham, and Whitehouse, Ref. 2.)

vessels circumventing a stenoses provides a marker of the hemodynamic and functional importance of the disease (Fig. 1). Existence of collaterals suggests a functionally important lesion in that pressure gradients of approximately 10 mmHg across a stenosis are necessary for their development, and this same degree of pressure change is associated with abnormal renin release from the kidney.

Pharmacoangiographic manipulation of the renal circulation may enhance the radiologic visualization of collateral vessels and allow documentation of otherwise equivocally important stenotic disease (14). Lesions may be considered functionally important if selective renal artery infusions of acetylcholine or epinephrine cause reversal of flow in nonparenchymal branches originating beyond the stenosis.

Standard aortography, performed in the anterior-posterior plane alone, may result in interpretive errors regarding the presence or absence of renal artery disease. Oblique views are often required to demonstrate both distal segmental dysplastic disease or proximal ostial atherosclerotic stenoses. In this regard, renal artery origins are perhaps best demonstrated using right posterior oblique projections (15).

Digital Subtraction Arteriography

Computerized enhancement of radiographic images following intravenous administration of contrast agents has been proposed to be an accurate means of screening for renovascular hypertension (16,17). The sensitivity of these studies is approximately 85%, with ostial or segmental disease in many cases not being evident because of the limited resolution of existing technology or the presence of overlying intestinal vessels. The specificity of such studies is approximately 95%, with false positives occurring infrequently among hypertensive patients with nonrenovascular disease. An important use of digital subtraction arteriography relates to intraarterial administration of contrast agents that, when performed in a selective fashion, lessens the risk of contrast nephrotoxicity and in contrast to intravenous studies provides better definition of the proximal segmental renal vessels.

Renin Assays

Renin is a proteolytic enzyme released from cells in the juxtaglomerular apparatus of the kidney. In patients with renovascular hypertension, this occurs as a consequence of baroreceptor responses to decreased renal artery blood pressure. Other stimuli such as increased sympathetic nervous system activity, low sodium, and low intracellular calcium may also contribute to renin release. Renin acts on renin substrate, an alpha$_2$-globulin produced in the liver, to form angiotensin I. This latter substance is converted to angiotensin II by a converting enzyme. Angiotensin II also causes the adrenal gland to produce greater amounts of aldosterone, thus increasing sodium retention and contributing to the volume element of renovascular hypertension.

Documentation of excessive renin activity seems logical in defining the presence of renin-mediated hypertension. Unfortunately, peripheral plasma renin activity has not proven to be a reasonable diagnostic study in cases of suspected renovascular hypertension. Approximately 15% of essential hypertensives have high circulating peripheral renins, and nearly 33% of proven renovascular hypertensives exhibit normal peripheral renin activity. Some of the latter patients might be identified as having abnormal renin activity if their peripheral renin levels were indexed to simultaneous urinary sodium excretion. However, the latter requires very careful regulation of sodium intake as well as drug therapy, and has never received much use in clinical practice.

Renal Vein Renin Ratio (RVRR)

Comparison of renin activity from the effluent venous blood from one kidney to that of the other kidney is important in evaluting unilateral renal artery stenotic disease. Measurement of renin activity from venous blood of each kidney in essential hypertensives has revealed that the kidneys both contribute an average of 24% more renin in their effluent venous blood than exists in their arterial blood supply (18). Thus, together both kidneys contribute 48% more renin in their venous output than is present in their arterial input. Variances of individual RVRR may range from 1.0 to 1.48. An abnormal RVRR, by definition, exists when this value becomes greater than 1.48. Compounding the physiologic disparities of RVRR are errors inherent in contemporary renin radioimmunoassays, the latter usually quantitating angiotensin I levels. Because of these errors, a RVRR actually approaching 2.00 may become necessary to assure the existence of excessive renin secretion (19-21).

RVRRs are of limited usefulness in the assessment of renovascular hypertension (Fig. 2). Two clinical situations compromise the validity of the RVRR as an indicator of renovascular hypertension. The first occurs in approximately 15% of cases where, because of advanced bilateral disease, renin production from both kidneys is abnormally elevated, but is equally high for both kidneys. In these instances the RVRR approaches 1.0, despite renin hypersecretion. The second situation occurs in patients with an unstimulated renin-angiotensin system. In these cases minimal variances in basal physiologic secretion during the course of samplings may result in high ratios that for practical purposes are of no clinical relevance. This may be lessened by stimulation of the renin-angiotensin system prior to blood sampling. This is usually accomplished by (a) reductions of sodium intake to no more than 20 mEq/day for 3 days, (b) administration of a natriuretic drug for 3 days, and (c) sampling of renal vein blood flow from the patient in the upright position. It should be obvious that agents inhibiting renal renin release, such as β-adrenergic blockers, should be discontinued prior to sampling blood for these

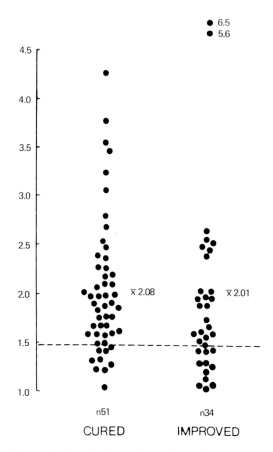

Figure 2 Renal vein renin ratios in 85 patients with renovascular hypertension who responded to surgical intervention. Differences between cured and improved categories were not present. Note: 18% of cured and 32% of improved patients had ratios less than 1.48. (Reproduced, with permission, from Stanley, Gewertz, and Fry, Ref. 21.)

assays. On the other hand, use of angiotensin-converting enzyme inhibitors may make renin data more reliable as a diagnostic test (22).

Renal/Systemic Renin Index (RSRI)

This index provides a means to document an individual kidney's contribution to total circulating renin (21). The RSRI lessens the errors inherent to the RVRR. The index is calculated by subtracting systemic renin activity from that of the renal vein and dividing the remainder by the systemic renin activity. Unilateral hypersecretion occurs when the RSRI is greater than 0.48. Functionally important disease also exists when the sum of the RSRI from both kidneys is greater than 0.48, even though an individual kidney's RSRI is less than 0.48. In cases with unusually high levels of circulating renin, the upper limits of a normal RSRI are less than 0.48 (18). The value of ischemic kidney hypersecretion (RSRI greater than 0.48) and contralateral renin suppression (RSRI less than 0.24, approaching 0.0) in discriminating between patients cured versus those improved following operation has been clearly documented (Fig. 3) (5,21,23). However, because of inconsistencies in patient preparation, variations in radioimmunoassay, and sampling errors, the diagnostic sensitivity of RSRI data is far from perfect. Approximately

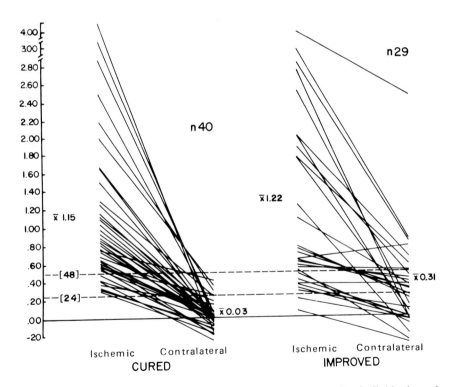

Figure 3 Renal/systemic renin indices in 69 patients comparing individual renal vein activity to systemic renin activity. Mean ischemic kidney hypersecretion in cured versus improved groups (1.15 and 1.22, respectively) did not prove to be statistically different. Contralateral suppression of renin activity was obvious in cured (0.03) group and nonexistent in improved (0.31) group. Differences in degree of suppression proved significant ($p < 0.01$). (Reproduced with permission from Stanley and Fry, Ref. 5.)

10% of known renovascular hypertensives fail to exhibit ischemic kidney hypersecretion and 8% of patients who are cured fail to exhibit contralateral kidney renin suppression (5). Thus, although the RSRI represents an important refinement in the interpretation of renin activity in patients suspected of having renovascular hypertension, rigid application of RSRI data to clinical decision making is inappropriate.

Angiotensin II Antagonists

Renin-dependent hypertension may be documented by competitively blocking angiotensin II receptor sites with agents such as saralasin (P113,1-Sar,8-Ala angiotensin II) (24-28). The effects of these competitive antagonists are decreased vascular smooth muscle contractility, subsequent falls in peripheral resistance, and decreased blood pressure. Criteria of positive saralasin tests usually involve 5-15 mmHg diminutions in the blood pressure. Blood pressure responsiveness to saralasin infusions are markedly affected by sodium balance. Unfortunately, the sensitivity of contemporary testing is only 75% with a specificity of approximately 85% (6). Because of these factors, the use of angiotensin II competitive antagonists is limited in screening patients for renovascular hypertension.

Angiotensin-Converting Enzyme Inhibitors

It was originally hoped that the presence of renovascular hypertension could be documented by inhibiting converting enzyme and quantitating subsequent diminutions in blood pressure (29). This would seem to be a more sensitive means of detecting angiotensin II-dependent blood pressure elevations than testing with agents like saralasin. Unfortunately, the specificity of diagnostic studies with converting enzyme inhibitors has proven unacceptable. This is primarily because drops in blood pressure following administration of these agents occur in all nonrenovascular hypertensives. This phenomenon is a reflection of the fact that converting enzyme is identical to kinase II, the latter being responsible for the degradation of bradykinin. Thus, converting enzyme inhibitors cause accumulation of the vasodepressor bradykinin, as well as reductions in angiotensin II. The limited usefulness of these agents in diagnostic testing does not lessen their value in therapy. However, an important complication of the therapeutic use of converting enzyme inhibitors is deterioration of renal function in patients whose entire renal mass is at risk because of stenotic disease. Such occurs in patients with bilateral renal artery occlusive lesions or in those with a solitary kidney harboring a stenotic renal artery (30). Whenever abrupt deterioration in renal function accompanies the use of converting enzyme inhibitors, renovascular hypertension should be suspected.

It should be obvious from the aforementioned discussion that most contemporary diagnostic and prognostic studies in patients suspected of renovascular hypertension have limitations. Although the specificity of many tests appears high, the sensitivity is such that given the low prevalence of renovascular hypertension in the general population, these studies have very limited predictive value as screening tests. A reasonable approach in attempting to establish the diagnosis of renovascular hypertension might be to use a scoring system combining: (a) one study related to renal excretion such as hypertensive urography, split renal function tests or isotopic renography, (b) another test relating to anatomic studies such as conventional arteriography or digital subtraction arteriography, and (c) a physiologic test concerning angiotensin II generation, such as peripheral renin activity related to urinary sodium, renal/systemic renin indices, or depressor responses to angiotensin II antagonists. Unfortunately, a scoring system using various combinations of studies assessing these different aspects of renal ischemia has not been forthcoming. Interestingly, most large clinical series report overall beneficial outcomes following operative therapy in excess of 90% (31). Given the limited sensitivity of current diagnostic testing, this raises the issue as to the likelihood that hypertensive patients with renovascular occlusive lesions are going unrecognized.

Documentation of renin-dependent hypertension and functionally important renal ischemia is but one factor in predicting the therapeutic outcome of surgical therapy. A second factor, often overlooked, is the realization that patients with renovascular disease may also be afflicted with essential hypertension. Elimination of stenotic renal artery disease in these cases clearly will not have an effect on the essential hypertension. Thus, among older patients where essential hypertension is relatively common, one cannot expect the same salutary response to surgical treatment occurring in younger patients where essential hypertension is uncommon (32-34). In this regard, relatively consistent differences in therapeutic outcomes have been observed in four major subgroups of renovascular hypertension (Table 4). The greatest benefits occur among pediatric patients, in whom 97% exhibit a favorable response to operative treatment, followed by a 94% benefit in adults with fibrodysplasia, a 91% response in adults with atherosclerosis when the only manifestation of their disease is secondary hypertension, and a 72% beneficial response in patients having atherosclerotic lesions with clinically overt extrarenal disease being evident at the time their renovascular disease is treated (34).

Renal revascularization in select cases may contribute to improved renal function and is of practical clinical importance (35-37). Because of the high incidence of bilateral renal artery occlusive disease and the known potential progression of all forms of these lesions, routine nephrectomy in the face of renal insufficiency is clearly undesirable. Most patients with impaired function due to diminished blood flow have severe stenotic lesions, with total renal artery occlusion often resulting as the end-stage of their disease. Secondary hypertension and renal insufficiency as a complication of chronic total renal artery occlusion may occur in as many as 60-75% of these cases (38,39). The care of such patients has generated controversy regarding means of differentiating viable, revascularizable kidneys maintained by collateral blood flow, from those having sustained irreversible

Table 4 Surgical Treatment of Renovascular Hypertension[a]

Subgroup	Number of Patients	Primary Operative Procedures		Operative Outcome[b]			Surgical Mortality[c]
		Arterial Reconstruction	Nephrectomy	Cured	Improved	Failure	
Fibrodysplasia, pediatric	34	39	2	85%	12%	3%	0%
Fibrodysplasia, adult	144	160	6	55%	39%	6%	0%
Atherosclerosis, focal renal artery disease	64	63	3	33%	58%	9%	0%
Atherosclerosis, overt generalized disease	71	70	6	25%	47%	28%	8.5%

[a]Results in specific patient subgroups, University of Michigan Experience, 1961-1980. Represents results of 405 operations (346 primary, 59 secondary) (34).
[b]Effect of operation on blood pressure defined as *Cured* if blood pressures were 150/90 mmHg or less for a minimum of 6 months, during which no antihypertensive medications were administered (lower pressure levels were utilized in evaluating pediatric patients). *Improved* if normotensive while on drug therapy, or if diastolic blood pressures ranged between 90 and 100 mmHg, but were as least 15% lower than preoperative levels. None of the improved patients were receiving converting enzyme inhibitors. *Failure* if diastolic blood pressures were greater than 90 mmHg but less than 15% lower than preoperative levels, or if they were greater than 110 mmHg.
[c]Surgical mortality includes all deaths within 30 days of operation.

ischemic damage. Renal revascularization and preservation of kidney parenchyma are commendable in the former instance, whereas nephrectomy may be more appropriate in the latter setting. A number of factors regarding revascularization and nephrectomy deserve comment.

Decreased kidney size is a known consequence of renal ischemia. This may be a reflection of simple reductions in renal blood volume, reversible atrophy, or progressive cellular damage and fibrosis in advanced cases. Size alone is not a valid criterion by which to predict the response to surgical therapy. Indeed, many small kidneys, less than 9.5 cm in length, may be successfully revascularized with nearly 50% exhibiting improved renal function and approximately 90% a lessening of the hypertensive state (38). The absolute minimum length of a retrievable ischemic kidney has not been defined, but may be in the range of 7.0 cm. Kidneys smaller than this have probably incurred irreparable cortical injury. Intraoperative biopsy has been undertaken in an attempt to define irreversible changes of ischemia, including obliteration of all glomeruli, interstitial fibrosis, and loss of tubules. Random biopsies of the kidney, and even directed biopsies toward areas of ischemic injury, unfortunately may reveal mixtures of changes including those of reversible atrophy. Because of such inconsistencies, biopsies alone are rarely the basis for choosing between nephrectomy and revascularization. Intraoperative arteriography is another useful but infrequently used method of assessing the potential for successful renal revascularization. Evidence of severe intraparenchymal artery obstructions, extensive "pruning" of cortical vessels due to nephrosclerosis, or multiple infarctions lend support to the performance of nephrectomy rather than revascularization. Although clinical experience is limited, intraoperative arteriography, even with its potential risk of contrast nephrotoxicity, is more appropriate than the casual performance of nephrectomy.

Benefits of renal revascularization regarding renal function are greater in cases of more advanced functional impairment. In certain instances, improved postoperative renal function may be a more direct effect of better control of preexisting hypertension than enhanced blood flow to the kidney. Such is certainly the explanation for improved renal function in patients undergoing unilateral nephrectomy (38). In treating the azotemic patient with renal artery occlusive disease, small kidney size and lack of a nephrogram or absent distal vessels on preoperative arteriographic studies should not deter surgical exploration with an attempt to undertake renal artery reconstruction if a viable, salvageable kidney is determined to be present at the time of operation.

Clearly, optimal therapy of renovascular occlusive disease follows accurate documentation of the functional importance of the stenotic lesion and proper performance of the renal revascularization. Primary nephrectomy should never exceed 5% in contemporary practice, and should occur only when irreparable ischemic injury in the form of infarcts or unreconstructable intraparenchymal vascular disease exists.

RENAL ARTERY ANEURYSMAL DISEASE

Renal artery aneurysms are an unusual vascular disease with apparent frequencies of 0.1% in the general population and 2.5% in hypertensive patients undergoing arteriographic studies for suspected renovascular disease (40). Aneurysms have been noted in 9.2% of a more selected population, namely those with renal artery fibrodysplastic stenoses (41). Considerable speculation persists concerning the clinical importance of these aneurysms, especially regarding: (a) morbidity attributable to intact aneurysms, (b) their association with renovascular hypertension, and (c) their risk of rupture (40,42,43).

Women are afflicted with renal artery aneurysms more often than men, but no sex predilection exists when patients with coexisting arterial fibrodysplastic disease are excluded. The vast majority of renal artery aneurysms are asymptomatic. Abdominal or flank pain, hematuria, and abdominal bruits have been attributed to these aneurysms, but rarely occur with uncomplicated disease. Similarly, renal artery aneurysms themselves are an uncommon cause of elevated blood pressure. However, occasionally aneurysmal thrombus propagates and occludes the adjacent artery or embolizes distally, with subsequent development of renal ischemia and renovascular hypertension. Thrombosis or thromboembolism occurs in less than 5% of these aneurysms (40). Rarely, compression of adjacent arteries by large extrarenal aneurysms may be the cause of renovascular hypertension. On the other hand, nearly 80% of patients with renal artery macroaneurysms are hypertensive, a fact that suggests that blood pressure elevations may contribute to the evolution of these aneurysms.

Rupture of renal artery aneurysms occurs with equal frequency into extraparenchymal tissues and adjacent renal veins. Rupture is uncommon, affecting less than a few percent of cases (40,43). Increased risk of rupture with aneurysms greater than 1.5 cm in diameter, noncalcified aneurysms, or in patients with diastolic hypertension is a logical, but unproven tenent. Aneurysmal rupture during the course of pregnancy is an exception to the otherwise benign nature of most lesions, with a maternal mortality approaching 80% and fetal death occurring in nearly all cases (44-46).

Indications for operative intervention of renal artery macroaneurysms include: (a) all symptomatic lesions, (b) aneurysms occurring coincidentally with functionally important renal artery stenotic disease, (c) aneurysms documented to harbor thrombus, especially if distal embolization is present, and (d) aneurysms occurring in all women of child-bearing age who might possibly conceive in the future. Large aneurysms, namely those greater than 2.0 cm in diameter, represent a relative indication for operative therapy, although there is no definitive evidence relating increased aneurysmal size to an increased risk of rupture.

Noninvasive Imaging

Renal artery aneurysms have been suspected following recognition of signet-ring calcifications on plain abdominal roentgenograms in approximately 15% of cases. Similar findings or indentations of the renal collecting system during intravenous urography account for recognition of an additional 15% of cases. Abdominal ultrasonography and computerized axial tomography may also reveal renal artery aneurysms, but inasmuch as the mean diameter of these aneurysms is 1.3 cm (40), such studies may not be sensitive enough to detect the presence of smaller aneurysms.

Conventional and Digital Subtraction Arteriography

Conventional arteriographic examinations for nonaneurysmal renal disease, such as renovascular hypertension or hematuria, has resulted in unanticipated documentation of renal artery aneurysms in approximately 50% of reported cases. Arteriographic studies for nonrenal disease have led to documentation of these aneurysms in an additional 10% of cases. The sensitivity and specificity of conventional arteriographic studies regarding renal artery macroaneurysms is well over 95%. False-positive studies occur occasionally when segmental vessels are viewed end-on-end, and appear to represent globular vascular structures similar to intraparenchymal aneurysms. False-negative studies occur in rare patients who have thrombosed lesions preventing accumulation of contrast within the aneurysm. The accuracy of digital subtraction arteriography in these cases is limited because of its lack of resolution of smaller vessels, where these aneurysms usually arise.

Among patients suspected of renovascular hypertension secondary to distortion of perianeurysmal vessels or thromboembolic complications of their aneurysm, arteriographic studies may demonstrate the occlusive process and are important in planning appropriate operative therapy. In equivocal cases it may be important to document the functional importance of these potential ischemic complications by establishing the presence of collateral vessels about the obstruction, excessive renin release, or angiotensin-dependent hypertension before operative treatment is undertaken.

The objective of surgical therapy for renal artery aneurysms is aneurysmectomy without loss of renal tissue or compromise of normal renal blood flow. Nephrectomy has proven an untenable therapeutic modality in these cases unless all other operative efforts fail, including ex vivo attempts at aneurysmectomy and renal artery reconstruction. Surgical intervention should be approached cautiously in patients harboring small renal artery aneurysms because of the known 10-15% incidence of nephrectomy associated with operative therapy, and the apparent low incidence of life-endangering and kidney-threatening rupture of otherwise bland renal artery aneurysms.

REFERENCES

1. Simon N, Franklin SS, Bleifer KH, Maxwell MH: Clinical characteristics of renovascular hypertension. J Am Med Assoc 220:1209-1218, 1972.
2. Stanley JC, Graham LM, Whitehouse WM Jr: Limitations and Errors of Diagnostic and Prognostic Investigations in Renovascular Hypertension. In Bernhard V, Towne J (ed): Complications in Vascular Surgery, Grune & Stratton, New York, 1985, pp. 213-227.
3. Bookstein JJ, Abrams HL, Buenger RE, Lecky J, Franklin SS, Reiss MD, Bleifer KH, Klatte EC, Varady PD, Maxwell MH: Radiologic aspects of renovascular hypertension. 2. The role of urography in unilateral renovascular disease. J Am Med Assoc 220:1225-1230, 1972.
4. Bookstein JJ, Maxwell MH, Abrams HL, Buenger RE, Lecky J, Franklin SS: Cooperative study of radiologic aspects of renovascular hypertension. Bilateral renovascular disease. J Am Med Assoc 237:1706-1709, 1977.
5. Stanley JC, Fry WJ: Surgical treatment of renovascular hypertension. Arch Surg 112:1291-1297, 1977.
6. Grim CE, Luft FC, Weinberger MH, Grim CM: Sensitivity and specificity of screening tests for renal vascular hypertension. Ann Intern Med 91:617-622, 1979.
7. Thornbury JR, Stanley JC, Fryback DG: Hypertensive urogram: A nondiscriminatory test for renovascular hypertension. Am J Roentgenol 138:43-49, 1982.
8. Dean RH, Foster JH: Criteria for the diagnosis of renovascular hypertension. Surgery 74:926-930, 1973.
9. Dean RH, Rhamy RK: Split renal function studies in renovascular hypertension. In Stanley JC, Ernst CB, Fry WJ (eds): Renovascular Hypertension, W B Saunders Co, Philadelphia, 1984, pp. 135-145.
10. Giese J, Mogensen P, Munck O: Diagnostic value of renography for detection of unilateral renal or renovascular disease in hypertensive patients. Scand J Clin Lab 37:307-310, 1975.
11. Keim HJ, Johnson PM, Vaughan ED Jr, Beg K, Follett DA, Freeman LM, Laragh JH: Computer-assisted static/dynamic renal imaging: A screening test for renovascular hypertension? J Nucl Med 20:11-17, 1979.
12. Machay A, Eadie AS, Cumming AMM, Graham AG, Adams FG, Norton PW: Assessment of total and divided renal plasma flow by ^{123}I-hippuran renography. Kidney Internat 19:49-57, 1981.
13. Franklin SS, Maxwell MH: Clinical work-up for renovascular hypertension. Urol Clin N Am 2:301-310, 1975.
14. Bookstein JJ, Walter JF, Stanley JC, Fry WJ: Pharmacoangiographic manipulation of renal collateral blood flow. Circulation 54:328-334, 1976.
15. Gerlock AJ, Goncharenko V, Sloan OM: Right posterior oblique: The projection of choice in aortography of hypertensive patients. Radiology 127:45-48, 1978.
16. Hillman BJ: Digital imaging of the kidney. Radiol Clin N Am 22:341-364, 1984.

17. Havey RJ, Krumlovsky F, delGreco F, Martin HG: Screening for renovascular hypertension. Is renal digital-subtraction angiography the preferred noninvasive test? J Am Med Assoc 254:388-393, 1985.

18. Sealy JE, Buhler FR, Laragh JH, Vaughan ED Jr: The physiology of renin secretion in essential hypertension. Estimation of renin secretion rate and renal plasma flow from peripheral and renal vein renin levels. Am J Med 55:391-401, 1973.

19. Marks LS, Maxwell MH, Varady PD, Lupu AN, Kaufman JJ: Renovascular hypertension: Does the renal vein renin ratio predict operative results? J Urol 115:365-368, 1976.

20. Marks LS, Maxwell MH: Renal vein renin: Value and limitations in the prediction of operative results. Urol Clin N Am 2:311-325, 1975.

21. Stanley JC, Gewertz BL, Bove EL, Sottiurai VS, Fry WJ: Arterial fibrodysplasia: Histopathologic character and current etiologic concepts. Arch Surg 110:561-566, 1975.

22. Thibonnier M, Joseph A, Sassano P, Guyenne TT, Corvol P, Raynaud A, Seurot M, Gaux JC: Improved diagnosis of unilateral renal artery lesions after captopril administration. J Am Med Assoc 251:55-60, 1984.

23. Vaughan ED, Buhler FR, Laragh JH, Sealey JE, Baer L, Bard RH: Renovascular hypertension: Renin measurements to indicate hypersecretion and contralateral suppression, estimate renal plasma flow, and score for curability. Am J Med 55:402-414, 1973.

24. Buda JA, Baer L, Arora SP, Parra-Carrillo JZ, Radichevich I: Evaluation of surgical response in renovascular hypertension using angiotensin II blockade. Surgery 84:664-670, 1978.

25. Krakoff LR, Ribeiro AB, Gorkin JU, Felton KR: Saralasin infusion in screening patients for renovascular hypertension. Am J Cardiol 45:609-613, 1980.

26. Marks LS, Maxwell MH, Kaufmann JJ: Renin, sodium, and vasodepressor response to saralasin in renovascular and essential hypertension. Ann Intern Med 87:176-182, 1977.

27. Streeten DHP, Phil D, Anderson GH, Freiberg JM, Dalakos TG: Use of an angiotensin II antagonist (saralasin) in the recognition of angiotensinogenic hypertension. N Engl J Med 292:657-662, 1975.

28. Wilson HM, Wilson JP, Slaton PE, Foster JH, Liddle GW, Hollifield JW: Saralasin infusion in the recognition of renovascular hypertension. Ann Intern Med 87:36-42, 1977.

29. Case DB, Wallace JM, Keim HJ, Weber MA, Drayer JIM, White RP, Sealey JE, Laragh JH: Estimating renin participation in hypertension: Superiority of converting enzyme inhibitor over saralasin. Am J Med 61:790-796, 1978.

30. Hricik DE, Browning PJ, Kopelman R, Goorno WE, Madias NE, Dzau VJ: Captopril-induced renal insufficiency in patients with bilateral renal-artery stenosis or renal-artery stenosis in a solitary kidney. N Engl J Med 308:373-376, 1983.

31. Stanley JC, Ernst CB, Fry WJ: Surgical Treatment of Renovascular Hypertension: Results in Specific Patient Subgroups. In Stanley JC, Ernst CB,

Fry WJ (eds): Renovascular Hypertension, W B Saunders, Philadelphia, 1984, pp. 363-371.

32. Stanley JC, Fry WJ: Pediatric renal artery occlusive disease and renovascular hypertension. Etiology, diagnosis, and operative treatment. Arch Surg 116: 669-676, 1981.

33. Stanley JC, Fry WJ: Renovascular hypertension secondary to arterial fibrodysplasia in adults: Criteria for operation and results of surgical therapy. Arch Surg 110:922-928, 1975.

34. Stanley JC, Whitehouse WM Jr, Graham LM, Cronenwett JL, Zelenock GB, Lindenauer SM: Operative therapy of renovascular hypertension. Br J Surg 69:S63-S66, 1982.

35. Dean RH, Englund R, Dupont DW, Meacham PW, Plummer WD Jr, Pierce R, Ezell C: Retrieval of renal function by revascularization. Study of preoperative outcome predictors. Ann Surg 202:367-375, 1985.

36. Novick AC, Pohl MA, Schreiber M, Gifford RW Jr, Vidt DG: Revascularization for preservation of renal function in patients with atherosclerotic renovascular disease. J Urol 129:907-912, 1983.

37. Ying CY, Tifft CP, Gavras H, Chobanian AV: Renal revascularization in the azotemic hypertensive patient resistant to therapy. N Eng J Med 311:1070-1075, 1985.

38. Whitehouse WM Jr, Kazmers A, Zelenock GB, Erlandson EE, Cronenwett JL, Lindenauer SM, Stanley JC: Chronic total renal artery occlusions: Effects of treatment on secondary hypertension and renal function. Surgery 89:753-763, 1981.

39. Lawson JD, Hollifield JH, Foster JH, Rhamy RK, Dean RH: Hypertension secondary to complete occlusion of the renal artery. Am Surg 44:642-649, 1978.

40. Stanley JC, Rhodes EL, Gewertz BL, Chang CY, Walter JF, Fry WJ: Renal artery aneurysm: Significance of macroaneurysms exclusive of dissections and fibrodysplastic mural dilations. Arch Surg 110:1327-1333, 1975.

41. Stanley JC, Gewertz BL, Bove EL, Sottiurai VS, Fry WJ: Arterial fibrodysplasia: Histopathologic character and current etiologic concepts. Arch Aurg 110:561-566, 1975.

42. Hubert JP Jr, Pairolero PC, Kazmier FJ: Solitary renal artery aneurysm. Surgery 88:557-565, 1980.

43. Tham G, Ekelund L, Herrlin K, Lindstedt EL, Olin T, Bergentz SE: Renal artery aneurysms. Natural history and prognosis. Ann Surg 197:348-352, 1983.

44. Burt RL, Johnson FR, Silverthorne RG, Lock FR, Dickerson AJ: Ruptured renal artery aneurysms in pregnancy: Report of a case with survival. Obstet Gynecol 7:229-233, 1956.

45. Cohen SG, Cashdan A, Burger R: Spontaneous rupture of a renal artery aneurysm during pregnancy. Obstet Gynecol 39:897-902, 1972.

46. Hidai H, Kinoshita Y, Murayama T, Miyai K, Matsumoto A, Ide K, Sato S: Rupture of renal artery aneurysm. Eur Urol 11:249-253, 1985.

9

The Use of Ultrasound and Computerized Tomographic Scanning in the Diagnosis of Vascular Pathology

LARRY R. WILLIAMS
University of South Florida
Tampa, Florida

Veterans Administration
  Medical Center
Bay Pines, Florida

ROBERT L. VOGELZANG
WILLIAM R. FLINN
Northwestern University
  Medical School
Chicago, Illinois

JAMES S. T. YAO
JOHN J. BERGAN
Northwestern University
  Medical School
Chicago, Illinois

WALTER J. McCARTHY III
Northwestern University Medical School and
Veterans Administration
  Lakeside Medical Center
Chicago, Illinois

GAIL SANDAGER
Columbus Hospital
Columbus, Ohio

Ultrasonic and computerized tomographic (CT) definition of vascular structures provide a wide variety of images from virtually every vascular segment. Real-time, ultrasound, B-mode scanning of carotid arteries has become a standard procedure in modern vascular laboratories. Ultrasonic examination of the aorta, primarily to evaluate abdominal aortic aneurysms, provided the first truly noninvasive assessment of aortic pathology. Computerized tomography has rapidly advanced as a key modality for precise measurement of anatomy in a cross-sectional plane, and provides a dimension not approached by most other imaging techniques. Carotid scans will be discussed elsewhere in the text. This chapter will concern itself with imaging of other vascular structures by ultrasound and CT, including those where these techniques are in a more developmental stage.

133

ULTRASOUND

Ultrasonic examination of the abdominal aorta has been available for over 20 years, and is used primarily for the detection and sizing of abdominal aortic aneurysms (1-4). The technique requires very little specific patient preparation, is convenient on an out-patient basis, and is relatively inexpensive. Since intravenous or oral contrast agents are not necessary, the risk of ultrasonic examination is practically non-existent.

Certain limitations specific to ultrasound include the inability to visualize the thoracic aorta due to the surrounding air-filled lungs and bony thoracic cage. The procedure is dependent at times upon the experience of the technologist performing the examination, and hard copies of the evaluation often lack detail. Increased bowel gas prevents penetration by the sound waves and at times deeper structures are difficult to image; however, with newer, multiple-frequency probes available, this has become less of a problem.

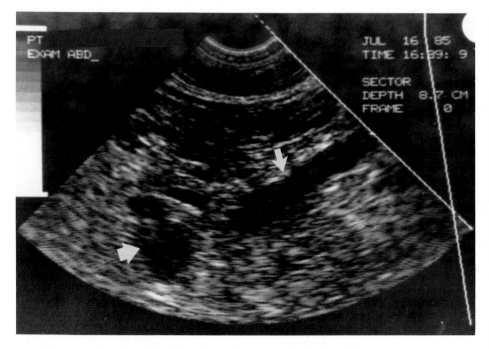

Figure 1 Abdominal ultrasound showing normal-sized aorta (small arrow) and celiac artery aneurysm (large arrow).

The Abdominal Aorta and Its Visceral Branches

Ultrasound provides an ideal method for screening for suspected abdominal aortic aneurysms. It has proven valuable for following patients with small aneurysms in whom an aortic operation has not been performed. Using current B-mode instrumentation, the celiac and superior mesenteric arteries are usually seen when evaluating the intraabdominal aorta and, with experience, considerable anatomic detail can be demonstrated in these branches. Aneurysms of the celiac and mesenteric arteries can be defined and measured and there is an increasing success in evaluating stenosis of these branches (Fig. 1).

By combining spectral analysis of pulsed Doppler signals with B-mode examination, it is possible to measure flow in both the superior mesenteric and celiac arteries. Jager studied preprandial and postprandial arterial flow in normal volunteers and found an increase of 3.7-fold in superior mesenteric artery flow following a test meal (5). Nicholls has compared duplex scanning to lateral arteriography in four patients with intestinal angina (6). The postprandial loss of diastolic reversed flow had a significant correlation with high-grade stenosis by angiography. This technique has important potential in scanning patients with suspected chronic intestinal ischemia and possibly in the evaluation of acute superior mesenteric artery occlusion.

The renal arteries can be imaged by ultrasound and studied by spectral analysis as well. Left lateral decubitus scanning aids in the detection of lesions at the origins of these vessels and also allows examination of renal parenchyma (7). Renal arteries are more difficult to image than the celiac and superior mesenteric vessels, especially in obese patients and in the presence of extensive intestinal gas. However, Norris successfully scanned both renal arteries in 113 of 120 patients and found ultrasound 97% specific for lesions greater than 60% stenotic by angiography (8).

Upper Extremity

Because the arteries and veins of the upper extremity are superficial, they are ideal for B-mode imaging (9). The subclavian artery can be successfully evaluated when the presence of an aneurysm is suspected (Fig. 2). This is usually related to thoracic outlet narrowing and may have been suspected based on the presence of a bruit or because of distal embolization. It is also possible to evaluate extra anatomic bypass grafts in this area, including axillofemoral grafts and carotid to subclavian reconstructions (10) (Fig. 3). It is not difficult to scan along the entire brachial artery, and this is useful in evaluating thrombosis or false aneurysm following transbrachial arterial catheterization or other trauma.

Hemodialysis arteriovenous fistulae can be evaluated periodically and it is possible to define hemodynamic incongruities along the shunt before they cause occlusion (11). Both the native arm veins and arteries can be imaged in addition to the

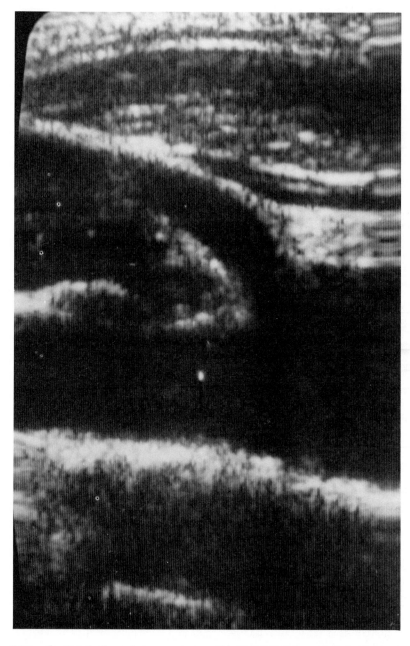

Figure 2   Subclavian artery aneurysm with laminated thrombus lining the aneurysm.

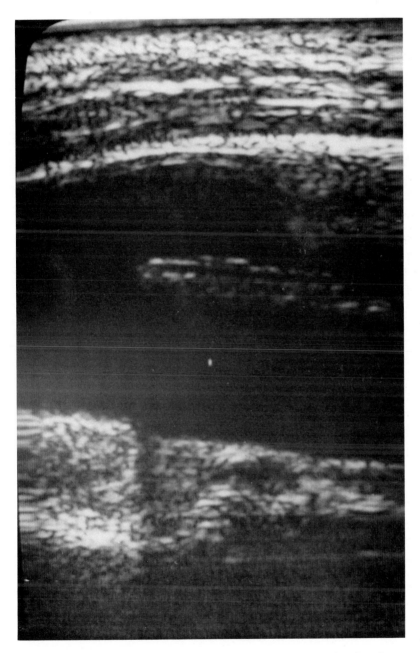

Figure 3 Scan of carotid artery to subclavian artery bypass showing the anastomosis of the PTFE graft to the common carotid artery.

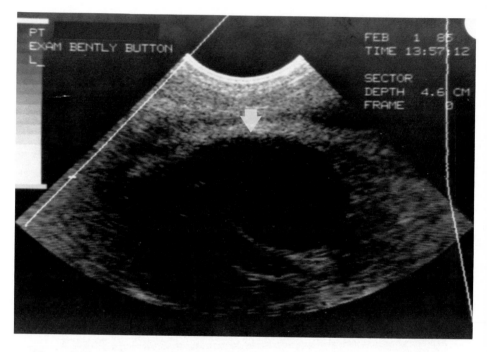

Figure 4 Scan of an angio-access prosthesis with an anastomotic pseudoaneurysm (arrow).

actual prosthetic A-V shunt (Fig. 4). The ultrasound can also provide preoperative imaging of the arterial anatomy before hemodialysis access surgery. Congenital arteriovenous malformations may be scanned to define their limits. The B-mode scan can delineate aneurysms and occlusions of the ulnar and radial arteries and even their continuation distal to the wrist.

Lower Extremity

Arterial and venous real-time B-mode scanning of the lower extremities has multiple practical applications. Some studies show B-mode scanning to correlate well with standard angiography in the evaluation of iliac and common femoral occlusive disease, providing accurate stenosis location and residual lumen size (12). It is also possible to trace the entire length of bypass grafts originating in the femoral area and evaluate their distal and proximal anastomoses. It is particularly practical to image "in situ"-type saphenous vein reconstructions because the grafts are in the subcutaneous position.

Evaluation of the popliteal space by ultrasound has been a part of clinical practice for over 10 years and remains an excellent screening test for popliteal aneurysms

(13,14). Although the ultrasound has been used with success to diagnose most periarterial masses in the popliteal space, including Baker's cysts (15), popliteal entrapment, adventitial arterial cysts, and aneurysms, CT scanning has become very helpful in confusing cases.

Complications and abnormalities following arterial bypass grafting are often amenable to B-mode investigation (16,17). Perigraft serum collections can usually be differentiated from anastomotic aneurysms. False aneurysms at prosthetic suture lines are usually well defined by B-mode (Fig. 5). The ultrasound is accurate in detecting perigraft fluid collections that are virtually never apparent on arteriography. Fluid collection is often useful evidence when evaluating a graft suspected of being infected.

The lower extremity venous system also lends itself to direct imaging. Vein patency, the presence of intravenous thrombus, and even the competence of vein valves have been demonstrated by venous scanning (Fig. 6) (18). These exciting applications will, with experience, become useful clinical parameters and may provide sufficient information to direct operative intervention.

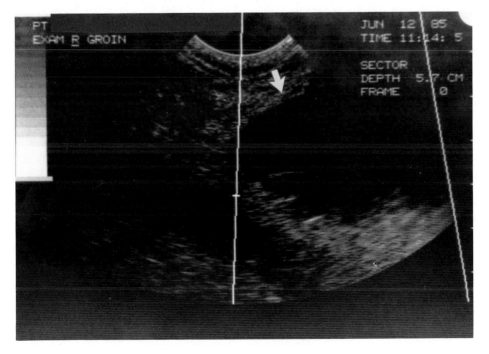

Figure 5   Longitudinal scan of a traumatic femoral artery false aneurysm (arrow).

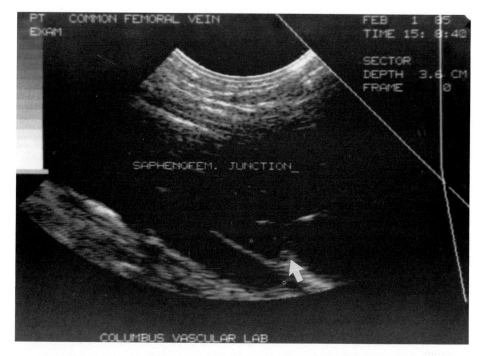

Figure 6 Longitudinal scan of the saphenofemoral junction illustrating a competent valve in the saphenous vein (arrow).

COMPUTERIZED TOMOGRAPHY

Computerized tomography (CT) has now taken a central role in vascular imaging by virtue of its unique cross-sectional display and unparalleled contrast resolution. Recent advances in spatial resolution and scan time allow near anatomic depiction of the vessel wall and surrounding structures. Current scanners operating at scan times of 2 sec produce minimal artifact due to bowel gas or metal clips. CT has been found to be an extremely useful adjunct to arteriography in a wide variety of vascular disease processes. In certain instances, it has been found that CT effectively replaces arteriography by providing superior definition of anatomic details or sufficient information to direct operative intervention.

Indications

Indications for CT may be appropriately divided into studies performed in the preoperative period and those related to postoperative problems and/or complications. In the preoperative period, CT is useful for the routine workup of all types of aneurysms, including atherosclerotic and mycotic (19-21). CT provides clear anatomic

definition of the aorta in patients with acute abdominal pain and question of aortic
aneurysm. It is likewise valuable in patients having known aneurysms with a change
in clinical status suggesting expansion, leakage, or rupture (22). Other indications
include complex atherosclerotic occlusive disease with distal embolization, trauma
with suspected rupture, and aortic dissection (23,24).

Postoperatively, CT has been found to be most useful in patients with complications of previously placed arterial grafts and those patients who have clinically
apparent simple graft occlusion. CT is probably not indicated unless repeated graft
occlusions mandate a search for alternate sources of that occlusion, e.g., emboli.
CT has proven effective in the detection of aortoiliac graft infection where the extent of the infection in the perigraft region is usually easily seen (25). Aortoenteric
fistula, previously an extremely difficult diagnosis to make on imaging, can now
be reliably detected using CT (26,27). Anastomotic pseudoaneurysm formation,
which may or may not be associated with infection, is usually easily seen as well.

Methods

In the vast majority of patients, high-quality CT of the vascular system demands
scanners capable of fast (less than 5 sec) scan time with variable slice thickness or
collimation. In most cases, intravenous contrast material is administered to opacify
patent vascular lumens and to provide distinction from surrounding intraluminal
thrombus, to identify vascular occlusion, and to aid in identification of branch
vessel origins. Differentiation of vessels from surrounding inflammation or hemorrhage can also be made. Although contrast administration is strongly recommended,
CT should not be withheld in patients with documented contrast allergy or renal
failure, since extremely useful information is still provided.

There are numerous methods of intravenous contrast administration. While
slow drip infusion or a single 50-ml bolus of contrast at the beginning of the examination may provide adequate CT scans for certain purposes, this is *not* satisfactory for adequate visualization of arterial structures. Dynamic scanning using
repeated boluses of contrast material may be used, however, it is cumbersome.
A technique we have found useful involves the injection of a bolus of 50 ml of
60% contrast material followed by pressurized infusion of 300 ml of 30% contrast material. The resulting scans give good arterial opacification throughout
the length of the study, which usually involves 20-25 slices.

Oral contrast is also administered in most elective cases to differentiate bowel
loops from fluid collections and hematomas. Administration of 30 oz of a dilute
barium suspension 1 hr prior to the study is followed by 15 oz of suspension 15
min prior to the study. This provides sufficient contrast in the small intestine and
stomach so that bowel can be easily differentiated from arterial structures.

Slice collimation (thickness) should be 10 mm, with slice spacing between 10
and 20 mm, depending on the clinical situation. In a routine search for abdominal
aortic aneurysm, slice spacing of between 15 and 20 mm is satisfactory. When finer

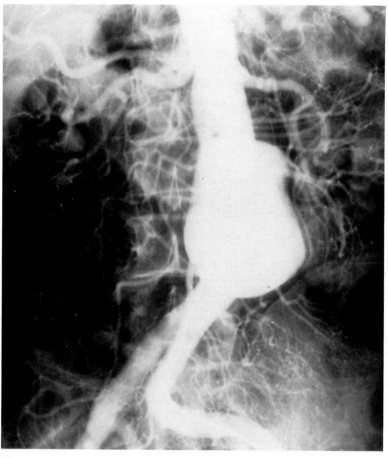

(a)

Figure 7 Typical appearance of abdominal aortic aneurysm. Angiogram (a) demonstrates large infrarenal saccular aneurysm. CT (b) demonstrates aneurysm containing opacified lumen (*) and surrounding low-density mural thrombus (arrows). The identification of thrombus allows more accurate sizing of the aneurysm.

anatomic detail is necessary, however, 5-mm collimation with overlapping slice spacing is indicated. It is thus very important to maintain careful control over the performance of the examination to insure adequate coverage of an area of abnormality.

Other techniques that may be used selectively include injection of sinus tracts or fistulae in search of graft infection, or aspiration of fluid or the perigraft space

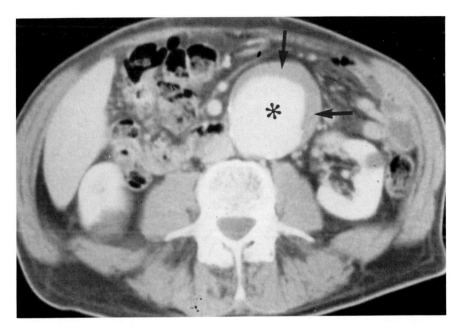

(b)

under CT guidance to determine the character or presence of fluid and obtain material for culture or chemical analysis (28).

Preoperative Evaluation

A therosclerotic aneurysms are ideally screened with CT. CT not only determines aortic aneurysm size more accurately than angiography because it demonstrates mural thrombus, but also determines renal artery involvement and iliac artery involvement with equal efficacy. In the rare situation in which CT is equivocal for involvement of the renal or the iliac arteries, arteriography may be added. Experience at Northwestern University, supported by reports from other institutions, documents that operative repair of the majority of abdominal aortic aneurysms can be adequately planned with computerized tomography as the only preoperative diagnostic method (29).

The CT appearance of aneurysms is characteristic (Fig. 7). A low-density mural thrombus with a calcified arterial wall is easily identified surrounding the enhanced lumen. The lumen itself may be somewhat eccentrically located. Although the renal arteries may not be seen in each instance, their level is well identified by visualization of the larger renal veins. Identification of the precise status of the suprarenal aorta in patients with a known or suspected thoracoabdominal aneurysm is easily

provided by CT. Rarely, in infrarenal aneurysms, tortuosity and kinking may mis-
leadingly suggest renal artery involvement. In such cases, arteriography is indicated.
While similar situations may arise with questionable common iliac arterial involvement, this is easily dealt with at operation.

CT is particularly well suited to the popliteal segment where atherosclerotic
aneurysms may present with thrombosis and distal occlusion. In these situations,
arteriography may reveal only femoropopliteal occlusion, while CT can easily provide identification of the presence, diameter, and longitudinal extent of the aneurysms. Since popliteal aneurysms are frequently bilateral, diagnosis of unsuspected aneurysms (30,31) (Fig. 8) on the contralateral side may also be made.
Other less common aneurysms, previously difficult to diagnose, are also amenable
to CT screening. These include visceral, internal iliac, and even coronary artery aneurysms.

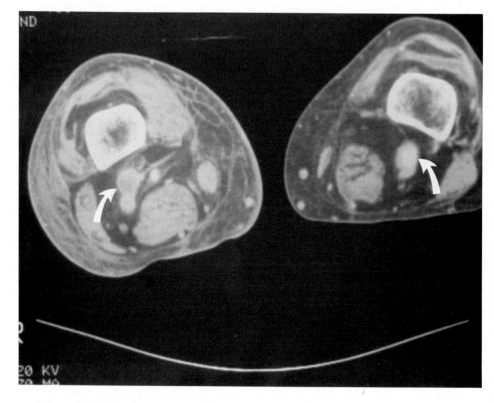

Figure 8 Popliteal aneurysm. Bilateral popliteal artery aneurysms (curved arrows).
The right-sided aneurysm is thrombosed.

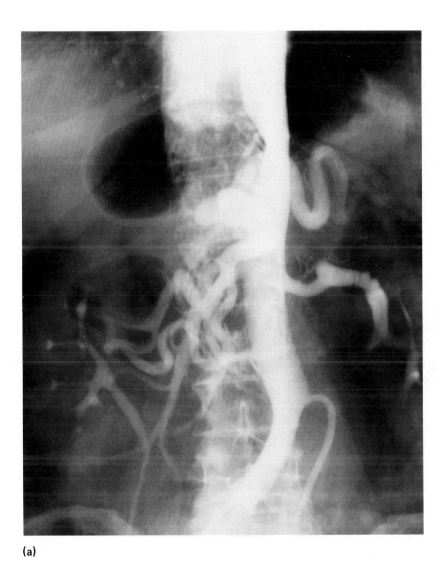

(a)

Figure 9 Aortic dissection. Chronic distal abdominal aortic dissection. Aortography (a) demonstrates compressed true lumen with visceral branches arising from it. CT (b) demonstrates compressed true lumen (*) filling the superior mesenteric artery (curved arrow). Larger false lumen (straight arrow) also contains some thrombus.

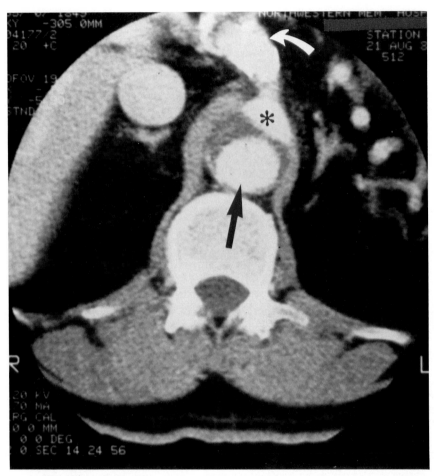

(b) *(Figure 9, continued)*

In patients in whom the presence of complications of abdominal aortic aneurysm is uncertain, CT should be obtained immediately for diagnosis. CT is clearly the ideal method for detection of contained rupture or retroperitoneal leakage. Characteristic aortic wall disruption or periaortic hematoma are diagnostic, whereas periaortic haziness is suggestive of aneurysm leakage. Inflammatory aneurysms can, in addition, be diagnosed on CT due to the increased aortic wall thickness, periaortic inflammation, and the adherence of the overlying duodenum to the aneurysm.

Occasionally, thoracic aortic dissections with extension to the abdomen may present with abdominal symptoms. CT is again an ideal method to detect the presence of dissection and the degree of extension (32) (Fig. 9). Renal involvement or

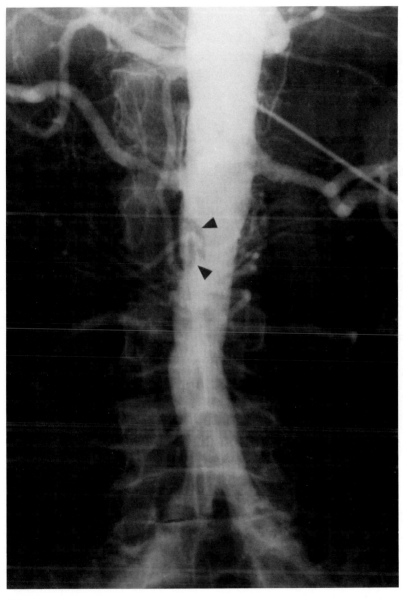

(a)

Figure 10 Aortic atherosclerosis. Translumbar aortogram (a) shows bulky infra-renal atherosclerosis (arrowheads). CT (b) shows slightly more extensive plaque disease but did not significantly change diagnostic considerations or potential therapy.

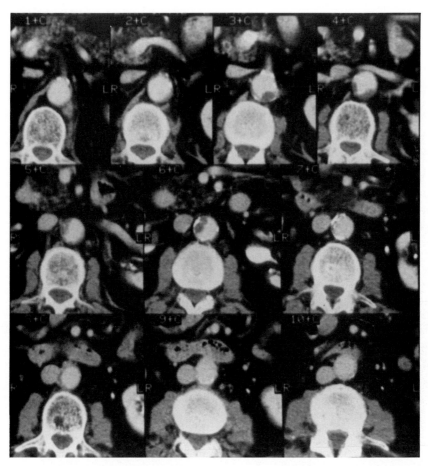

(b) *(Figure 10, continued)*

occlusion and, occasionally, celiac or superior mesenteric artery involvement may be shown.

CT evaluation of routine atherosclerotic disease has not been particularly help-ful in our experience, with aortoiliofemoral arteriography remaining the diagnostic tool of choice. While angiography identifies luminal caliber and irregularity more accurately than CT, mural thrombus, atherosclerotic plaque thickness, and intra-luminal projection are better demonstrated by CT (Fig. 10).

Limitations of CT in the evaluation of arterial occlusive disease include the tendency to underestimate luminal size due to calcification, as well as inaccurate assessment of vessels that are tortuous or nonperpendicular to the section plane.

Postoperative Evaluation

CT has proven extremely valuable in the evaluation of postoperative graft complications. Grafting procedures of the aortoiliac segment are usually of great reliability and are relatively complication free. Complications that may develop, however, include graft infection and/or subsequent graft-enteric fistula and graft thrombosis. CT offers significant help in the postoperative period in these complex situations (33-38).

The normal appearance of aortic grafts is fairly characteristic. An end-to-side proximal aortic anastomosis appears as a diseased calcified aorta seen posteriorly to a contrast-enhancing tubular graft, which may have slightly opaque walls. More distally, the iliac limbs appear anterior to their respective native arteries. The patent grafts enhance well with contrast material. End-to-end proximal anastomoses may be seen as a continuation of the native aorta in which the contrast in the graft may be seen arising in front of the obliquely divided native vessel. Aortic aneurysm repair gives a very characteristic appearance consisting of a calcified peripheral wall with low-density thrombus surrounding a contrast-enhancing, higher-density graft. In the initial postsurgical period, air or fluid is usually seen in or around the graft. Differentiation of simple hematoma from infection is usually based on clinical

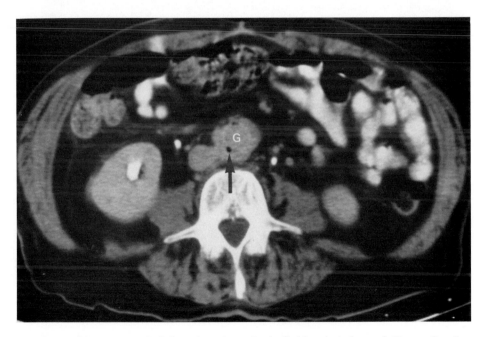

Figure 11 Aortic graft (G) with periprosthetic fluid and air (arrow) diagnostic of graft infection.

grounds in the immediate postoperative period, with persistence of air beyond 6 weeks consistent with infection (38) (Fig. 11).

Previously, identification of graft infection was based almost entirely on clinical grounds and/or suggestive angiographic signs. CT currently possesses great sensitivity for detection of aortic or infrainguinal graft infections, demonstrating perigraft fluid, thickening, or air associated with graft occlusion and sometimes with anastomotic aneurysm (Fig. 12). Draining sinuses can also be seen on CT, with extension of the tract to the graft demonstrated by injection of dilute contrast material into the sinus.

CT is particularly valuable for detection of complications at the proximal aortic anastomotic site, including pseudoaneurysms and graft-enteric fistulae. CT can easily differentiate between anastomotic aneurysm and simple prominence of the

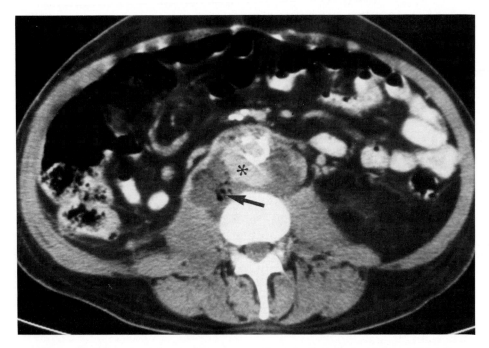

Figure 12 Mycotic abdominal aneurysm. Chronically infected infrarenal aortic aneurysm with contained rupture. Note calcified native aorta with opacified blood (*) within contained rupture. Extensive low-density clot with gas (arrow) surrounds the aorta, as well.

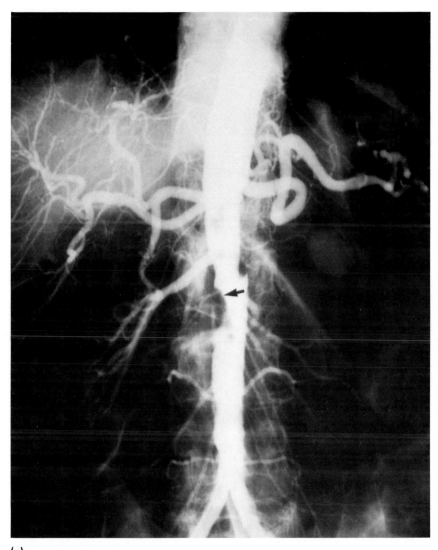

(a)

Figure 13 Aortic thrombus. Aortogram (a) shows occlusion of the left renal artery and fairly bulky intraluminal thrombus (arrow). CT (b) nicely demonstrates low-density thrombus (*), as well as infarcted left kidney (K). CT demonstrated the abnomality equally as well as angiography and added significant information about the status of the left kidney.

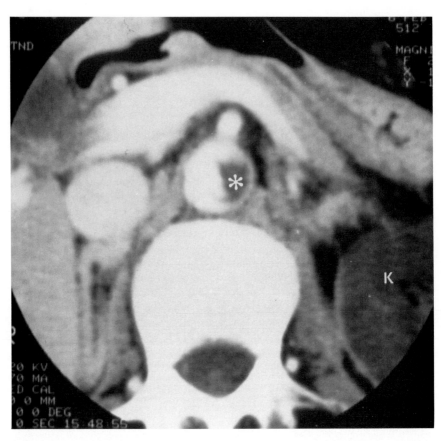

(b) (*Figure 13, continued*)

anastomotic site, both intraabdominally and peripherally, by demonstrating the native artery, graft, and contained thrombus (Figs. 13, 14).

CT has been found to be superior to other modalities in the detection of abdominal abscesses and retroperitoneal fluid collections associated with aortic operative procedures (39). Postoperative urinary leakage due to ureteral injury, other abdominal infectious processes, or abscess not related to the aortic graft, as well as hematomas, are adequately evaluated by CT (40). In addition to identification of the relationship of fluid collections to the aortic graft, percutaneous catheter drainage can often be appropriately guided.

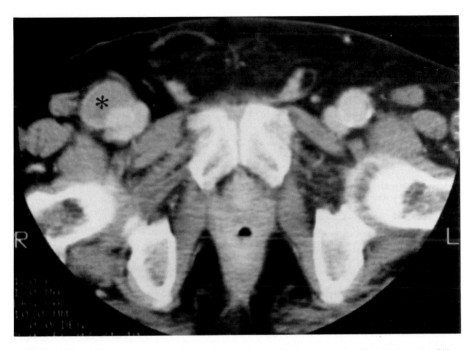

Figure 14 CT demonstrating large femoral pseudoaneurysm in the right groin (*).

REFERENCES

1. Goldberg BB, Ostrum BJ, Ishand HJ: Ultrasonic aortography. J Am Med Assoc 198:353, 1966.
2. Gooding GAW: B-mode imaging of the aorta and the iliac and femoral vessels. In Zwiebel WJ (ed): Introduction to Vascular Ultrasonography, Grune and Stratton, New York, 1982.
3. Leopold GR, Goldberger LE, Bernstein EF: Ultrasonic detection and evaluation of abdominal aortic aneurysms. Surgery 72:939, 1972.
4. Winsberg F, Cole-Beuglet C, Mulder DS: Continuous ultrasound "B" scanning of abdominal aortic aneurysms. AJR 121:626, 1974.
5. Jager K, Bollinger A, Valli C, et al: Measurement of mesenteric blood flow by duplex-scanning. In Proc. of San Diego Symposium on Noninvasive Diagnostic Techniques in Vascular Disease, p. 60, February, 1985.
6. Nicholls SC, Kohler TL, Martin R, Strandness DE: Use of hemodynamic parameters in the diagnosis of mesenteric insufficiency. In Proc. of San Diego Symposium on Noninvasive Diagnostic Techniques in Vascular Disease, p. 59, February, 1985.

7. Norris CS, Pfeiffer JS, Rittgers SE, Barnes WB: Noninvasive evaluation of renal artery stenosis and renovascular resistance. J Vasc Surg 1:192, 1984.

8. Isikoff MB, Hill MC: Sonography of the renal arteries: Left lateral decubitus position. AJR 134:1177, 1980.

9. Payne K, Blackburn D, Peterson L, et al: B-mode imaging of the arteries of the hand and upper extremity. Bruit, in press.

10. Gooding GAW, Etteney DJ: Donography of axillofemoral and femorofemoral subcutaneous arterial bypass grafts. AJR 144:1005, 1985.

11. Scheible W, Skram C, Leopold GAW: High resolution real-time sonography of hemodialysis vascular access complications. AJR 134:1173, 1980.

12. Wetzner SM, Kiser LC, Bezreh JS: Duplex ultrasound imaging: vascular applications. Radiology 150:507, 1984.

13. Scott WW, Penelope PS, Sanders RC: B-scan ultrasound in the diagnosis of popliteal aneurysms. Surgery 81:436, 1977.

14. Collins GJ, Rich NM, Phillips J, et al: Ultrasound diagnosis of popliteal artery aneurysms. Am Surg 42:853, 1976.

15. McDonald DG, Leopold GR: Ultrasound B-scanning in the differentiation of Baker's cyst and thrmbophlebitis. Br J Rad 45:729, 1972.

16. Gooding GAW, Etteney DJ, Goldstone J: The aortofemoral graft: Detection and identification of healing complications by ultrasonography. Surgery 89:94, 1981.

17. Wolson AH, Kaupp HA, McDonald K: Ultrasound of arterial graft surgery complications. AJR 133:869, 1979.

18. Sandager G, Williams LR, McCarthy WJ, Flinn WR, Yao JST: Assessment of venous valve function by duplex scan. Bruit, in press.

19. Eriksson I, Hemmingsson A, Lindregn PG: Diagnosis of abdominal aortic aneurysms by aortography: cvmputer tomography and ultrasound. Acta Radiol Diag 21:209-214, 1980.

20. Larson EM, Albrechisson U, Christenson JT: Computed tomography versus aortography for preoperative evaluation of abdominal aortic aneurysm. Acta Radiol Diag 25:95-100, 1981.

21. Anderson PE, Lorentzen JE: Comparison of computed tomography andaortography in abdominal aortic aneurysms. J Computer Assisted Tomogr 7(4):670-673, 1983.

22. Rosen A, Korobkin M, Silverman, PM, Moore AV, Jr, Dunnick NR: CT diagnosis of ruptured abdominal aortic aneurysm. AJR 143:265-258, 1984.

23. Egan TJ, Neiman HK, Herman RJ, Malave SR, Sanders JH: Computed tomography in the diagnosis of aortic aneurysm dissection or traumatic injury. Radiology 136:141-146, 1980.

24. Heiberg E, Wolverson MK, Sundaram M, Shields JB: CT in aortic trauma. AJR 140:1119-1124, 1983.

25. Mark AS, McCarthy SM, Moss AA, Price D: Detection of abdominal aortic graft infection: Comparison of CT and in labeled white blood cell scans. AJR 144:315-318, 1985.

26. Mark AS, Moss AA, McCarthy S, McCowin M: CT of aortoenteric fistulas. Invest Radiol 20:272-275, 1985.

27. Kukora JS, Rushton FW, Cranston PE: New computed tomographic signs of aortoenteric fistula. Arch Surg 139:251-253, 1984.
28. Cunat JS, Haaga R, et al: Periaortic fluid aspiration for recognition of infected graft. AJR 139:251-253, 1982.
29. Williams LR, Flinn WR, McCarthy WJ, Bergan JJ, Yao JST: Use of computerized tomography in the management of complex aortic problems. J. Vasc Surg (in press).
30. Friesen G, Ivins JC, Janes JM: Popliteal aneurysms. Surgery 51:90, 1962.
31. Wychulis AR, Spittell JA, Jr, Wallace RB: Popliteal aneurysms. Surgery 68: 942, 1970.
32. Parienty RA, Couffinhal JC, Wellers M, Farge C, Pradel J, Dologa M: Computed tomography versus aortography in diagnosis of aortic dissection. Cardiovasc Intervent Radiol 5:285-291, 1982.
33. Davis JH: Complications of surgery of the abdominal aorta. Am J Surg 130: 523-527, 1975.
34. Vollmar JF, Heyden B: Experiences with reconstructive surgery of the aorto-iliac segment. In Bergan JJ, Yao JST (eds): Surgery of the Aorta and Its Body Branches, Grune & Stratton, New York, pp. 243-261, 1979.
35. Bunt TJ: Synthetic vascular graft infections. I. Graft infections. Surgery 93: 733-746, 1983.
37. Bunt TJ: Synthetic vascular graft infections. II. Graft-enteric erosions and graft-enteric fistulas. Surgery 94:1-9, 1983.
38. Mark A, Moss AA, Lusby R, Kaiser JA: CT evaluation of complications of abdominal aortic surgery. Radiology 145:409-414, 1982.
39. O'Hara PJ, Borkowski GP, Hertzer NR, O'Donovan PB, Brighan SL, Beven EG: Natural history of periprosthetic air on computerized axial tomographic examination of the abdomen following abdominal aortic aneurysm repair. J Vasc Surg 1:429-433, 1984.
40. Meuller PR, Simeone JF: Intra-abdominal abscesses: Diagnosis by sonography and computed tomography. Radiologic Clinics of North America 21(3):425, 1983.

10

Ancillary Techniques in Diagnostic Angiography

ROBERT L. VOGELZANG
Northwestern University Medical School
Chicago, Illinois

OPTIMIZING THE PERIPHERAL ARTERIOGRAPHIC EXAMINATION

The efficacy and durability of vascular bypass procedures in the lower extremities can be predictably related to the status of distal vascular runoff, particularly in regard to the patency of the pedal arches (1,2,3). Although the distal vessels may be assessed on an intraoperative arteriogram, accurate preoperative arteriography is essential to the ability to make sound clinical judgments, particularly with regard to a decision for standard femoral popliteal grafting or distal tibial bypass. Arteriography of the lower extremities, however, is often looked upon by radiologists and surgeons as a necessary but somewhat tedious and uninteresting part of the practice of vascular radiology. Nowhere is this lack of interest more obvious than in the failure of many vascular radiologists to obtain good visualization of all segments of the arterial tree that may contribute to vascular disease. This includes, during the lower extremity arteriographic examination, visualization of the entire abdominal aorta as well as the entire course of tibial vessels beyond the popliteal trifurcation. Demonstration of the pedal arches is also an ideal that should be strived for. In the examination of the upper extremity, complete visualization of the proximal vessels, i.e., subclavian and innominate arteries, including their origins, is of vital significance. Examination of both upper extremities is likewise important in most cases since processes producing ischemia may well be bilateral. Optimum arteriography of the hands also demands careful attention to detail (4).

157

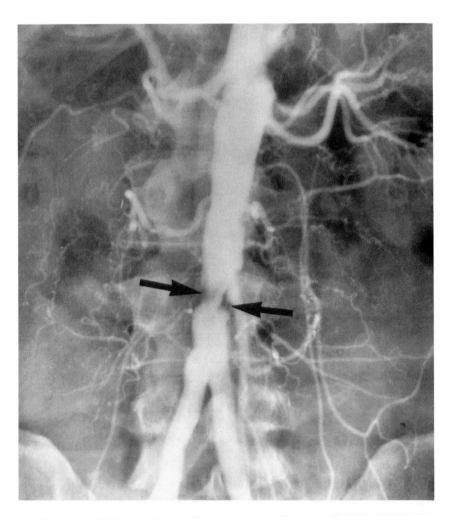

Figure 1 Isolated infrarenal aortic stenosis (arrows) was responsible for lower extremity claudication and impotence in this 56-year-old man. Lower extremity arteriography that had not included aortography missed this abnormality on a previously performed arteriogram.

Lower Extremity Arteriography

Aortography obviously should always be included as an integral part of the lower extremity examination, except when limited examinations such as postoperative evaluation for a graft are required or when contrast limitations intervene. Significant aortic atherosclerosis may be a cause of atheroembolization (5-9). Unsuspected abdominal aortic aneurysms may also be uncovered. Identification of these "silent" abnormalities will obviously influence clinical decision-making since an aortic aneurysm may mandate aortobifemoral grafting in a patient who could otherwise have transluminal angioplasty performed upon a single isolated iliac stenosis. An isolated aortic stenosis may cause extremity vascular symptoms as well (Fig. 1). Questionable areas of abnormality should be evaluated with oblique filming for which intraarterial digital recording of contrast material is ideal.

It is in visualization of the distal tibial and foot bessels that attention to detail plays a major role. Several methods exist to obtain accurate arteriographic recordings of the distal tibial and pedal vessels. These are outlined below.

High-Dose Examination Without the Use of Vasodilators

After performance of the aortogram, evaluation of the entire vascular supply to the lower extremities can be performed by "flooding" the extremities with approximately 100 cc of contrast delivered at a rate of 8-9 cc/sec. This prolonged injection of contrast essentially replaces the blood volume with contrast and yields good arteriographic contrast density throughout the vessels. Recording of the various limb segments can be done using a "long-leg" changer with a 6 ft (72 in.) tube-to-film distance. Three to four exposures are taken during injection and the results are usually quite good. Alternately, in most current all-purpose angiographic suites, a shifting-table method is used whereupon, after an appropriate delay of 3-4 sec, the various segments of the lower extremity are visualized by moving the patient beneath the stationary x-ray tube. By shifting the table four times, distal vessels can be visualized nicely in the majority of patients. In our hands this latter method is most commonly responsible for good visualization of the distal tibial and pedal vessels. The feet, however, are not necessarily optimally positioned since they are usually in an anteroposterior or slightly oblique lateral position. This may result in superimposition of vessels over bones and in the feet not allow complete visualization of the pedal arches and anastomoses. In those situations in which visualization of the distal vessels is not considered adequate, the examination is not complete without a separate injection for visualization of the feet. At this point, several methods can be used to augment distal vascular visualization since the small vessels of the feet can be resistant to contrast flow, which may be very slow through even normal-sized arteries. These are outlined below.

Intraarterial Vasodilators and Reactive Hyperemia

The most commonly used intraarterial vasodilators include papaverine, tolazoline, and nitraglycerin (10-13). Reactive hyperemia, which is obtained after the tourniquet occlusion of arterial flow for 5-10 min may also be used (14,15). We recently evaluated various methods of augmenting distal visualization of the feet at Northwestern University when we compared tolazoline at a dose of 50 mg injected at the aortic bifurcation with nitroglycerin (200 μg) and reactive hyperemia. We found that superior visualization was obtained with nitroglycerin. Reactive hyperemia

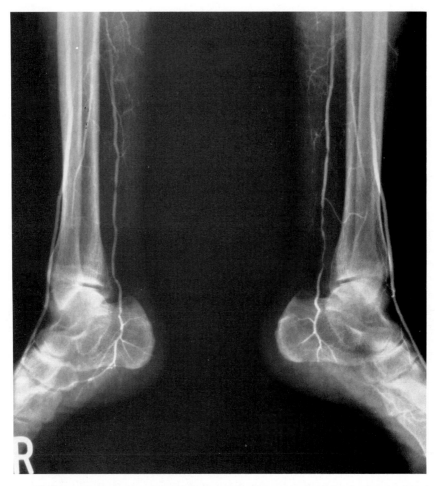

Figure 2   Bilateral visualization of distal tibial vessels routinely obtained with the use of intraarterial nitroglycerin.

was equal in many cases but nonresponders (10% in various reports) detracted from the utility of this technique (16). Tolazoline was clearly inferior to the other modalities. We currently are now routinely employing nitroglycerin in 200-μg doses for visualization of the lower extremities and this yields excellent results (Fig. 2).

Selective Femoral Popliteal Injection

In specific clinical situations such as trauma or preoperatively, particularly in plastic surgical procedures, the distal tibial vessels and feet must be examined in great detail

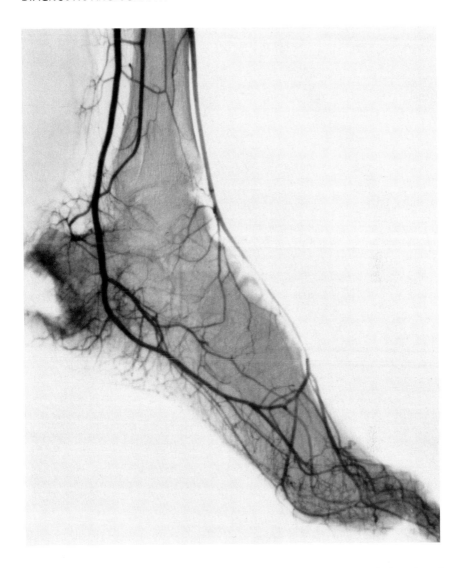

Figure 3 Selective distal popliteal artery injection with intraarterial nitroglycerin demonstrates excellent vascular anatomic detail in the foot.

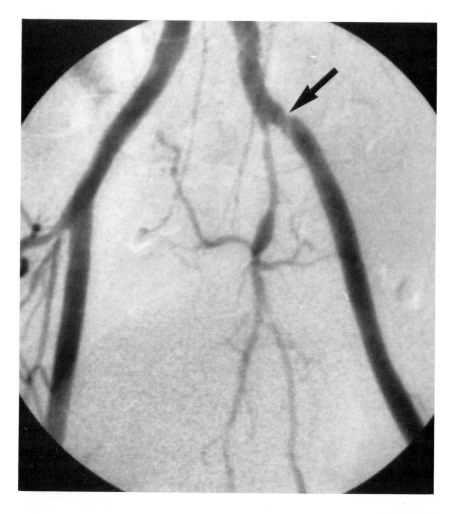

Figure 4   Oblique intraarterial digital subtraction examination of the iliac vessels reveals a band-like iliac stenosis (arrow). This lesion was not seen on conventional anterior posterior arteriogram.

and several projections. In these instances, selective catheterization of the distal superficial femoral artery or proximal popliteal vessel is required; upstream injections into the iliac system or even common femoral are not adequate. In the situation in which both feet must be examined, catheterization of both femoral arteries can be accomplished from a single puncture site. The contralateral side may be catheterized crossing the aortic bifurcation. The ipsilateral femoral artery is then selected by reversal of the catheter direction using a "loop" type catheter as described by Kadir et al. (17). Selective femoral catheter placement always gives excellent visualization of foot vessels (Fig. 3). Intraarterial nitroglycerin in a dose of 100 μg delivered immediately prior to injection is also required and is a routine part of our studies when distal femoral popliteal injection is made.

Digital Subtraction Techniques (DSA)

Digital recording of intraarterial contrast material is helpful, particularly in selective examination of the lower extremities (18-20) (Fig. 4). We have not, however, found it to be of significant aid when routine aortic bifurcation injections are used. Although the use of DSA may limit contrast dose somewhat, film arteriography with its larger field-of-view and better spatial resolution is the mainstay of diagnostic imaging. In addition, problems related to patient motion may degrade digital subtraction recording of intraarterial contrast material sufficiently to render that technique invalid. We personally have been somewhat frustrated with the ability of digital subtraction angiography to yield sufficiently detailed images, although it can certainly be helpful in certain circumstances.

Upper Extremity Arteriography

In most cases, examination of the upper extremity for ischemia demands a bilateral study when it is realized that ischemic symptoms in the hand may be related to atherosclerosis, collagen vascular disease, vibratory trauma, Raynaud's phenomenon, or Buerger's disease (4,21-24). These diseases may or may not be bilateral; the search for the etiology of upper extremity ischemia may be significantly aided when the process is noted to be unilateral or bilateral, the finding of ulilaterality or bilaterality further narrowing the differential diagnostic possibilities. The possibility of repetitive distal embolization should also be considered in any examination for upper extremity ischemia. For this reason, evaluation of the entire vascular supply is mandatory; thoracic aortography is routinely performed at the termination of the bilateral upper extremity study (Fig. 5).

Visualization of the hand is just as important. Nitroglycerin is the preferred vasodilating agent to maximize identification of all the vessels of the hand including digital arteries. Prolonged filming for 20 sec and placement of a selective catheter in the distal brachial artery to minimize contrast flow into muscular branches is also important (Fig. 6). The use of prostaglandin E_1 has also been advocated (25).

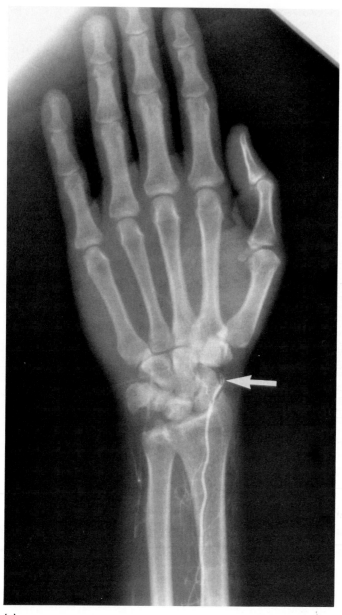

(a)

Figure 5 Proximal subclavian atherosclerosis with distal emboli. (a) Hand arteriography demonstrates radial and ulnar occlusion with small filling in the radial artery (arrow). (b) Thoracic aortography. Irregular plaque (arrow) in proximal left subclavian artery responsible for distal digital emboli.

164

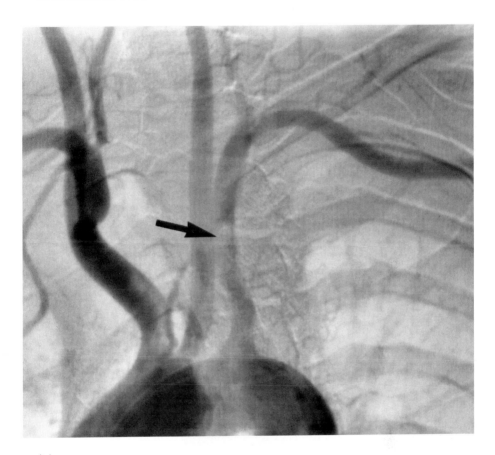

(b)

Upper Extremity Vascular Compression Syndromes and Their Angiographic Detection

Many neurovascular compression syndromes have been described, most of them involving the upper extremity at the thoracic outlet (25-30). Prior to surgical exploration for vascular compression, however, angiographic demonstration of the point of obstruction is vital. Several points must be considered prior to beginning arteriography. First, the demonstration of a vascular compression syndrome during blood flow testing or physical examination may be real but may to a large degree be dependent on normal anatomic (gravity dependent) position of the shoulder girdle muscles and thoracic outlet structures (31). A positive Adson's maneuver may be present on clinical examination but may be absent with a patient supine on the angiographic table, as we have encountered on several occasions. When it

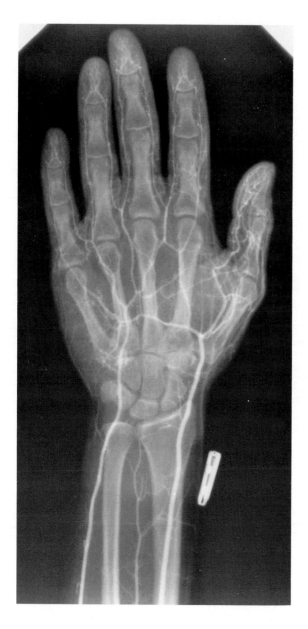

Figure 6 Normal hand arteriogram with complete visualization of all vascular anatomy including distal digital branches obtained with distal brachial artery injection and intraarterial nitroglycerin.

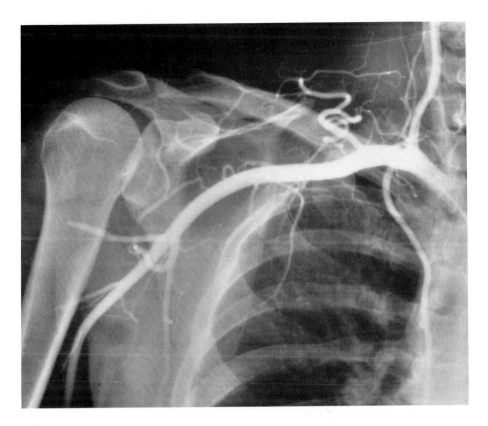

(a)

Figure 7   Right subclavian arteriogram in neutral position (a) is normal. Hyper-abducted position (b) reveals axillary occlusion (arrow) in the subcoracoid region secondary to pectoralis minor tendon compression.

does occur, examination of the distal pulse using Doppler instruments in the angiography suite is very helpful. The upper extremity is manipulated in the hyperabducted externally rotated position until the precise point of obliteration of the pulse is identified, whereupon arteriography is carried out (Figs. 7,8). The patient may also be asked to assume the position that he or she has felt to be the most symptomatic in the past; numbness or tingling of the hand is often reported by the patient in that position. Arteriography in the abducted and externally rotated position without attention to the character of the pulse or distal symptoms may result in a falsely negative examination.

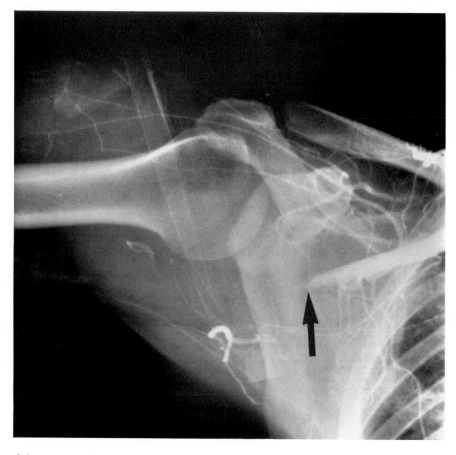

(b)

Newer Techniques in Digital Imaging

Digital subtraction arteriography was introduced with a great deal of enthusiasm for its future. Some believed that intravenously administered contrast with digitized recording of the arterial examination would virtually replace arteriography with the exception of specialized examinations or studies requiring subselective injections (32-34). A large amount of money was spent by radiologic manufacturers in bringing these products to the market place and within 1-2 years most radiology departments within the United States had some form of "digital." The volume of scientific publications on the subject increased dramatically and it appeared that, along with computed tomography and ultrasound, digital subtraction angiography

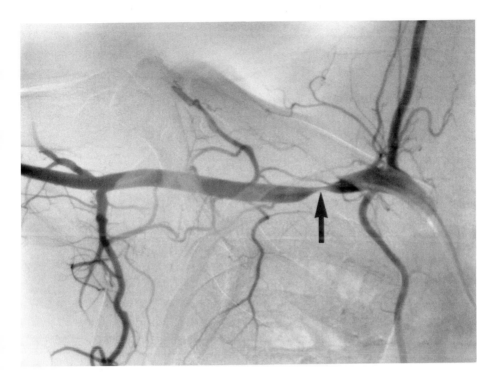

Figure 8 Typical proximal subclavian narrowing (arrow) secondary to a scalene anticus compression in a professional baseball pitcher.

was the "new kid on the block," with as much promise and expectation as any of the new modalities.

As practicing radiologists who did not have a vested interest in prompting or performing intravenous digital subtraction arteriography obtained the instrument the bubble burst. Many physicians, this one included, were frankly appalled at the image quality and lack of spatial resolution. Most importantly, patient motion artifact, such as swallowing artifact or inadvertent abdominal movements or peristalsis, could obliterate any chance at diagnostic images (Fig. 9). Although many high-quality images were produced, the uncertainty of the examination, particularly in regard to patients with poor cardiac output or those who could not cooperate, began to be an extraordinarily frustrating aspect of producing the examinations. Finally, the amount of contrast material administered during a routine examination often exceeded the amount given during standard arteriography by a factor of 2 or 3. The lack of adequate field size made it difficult to screen the lower extremities

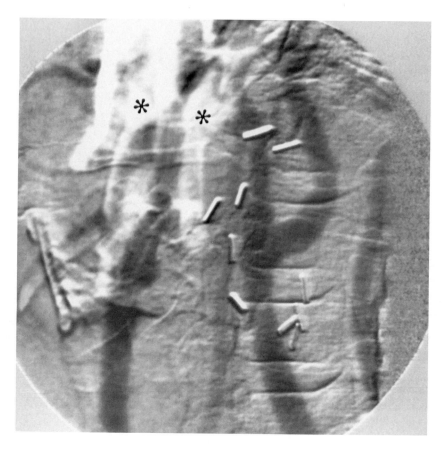

Figure 9   Intravenous digital subtraction examination of the carotid arteries. Complete obliteration of right carotid artery by swallowing artifact (∗).

and the abdomen adequately without a large number of injections. Digital imaging of intravenously administered contrast material rapidly became practically limited to carotid screening and evaluation of the renal arteries (32-36). One group of authors indicated that intravenous digital subtraction arteriography failed to detect multiple renal arteries in 17% of patients, further limiting its use (37). Peristaltic artifact often obscured the renal arteries, yielding significant numbers of false positives and negatives.

Reports in the vascular surgery literature have indicated the problems associated with intravenous digital subtraction arteriography of the carotid arteries (38,39) and these reports, as well as personal experience, have led many in vascular surgery to abandon the technique and return to clinical examination, duplex scanning of the carotids, and standard arteriography prior to surgery.

Coupled with the above-mentioned significant negatives of the technique was that early instruments lacked adequate spatial and/or contrast resolution. The images themselves were often grainy, fuzzy, and certainly not at all impressive when compared with film arteriography. Many of us within the field failed to understand the utility of intravenous digital subtraction arteriography in any capacity. The experience at our institution reflects the wider experience across the United States. At Northwestern University/Northwestern Memorial Hospital, where a large busy vascular surgery service exists, digital subtraction arteriography initially accounted for approximately 30-40 examinations per week. Over a 1-2-year period, we have seen that number of examinations decrease to less than eight per week on a regular basis. Our experience certainly is mirrored at other institutions.

It should be clear from the above brief history and opinions that intravenous digital subtraction arteriography is probably not a valid clinical tool for routine use. If available, the examination may provide information in selected cases, but in many of the instances arteriographers have virtually abandoned the technique and now recognize the true application of digital subtraction arteriography in the recording of intraarterial contrast material (18-20,39). In this setting, digital subtraction arteriography has substantial advantages and, when used in a judicious manner, can expedite examinations, reduce film costs and radiation exposure to the patient, as well as reduce contrast loads given to the patient during arteriography. The instrument is best utilized as a large electronic "box" of subtraction film yielding as it does rapid images and prompt patient throughput.

There are several areas in which the use of digital subtraction arteriography can augment and simplify the vascular radiologist's work. They are outlined below.

Augmentation of Arteriographic Examination
of the Extremities

As indicated previously, digital filming of the lower extremity vessels may aid in visualization of distal runoff (18). In addition, and just as importantly, digital filming may augment the conventional radiographic image when oblique views are required or an isolated abnormality requires reexamination. We routinely utilize the technique when oblique iliac arteriography is necessary to define stenoses more appropriately and when specific lesions such as popliteal aneurysms require a "second look" (Fig. 10). In cases of trauma, rapid screening of an extremity can be performed since the time required to expose and process films may be substantially reduced by the rapidity with which one receives images from the digital screen (40). Although some authors have advocated the use of digital recording of intraarterial contrast material as a substitute for the lower extremity examination, the majority of angiographic laboratories do not possess sufficiently large image intensifiers to visualize both lower extremities simultaneously as a standard 14-in. film can. As was previously mentioned, however, additional views may be quickly obtained using digital subtraction.

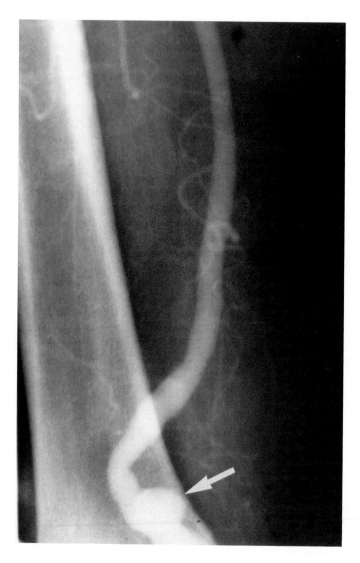

(a)

Figure 10 Conventional angiogram (a) demonstrates proximal portion of the popliteal aneurysm (arrow) whose distal portion was poorly demonstrated on films
over the knee. Intraarterial digital subtraction study (b) nicely demonstrates the
full extent of aneurysm.

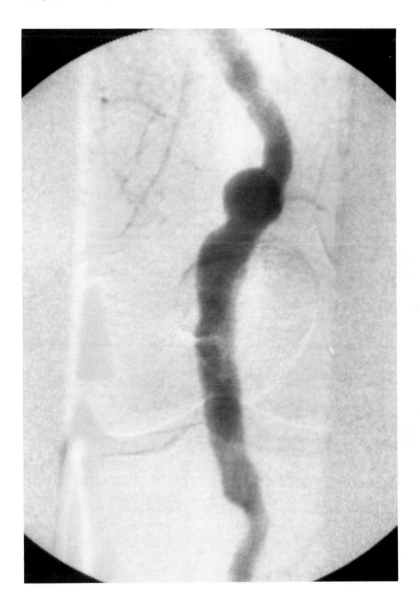

(b)

Use During Catheterization Procedures

Many digital units are equipped with a "road mapping" feature that permits super-imposition of an injected vessel upon a live fluoroscopic image. Catheter and guide-wire manipulation can then be made through tortuous vessels in "real-time," with appropriate manipulations being made to avoid stenoses. We have found this tech-nique to be particularly useful in angioplasty procedures where negotiation of high-

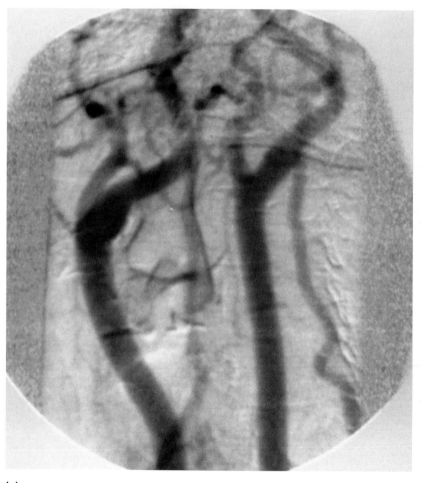

(a)

Figure 11 Examples of screening intraarterial examinations performed through a 4.0 French catheter in the aortic arch. Carotid views (a) and arch aortography (b) show good diagnostic quality.

grade irregular stenoses is of great importance in the safe performance of the technique (41).

Outpatient Arteriography

There has recently been a great deal of interest in screening carotid arteriography done via small 3.0 and 4.0 French catheters inserted via the right brachial approach. The technique has yielded good diagnostic quality examinations (Fig. 11) with very little risk to the patient. In brief, the technique involves catheterization of the right brachial artery at the antecubital fossa and manipulation of a thin guidewire up the

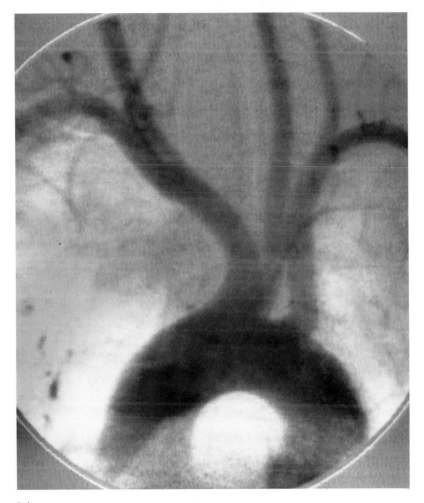

(b)

brachial artery followed by small (3.0 and 4.0 French) catheters capable of with-standing high flow rates (42). The technique appears to be safe with no significant brachial artery injuries, and the diagnostic quality of the examinations has been good. Other authors have reported similar results from the femoral or axillary routes (20). In all cases, accurate arteriographic screening for carotid artery disease is pos-sible, together with the economic savings realized by outpatient procedures. Small

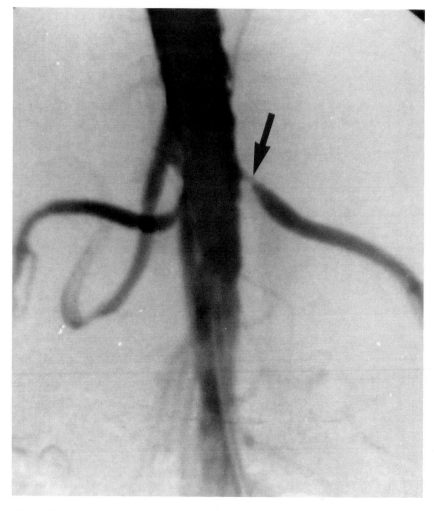

Figure 12 Intraarterial digital subtraction arteriography of the renal arteries shows good diagnostic quality and demonstrates a high-grade renal artery steno-sis (arrow).

catheters permit adequate hemostasis and a very low risk of postprocedural hematoma and/or vascular injury. We have experienced similar findings with screening for renovascular hypertension via the femoral approach in which 4.0 French catheters are inserted and the renal arteries are examined using digitally recorded contrast material (Fig. 12). Other applications certainly come to mind, but these two areas have been fairly fruitful and will probably continue to be widespread in their use as economic incentives continue to be brought to bear on diagnostic imaging.

Dose Limitation in Patients with Renal Failure

The use of intraarterial digital examination has resulted in significant contrast dose reduction in those patients who have preexisting renal failure and in the reduction of allergic potential in patients with allergy history. In renal failure an average screening intraarterial digital examination for renal artery stenosis will decrease the amount of contrast received to 25 ml or less. In allergic patients nonionic agents such as metrizamide, which have been shown to have little or no allergic tendency (43), can be used diluted to reduce the high cost of the agents.

Upper Extremity Venography

Upper extremity venography is usually recorded on film but routine evaluation of the subclavian and innominate veins, as well as superior vena cava, can be difficult since numerous flow defects and dilution of contrast material may limit its effectiveness. At Northwestern Memorial Hospital we now record virtually all upper extremity venograms on digital film, particularly the subclavian and innominate systems. The technique involves the use of distal arm injection of undiluted contrast material and filming during the subclavian and innominate phases of the study. The results have been excellent uniformly with clear identification of the innominate veins and demonstration of superior vena cava patency (Fig. 13). Clots can be distinguished as can chronic venous changes (Fig. 14). Most importantly, the use of digital examination can permit evaluation of an extremity in which only small butterfly needles can be inserted distally.

Digital Splenoportography

Conventional splenoportography was replaced in the late 1960s and early 1970s by arterial portography, a procedure that is certainly adequate for identifying the mesenteric venous anatomy. Splenoportography as practiced initially involved puncture of the spleen by a very large (18-gauge) sheathed needle with injection of contrast into the splenic pulp. The incidence of splenic hemorrhage and subsequent splenectomy was fairly high; some reduced the complication rate by plugging the tract with pledgets of surgical gelatin. Despite the theoretical and practical advantages of splenoportography the technique has failed to be widely applied since the

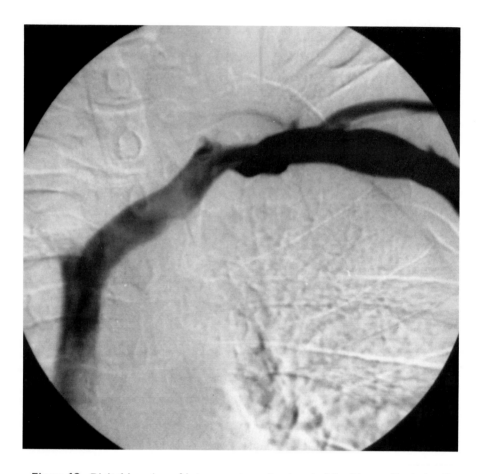

Figure 13 Digital imaging of intravenous contrast material with excellent visualization of the subclavian and innominate veins as well as the superior vena cava.

advent of arterial portography. Recently, however, we have explored the capabilities of the superior contrast resolution of DSA to perform digital splenoportography. In brief, the technique allows puncture of the spleen with a thin (21-gauge) needle, which is significantly less traumatic than the larger needle previously used. A smaller amount (15-20 ml) of contrast material is injected and the splenic and portal veins evaluated. In one case, the use of the technique identified portal thrombosis that was not well identified on arterial portography (Fig. 15). To date we have performed the procedure on 25 patients without complication. Another group reports similar findings (44).

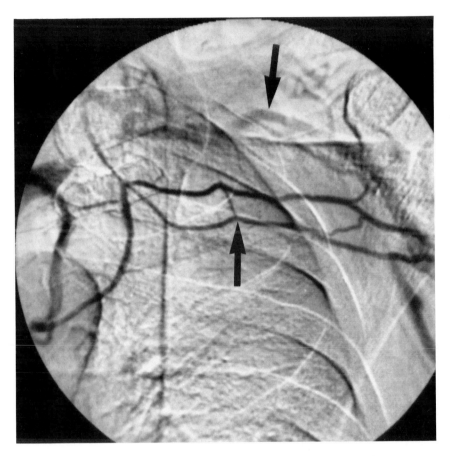

Figure 14 Chronic subclavian vein occlusion imaged with injection for 21-gauge needle in a small finger vein. There is subclavian vein occlusion. Chest wall collaterals (arrow) are identified.

Renal Venous Sampling in Hypertension

Although many patients have renal artery stenosis, not all of these will have renovascular hypertension (45). Renal venous sampling for determination of renin activity is the accepted standard for defining the functional significance of renal artery disease in hypertension. The test is widely used to predict the results obtained with angioplasty or surgery (46-49). When an abnormal ratio (1.5 or greater) of renin activity between the affected and normal kidney is seen and there is an anatomic abnormality, the diagnosis of renovascular hypertension is very strongly assured, particularly when there is evidence of suppressed renin secretion from the Many of the negative results are due to technical and/or laboratory failures; it is thus imperative that proper techniques for sampling be used to minimize the problems associated with the test.

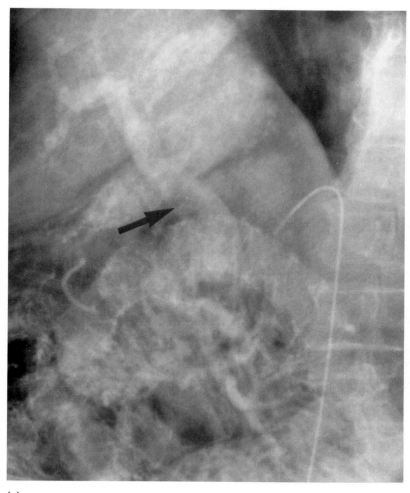

(a)

Figure 15 Splenic vein thrombosis with extension of thrombus into the portal vein. Venous phase of superior mesenteric arteriography (a) demonstrates the portal vein. A filling defect (arrow) was believed to represent flow artifact. The splenic vein was known to be occluded. Digital splenoportography (b, c) was then performed. Injection of contrast into the splenic pulp through a 21-gauge needle (b) demonstrates contrast within the splenic pulp (S) and splenic vein occlusion (arrow) with collaterals. Delayed filming over the portal vein (c) shows gastroepiploic collateral veins (arrow) and clot (white *) within the portal vein. The diagnosis was confirmed with computed tomography and substantiated at surgery.

normal kidney. Correction of the causative lesion can be expected to yield improvement or cure of hypertension in over 90% of patients. However, as many as 50% of patients will improve despite negative results if an antomic lesion is present (48).

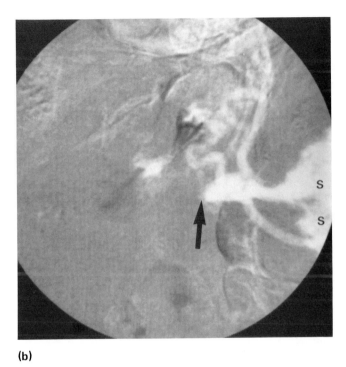

(b)

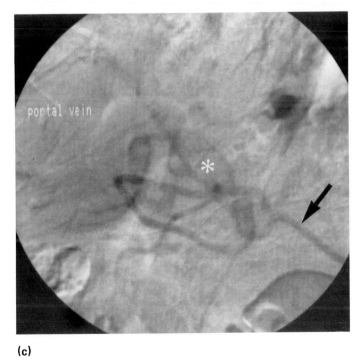

(c)

Technique

A rigid protocol should be used and stringent criteria applied to the performance of the test. Samples should be obtained only in hypertensive patients who have had an angiographically demonstrated renal artery stenosis or in those patients who had a previous attempt at correction of the lesion and require follow-up examination. Generally, a catheter with a shape appropriate for selective branch vessel catheterization should be used; of paramount importance is the ability to place the catheter tip deeply enough within the renal vein to withdraw samples undiluted by venous effluent from the cava or gonadal veins. There has been some controversy in the past over the timing of sampling in regard to angiography and whether simultaneous sampling of the veins is necessary. Harrington et al., however, documented convincingly that the accuracy of renin determination is not affected by arteriography immediately prior to the study or by the use of a single catheter to withdraw specimens sequentially as opposed to simultaneously (49).

Sampling is performed from both renal veins and the infrarenal inferior vena cava sequentially. Injection of small amounts of contrast to assure proper catheter placement should be done since contrast has not been shown to adversely affect the results of the study. The use of stimulation of renal vein renin production by exogenous means to increase the renal vein renin ratio is now also firmly accepted and, while numerous regimens have been proposed, including low sodium diet, postural techniques, and the use of drugs, clearly superior results have been demonstrated with the administration of captopril at 1 mg/kg dose levels. Sampling is performed 30-60 min following oral ingestion. The use of captopril is very effective and eliminates the need for withdrawal of antihypertensive medication prior to the study. Thibonnier et al. demonstrated an increase in sensitivity to 100% and an increase in the negative predictive value to 100% in a study involving 37 patients using captopril stimulation (50).

Sources of Sampling Error

Problems with catheter placement are probably the most common and most easily corrected errors associated with false-negative tests. Sampling error can be avoided by observing the following cautions: (a) The catheter must be within the renal vein and not in a lumbar vessel; contrast injection will reveal proper position. (b) Dilutional effects from nonrenal venous effluent can be avoided, particularly on the left, by placing the catheter tip deeply within the main renal vein beyond the point of entry of the gonadal vein. On the right the short renal vein may allow inferior vena cava dilution and deep placement is again necessary. There are many catheters designed that will allow this to be done, but the tip should be long enough to extend into the vein without excessive manipulation. (c) Multiple renal veins will be seen about 25% of the time on the right and 1-3% of the time on the left (46). We routinely probe the length of the vena cava paying particular attention to the right side for multiple veins that must be sampled. Circumaortic left renal vein can be a problem since the retroaortic vein can preferentially drain the lower pole (45). (d) Segmental renal disease as in intrarenal stenosis, juxtaglomerular tumor, infarction, hyperplasia, or hydronephrosis must be accurately assessed with the use of segmental venous sampling which will significantly increase the diagnostic accuracy in these patients (47,51,52). In such situations, specific catheters designed for segmental or subsegmental catheterization should be used. (e) Inappropriate specimen labeling, an obvious source of error, should be carefully avoided.

The key to accurate performance of renal vein renin sampling is in the avoidance of technical errors that cause problems related to dilution or nonsampling. These errors can be easily avoided and the accuracy of this valuable test increased.

REFERENCES

1. O'Mara CS, Flinn WR, Neiman HL, et al: Correlation of foot arterial anatomy with early tibial bypass patency. Surgery 89:743-752, 1981.
2. Nicholas GG, Latshaw RF: Femoropopliteal bypass grafting: Predictive value of preoperative angiography. Am J Surg 138:672-674, 1979.
3. McCurdy JR, Lain KC, Allgood RJ, et al: Angiographic determinants of femoropopliteal bypass graft patency: Ten year experience. Am J Surg 124: 789-793, 1972.
4. Yao JST, Neiman HL: Occlusive arterial disease below the inguinal ligament. In Neiman HL, Yao JST (eds): Angiography of Vascular Disease, Churchill Livingstone, New York, pp. 109-150, 1985.
5. Caravajal JA, Anderson RA, Weiss L, et al: Atheroembolism, an etiologic factor in renal insufficiency, gastrointestinal hemorrhages, and peripheral vascular diseases. Arch Intern Med 119:593-599, 1967.
6. Cranley JJ, Krause ES, Strasser ES, et al: Peripheral arterial embolism: Changing concepts. Surgery 55:57-72, 1964.
7. Kwaan JHM, Van der Molen R, Stemmer EA, Connoly JE; Peripheral embolism resulting from unsuspected atheromatous aortic plaques. Surgery 78:583-588, 1975.
8. Yao JST, Bergan JJ, Neiman HL: Arteriography for upper extremity and digital ischemia. In Neiman HL and Yao JST (eds): Angiography of Vascular Disease, Churchill Livingstone, New York, pp. 353-392, 1985.
9. Flinn WR, Harris JP, Rudo ND, et al. Atheroembolism as a cause of graft failure in femoral distal reconstruction. Surgery 90:698-706, 1981.
10. Jacobs JB, Hanafee W: The use of Priscoline in peripheral arteriography. Radiology 88:957-960, 1967.
11. Wilner HL, Kay R, Eisenbrey BA: Pharmacologic aids in angiography of the upper extremity. AJR 212:150-154, 1984.
12. Neubauer B: Intra-arterial tolazoline in angiography. Acta Radiol Diag 19: 793-798, 1978.
13. Carlson LA, Ericsson M, Erikson U: Prostaglandin E_1 (PGE_1) in peripheral arteriographies. Acta Radiol Diag 14:583-587, 1973.

14. Friedman H, Zeit RM, Cope C, Bernhard VM: Optimal use of tolazoline in arteriography. AJR 142:817-820, 1984.

15. Kahn PC, Boyer DN, Moran JM, Callow AD: Reactive hyperemia in lower extremity arteriography: An evaluation. Radiology 90:975-980, 1968.

16. Hishida Y: Peripheral arteriography using the reactive hyperemia. Japanese Circulation Journal 27:349-358, 1963.

17. Kadir S, Baassiri A, Barth KH: Technique for conversion of a retrograde into an antegrade femoral artery catheterization. AJR 136:430-431, 1981.

18. Kaufman SL, Chang R, Kadir S, Mitchell SE, White RI Jr: Intra-arterial digital subtraction angiography in diagnostic arteriography. Radiology 151:323-327, 1984.

19. Foley DW, Milde MW: Intra-arterial digital subtraction angiography. Radiologic Clinics of North America 23(2):293-319, 1985.

20. Bunker SR, Cutaia FI, Cable HF, Brown CW, Wolf EA, Jr, Ortega G, Blumoff, RL, Mozersky DJ: Femoral intra-arterial digital angiography: An outpatient procedure. AJR 141:593-596, 1983.

21. Bouhoutsos J, Morris T, Martin P: Unilateral Raynaud's phenomenon in the hand and its significance. Surgery 82:547, 1977.

22. Conn J, Bergan JJ, Bell JL: Hypothenar hammer syndrome: Posttraumatic digital ischemia. Surgery 68:1122, 1970.

23. Hirai M, Shionoya S: Arterial obstruction of the upper limb in Buerger's disease: Its incidence and primary lesion. Br J Surg 66:124, 1979.

24. Norton WL, Nardo JM: Vascular disease in progressive systemic sclerosis (scleroderma). Ann Intern Med 73:317, 1970.

25. Levy JM, Joseph RB, Bodell LS, Nykamp PW, Hessel SJ: Prostaglandin E_1 in hand angiography. AJR 141:1043-1046, 1983.

26. Kelly TR: Thoracic outlet syndrome: Current concepts of treatment. Ann Surg 190:657-661, 1979.

27. Dale WA, Lewis MR: Management of thoracic outlet syndrome. Ann Surg 181:575-585, 1975.

28. Fairbairn JF, Campbell JE, Payne WS: Neurovascular compression syndrome of the thoracic outlet. In Juergens, Spttel, and Fairbairn (eds): Peripheral Vascular Disease, W.B. Saunders, Philadelphia, p. 629, 1980.

29. Raff J: Surgery for cervical rib and scalenus anticus syndrome. J Am Med Assoc 157:219, 1955.

30. Lang E: Arteriographic diagnosis of thoracic outlet syndrome. Radiology 84:292, 1965.

31. Benzian SR, Mainzer R: Erect arteriography: Its uses in the thoracic outlet syndrome. Radiology 111:275-277, 1974.

32. Seeger JF, Carmody RF: Digital subtraction angiography of the arteries of the head and neck. Radiologic Clinics of North America 23(2):192-210, 1985.

33. Chilcote WA, Modic MT, Pavlicek WA, et al: Digital subtraction angiography of the carotid arteries: A comparative study in 100 patients. Radiology 139:287-295, 1981.

34. Christenson PC, Ovitt TW, Fisher HD III., et al: Intravenous angiography using digital video subtraction: Intravenous cervicocerebrovascular angiography. AJNR 1:379-386, 1980.
35. Strother CM, Sackett JF, Crummy AB, et al: Clinical application of computerized fluoroscopy: The extracranial carotid arteries. Radiology 136:781-783, 1980.
36. Hillman BJ, Ovitt TW, Nudelman S, et al: Digital video subtraction angiography of renal vascular abnormalities. Radiology 139:277-280, 1981.
37. Rabe FE, Smith EJ, Yune HY, et al: Limitations of digital subtraction angiography in evaluating potential renal doners. AJR 141:91-93, 1983.
38. Earnest F, Houser OW, Forbes GS, Kispert DB, Folger WN, Sundt TM: The accuracy and limitations of intravenous digital subtraction angiography in the evaluation of atherosclerotic cerebrovascular disease: Angiographic and surgical correlation. Mayo Clin Proc 58:735-746, 1983.
39. Summer DS, Porter DJ, Moore DJ, Winders RE: Digital subtraction angiography: Intravenous and intra-arterial techniques. J Vasc Surg 2(2):344-353, 1958.
40. Goodman PC, Jeffrey RB Jr., Brant-Zawadzki M: Digital subtraction angiography in extremity trauma. Radiology 153:61-64, 1984.
41. Katzen BT: Peripheral, abdominal, and interventional applications of DSA. Radiologic Clinics of North America 23(2):227-241, 1984.
42. Becker GJ, Hicks ME, Holden RW, Edwards MK, Jackson VP, Bendick PJ: Screening for occlusive vascular disease with intra-arterial DSA. Preliminary experience with a high flow 4-F catheter. Radiology 153:823, 1984.
43. Rapoport S, Bookstein JJ, Higgins CB, Carey PH, Sovak M, Lasser EC: Experience with metrizamide in patients with previous severe anaphylactoid reactions to ionic contrast agents. Radiology 143:321-325, 1982.
44. Braun SD, Newman GE, Dunnick NR: Digital splenoportography. AJR 144:1003-1004, 1985.
45. Abrams HL: Renal venography. In Abrams HL (ed): Abrams Angiography: Vascular and Interventional Radiology, Vol. II, Third ed., Little, Brown and Company, Boston, pp. 1327-1364, 1983.
46. Stanley JC, Gewertz BL, Fry WJ: Renal:systemic renin indices and renal vein renin ratios as prognostic indicators in remedial renovascular hypertension. J Surg Res 20:149-155, 1976.
47. Marks LS, Maxwell MH: Renal vein renin: Value and limitations in the prediction of operative results. Urologic Clinics of North America 2(2):311-325, 1975.
48. Bourgoignie J, Kurtz S, Catanzaro FJ, Serirat P, Perry HM: Renal venous renin in hypertension. Am J Med 48:332, 1970.
49. Harrington DP, Whelton PK, Mackenzie EJ, Russell RP, Kaufman SL, Barth, KH, White RI Jr., Walter WG: Renal venous renin sampling. Radiology 138:571-575, 1981.
50. Thinbonnier M, Joseph A, Sassano P, Guyenne TT, Carvol P, Raynaud A, Seurot M, Gaux JC: Improved diagnosis of unilateral renal artery lesions after captopril administration. J Am Med Assoc 251:56-60, 1984.

51. Lindstrom RR, Brosman SA, Paul JG, Bennett CM, Connor G, Barajas L: Segmental intrarenal catheterization in renin-mediated hypertension. J Urol 118: 10-12, 1977.
52. Korobkin M, Glickman MG, Schambelan M: Segmental renin vein sampling for renin. Radiology 118:307-313, 1976.

Part II
INTRAOPERATIVE METHODS

11

Pre-bypass Operative Arteriography

D. PRESTON FLANIGAN
University of Illinois College of Medicine at Chicago
Chicago, Illinois

Although infrainguinal bypass was once an infrequently performed procedure, today the procedure is commonly performed by nearly all surgeons treating lower extremity arterial occlusive disease. This increase in the application of the procedure has paralleled improved results as patient selection and operative techniques have been perfected. Currently, patency rates for tibial vessel bypasses are approaching those of aortofemoral bypass, suggesting that these distal procedures will be utilized even more so in the future (1). Because such excellent results can be achieved with distal bypass procedures, it seems clear that a substantial increase in limb salvage could be achieved in the dysvascular population if candidates for the procedure could be identified through visualization of the most distal lower extremity circulation. Traditionally, preoperative arteriography has been used to map arterial occlusive disease and provide the information necessary to help in the selection of the proper operative procedure. Visualization of the proximal lower extremity vascular system is usually not a problem using standard arteriographic techniques but good distal visualization can be a problem in cases of severe atherosclerosis. Patients requiring distal bypass usually have a greater degree of atherosclerotic occlusive disease than those requiring more proximal reconstructions, thus, the patients who require good distal arteriographic visualization are the ones in which it is most difficult to obtain.

To overcome this problem, many special arteriographic techniques have been developed. These techniques include delayed filming techniques, the use of epidural anesthesia, vasodilator injection, reactive hyperemia, and digital subtraction techniques (2-4). Yet, despite the use of these innovative procedures, many patients, who are subsequently shown to have patent distal vessels, do not have their lower leg and foot vasculature visualized preoperatively.

Inability to visualize a patent distal circulation in patients with critical ischemia can lead to unnecessary amputation. One method of avoiding this unfortunate
event is to explore the distal vessels in an attempt to find a suitable outflow bed.
This technique, although occasionally successful, is of limited use in that it only
defines local anatomy and does not provide the surgeon with prognostic information. Complete arteriographic visualization of the distal vasculature is necessary
for optimal results.

Several studies attest to the accuracy of completion operative arteriography
in the detection of technical errors made at operation (5-8). The technique is relatively safe and can be performed using portable equipment in any operating suite.
Only recently, however, has attention been directed toward the use of operative
arteriography prior to an anticipated bypass procedure to determine the feasibility
of bypass, provide prognostic information, and to help in the selection of the most
appropriate vessel for a distal graft anastomosis (9-12). We have optimistically
termed this procedure "pre-bypass operative arteriography" (10).

INDICATIONS

Initially, our indication for pre-bypass operative arteriography was failure to visualize a distal recipient vessel on preoperative arteriography in patients facing immediate major amputation. However, as the value of the technique and the excellent
visualization achievable with the technique became appreciated, the indications
were extended to any patient requiring distal bypass in whom the distal arteriographic visualization was not felt to be optimal. An additional indication for the
technique is in the patient who presents with an acutely occluded infrainguinal
bypass graft and critical ischemia. In these patients preoperative arteriography often fails to demonstrate the distal vasculature and can delay urgently needed revascularization. In such situations, immediate operation with graft thrombectomy
and subsequent operative arteriography through the graft will provide an excellent
delineation of the outflow bed.

One last situation in which we have employed the technique is in patients who
are undergoing proximal revascularization necessitating operative exposure of the
common femoral artery who have poor visualization of their distal vasculature on
preoperative arteriography and may need a subsequent outflow procedure. An arteriographic pre-bypass study of the infrainguinal vessels obtained at the time of
the inflow procedure will provide useful information should subsequent infrainguinal vascular reconstruction be required.

The number of patients requiring pre-bypass operative arteriography will vary
with the severity of disease seen in one's practice but also will depend upon the
quality of the preoperative arteriography available in one's institution.

TECHNIQUE

The excellent visualization seen with pre-bypass arteriography is a direct result of the technique employed. Although techniques vary, we believe that our excellent results are primarily the result of inflow occlusion and large volume contrast injection. Since operative arteriography usually does not provide the luxury of multiple timed exposures, the longer the vasculature is filled with contrast the more likely

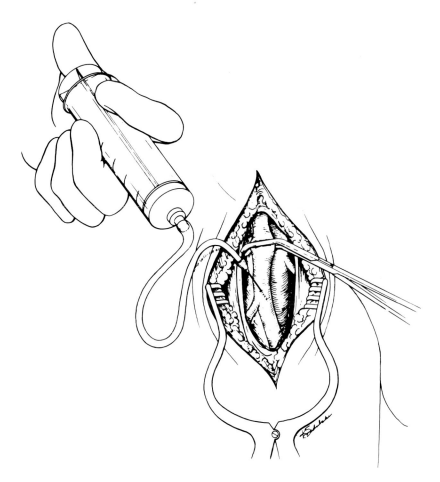

Figure 1 Technique of pre-bypass operative arteriography consisting of arterial dissection, inflow occlusion, arterial puncture, and hand injection. (From Flanigan DP, et al., Ref. 10, with permission.)

the single exposure necessitated by portable arteriography is to capture visualization of the distal circulation. Logically, one could expect operative techniques via the common femoral artery that do not employ inflow occlusion to be inferior to preoperative techniques since preoperative techniques have the advantage of multiple exposures.

Injections may be performed at any location, but they are most commonly performed at either the common femoral or popliteal levels. When a choice is available, the popliteal artery is preferred since good results are more often achievable at this level.

Regardless of the site of injection, the technique is similar except for timing, the size of the needle used, and the amount of contrast injected. Arterial dissection is performed at the preselected injection site and a proximal clamp is placed on the artery to occlude arterial inflow, as previously described by Fedde (13). A 19-gauge

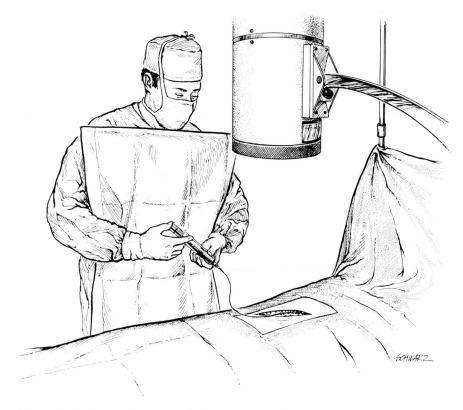

Figure 2   Radiation shield used during intraoperative arteriography. (From Sigel B, et al., Ref. 14, with permission.)

needle, attached to intravenous extension tubing and a hand-held syringe, is used to enter the common femoral or popliteal arteries (a 23-gauge needle is used for tibial artery injections) (Fig. 1). For femoral injections, 50-60-cc of undiluted Renografin 60 is injected rapidly and the film is exposed following a 7-sec delay. For popliteal (20-25 cc) and tibial (10-15 cc) injections, no delay is used. A 14 X 17-in. X-ray film is placed in a sterile clear plastic bag and placed immediately under the patient's leg. The film is usually turned diagonally to maximize the length of the extremity visualized by the roentgenogram. The surgeon stands behind a modified i.v. pole which is draped with a lead apron and covered with a sterile Mayo stand cover, as previously reported from our institution by Sigel et al., to minimize radiation exposure (Fig. 2) (14). The arteriogram is performed without heparinization and the proximal inflow-occluding clamp is released immediately after film exposure so as to minimize the time of exposure of the arterial intima to concentrated contrast material. The entire procedure consumes less than 10 min of operating room time exclusive of the time for arterial dissection.

UNIVERSITY OF ILLINOIS EXPERIENCE

Several hundred pre-bypass operative arteriograms have now been performed on our services at the University of Illinois and affiliated hospitals, but our techniques and results have not changed since our initial report in 1982 (10). During the initial study (August 1978 to July 1981), 31 patients evaluated for lower extremity arterial bypass had inadequate preoperative arteriographic studies despite the selected use of epidural anesthesia, delayed filming, vasodilator injection, selective arterial catheterization, and reactive hyperemia techniques. All patients were male with an average age of 62 years (range, 42-85 years). There was a 2.4:1 black-to-white racial ratio and 13 patients (42%) had diabetes mellitus. One patient underwent two bypass procedures. The indications for operation were claudication in four extremities (12%), severe rest pain in 14 extremities (44%), and gangrene in 14 extremities (44%). All patients with gangrene and one patient with rest pain were candidates for immediate major amputation should bypass not be possible. All but one patient underwent preoperative and postoperative segmental Doppler pressure measurements and waveform recordings.

Thirty-three pre-bypass operative arteriograms were performed prior to 32 operative procedures at the common femoral (n = 14), above-knee popliteal (n = 9), below-knee popliteal (n = 8), proximal posterior tibial (n = 1), and dorsalis pedis (n = 1) arteries. Injection sites were selected such that the incisions made for the performance of the arteriograms would also be appropriate sites for the performance of one of the anticipated bypass graft anastomoses. Eighteen contrast injections were performed in the vessel expected to be the site of the future proximal anastomosis whereas 15 injections were performed at the site of the anticipated distal anastomosis. Pre-bypass operative arteriograms were performed through the

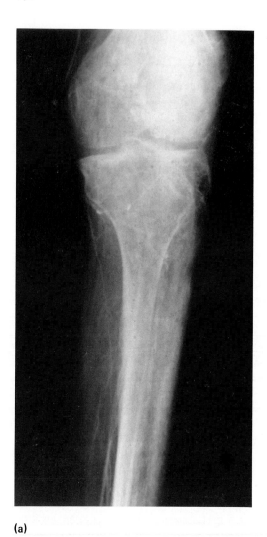

(a)

Figure 3 (a) Preoperative arteriogram demonstrating no filling of the popliteal or tibial vessels. (b) Pre-bypass operative arteriogram of the same extremity showing widely patent anterior tibial and peroneal arteries. (From Flanigan DP, et al., Ref. 10, with permission.)

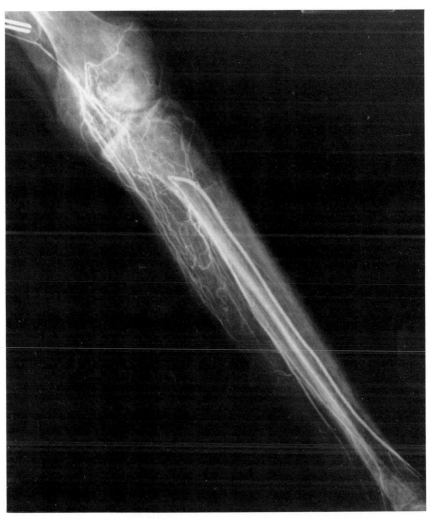

(b)

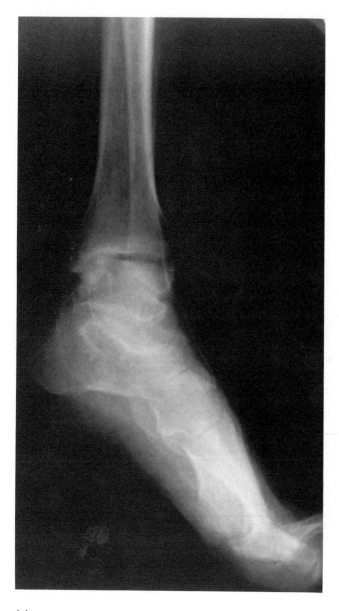

(a)

Figure 4 (a) Preoperative arteriogram showing only faint visualization of the dorsal pedal artery, posterior tibial artery and pedal arch. (b) Pre-bypass operative arteriogram of the same extremity showing patent anterior tibial, posterior tibial, and pedal arch vessels. (From Flanigan DP, et al., Ref. 10, with permission.)

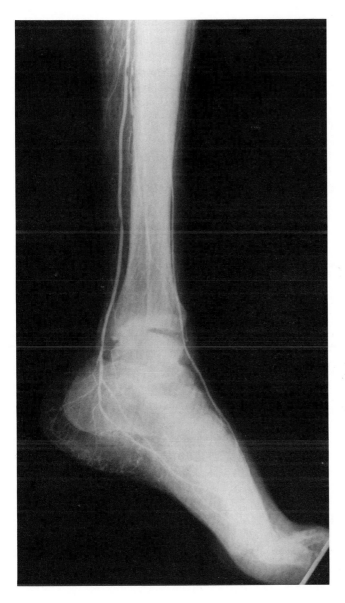

(b)

common femoral artery in the presence of a superficial femoral artery occlusion when the popliteal artery was not visualized preoperatively or the popliteal artery could be seen but delineation was poor. Popliteal injections were performed when the axial arteries were patent to the popliteal artery but popliteal runoff was inadequately visualized, or when the superficial femoral artery was occluded and the popliteal artery was visualized but felt to be a poor recipient vessel for a bypass and the popliteal runoff was poorly visualized. When the popliteal artery was well visualized preoperatively but the popliteal runoff was uncertain, injections were performed either at the common femoral or popliteal level depending upon the personal preference of the operating surgeon. The one instance of injection into the proximal posterior tibial artery was in a patient without visualization of the popliteal artery preoperatively (a pre-bypass operative femoral arteriogram was not attempted). The single dorsalis pedis pre-bypass operative arteriogram was performed to delineate better the pedal arch in a patient already having a popliteal pre-bypass operative arteriogram.

Pre-bypass operative arteriography was beneficial in 29 of the 32 extremities (91%). In 21 extremities (66%) bypasses were performed to vessels that were not visualized on preoperative arteriograms (Fig. 3). In eight extremities (25%) bypasses were performed to vessels that were visualized preoperatively but the pre-bypass intraoperative arteriogram showed better visualization of the vessels and the runoff, thus, allowing bypass to the best site on the optimal recipient artery (Fig. 4). In only three extremities (9%) was the intraoperative technique not beneficial as no additional arterial visualization was provided. Only one patient could not have a bypass because of nonvisualization of recipient vessels.

Distal anastomoses were performed to the popliteal (n = 16), anterior tibial (n = 4), posterior tibial (n = 7), peroneal (n = 2), and dorsalis pedis (n = 2) arteries. Mean ankle/brachial Doppler-derived pressure indices rose from 0.35 ± 0.25 preoperatively to 0.86 ± 0.26 postoperatively (n = 30). Overall, major amputation was avoided in 86% (24/28) of extremities suffering from rest pain or gangrene during the period of study. Ninety-three percent (14/15) of extremities otherwise facing immediate amputation were salvaged by employing the information provided by the pre-bypass operative arteriogram.

In only one patient did the arteriography necessitate an incision that was not necessary for the performance of a bypass. All injections were performed without complication and in no patient did the technique result in nonhealing of incisions at the injection sites or necessitate a more proximal amputation.

DISCUSSION

Dardik first emphasized the value of pre-bypass operative arteriography in 1975 (7). Other reports by Scarpato (9), Flanigan (10), Ricco (11), and King (12) followed in 1981, 1982, 1983, and 1984, respectively. The paucity of other reports probably only indicates the obvious value of the technique. Although the techniques have varied the results have been similar. In Scarpato's report only the popliteal artery was injected and inflow occlusion was not utilized. These authors found that when the procedure was applied routinely (including cases with "adequate" preoperative visualization) the operative study provided additional information most of the time. In 53% of limbs, better visualization was obtained and in 12% of patients the operative approach was altered.

The technique as reported by King employs inflow occlusion but calls for release of the clamp immediately following contrast injection. Both femoral and popliteal injections were employed, but the authors prefer the femoral route. King et al. were the first to point out the adjunctive value of pedal Doppler signals to find patent distal vessels, although the number of cases reported in which this was shown to be of benefit was small. Much like arterial exploration, the presence of a Doppler signal does not indicate the quality of the runoff bed. Likewise, inability to detect the signal could be secondary to technical problems and indicate the absence of a patent vessel when one is actually present. We have favored popliteal injection with inflow occlusion when possible and have not encountered false-negative arteriograms using this injection site but we recently have had false-negative studies when employing common femoral artery injection sites. The need for adjunctive Doppler studies in King's experience may be due to the preference for femoral injection sites.

The results of King's report is likewise encouraging. Of 26 preoperative arteriographic studies showing no distal visualization, 24 extremities underwent successful bypass and only two required amputation. Of 40 limbs having limited visualization of the distal vasculature on preoperative arteriograms, the site of the distal anastomosis was altered in eight. Interestingly, King et al. looked at comparative patency rates between bypasses performed with the benefit of pre-bypass operative arteriography and those with adequate preoperative studies and found no difference. This would seem to indicate that bypasses to arteries that are difficult to visualize do not result in inferior results.

Pre-bypass operative arteriography clearly provides information that often cannot be obtained from preoperative studies despite the use of special techniques. The technique is simple and almost uniformly provides excellent arteriograms, although, occasionally, alteration of exposure delay following injection is required when using the femoral approach.

Concern about contrast injury to the arterial intima leading to increased thrombosis has not been supported by a higher incidence of failure in the pre-bypass study group. Likewise, concerns about nonhealing incisions necessitated by the procedure have not been borne out. In our experience, only one patient had an unnecessary groin incision, which subsequently healed, and in King's report a similar experience with only two patients was encountered.

Radiation exposure should be of concern to the busy vascular surgeon, particularly if completion operative arteriography is also used. Scarpato has estimated an exposure of 0.1 rads/arteriogram and indicated that 75 studies could be done safely annually. The use of the sterile radiation shield as proposed by Sigel would seem advisable.

Some uncertainty exists regarding what consitutes an inadequate preoperative arteriogram. It is widely held that visualization of collateral vessels at a given level in the extremity, in the absence of visualized axial arteries at that level, indicates that the axial vessels are occluded. Although this is often true, we have seen many exceptions to this rule and would recommend that patients such as these not be subjected to amputation without an operative attempt at arteriographic visualization of the distal circulation.

REFERENCES

1. Taylor LM Jr, Phinney ES, Porter JM: Present status of reverse vein bypass for lower extremity revascularization. Presented to the 39th meeting of the Society for Vascular Surgery, Baltimore, Maryland, June 8, 1985.
2. Feins RH, Roedersheimer LR, Baumstark AE, et al: Predicted hyperemic angiography: A technique of distal arteriography in severely ischemic legs. Surgery 89:202, 1981.
3. Spigos DG, Akkaineni S, Tan W, et al: Epidural Anesthesia: An effective analgesia in aorto-ilio-femoral arteriography. Am J Radiology 134:335, 1980.
4. Crummy AB, Strother CM, Lieberman RP, et al: Digital video subtraction angiography for evaluation of peripheral vascular disease. Radiology 141:33, 1981.
5. Courbier R, Jausserman JM, Reggi M: Detecting complications of direct arterial surgery. Arch Surg 112:1115, 1977.
6. Dardik H, Ibrahim IM, Koslow A, et al: Evaluation of intraoperative arteriography as a routine for vascular reconstructions. Surg Gynecol Obstet 147: 853, 1978.
7. Dardik I, Ibrahim IM, Sprayregen S, et al: Routine intraoperative angiography. Arch Surg 110:184, 1975.
8. Pinkerton JA Jr: Operative arteriography: A new variation. Arch Surg 110: 841, 1975.
9. Scarpato R, Gembarowicz R, Farber S, et al: Intraoperative pre-reconstruction arteriography. Arch Surg. 116:1053, 1981.
10. Flanigan DP, Williams LR, Keifer T, et al: Prebypass Operative Arteriography. Surgery 92:627, 1982.
11. Ricco JB, Pearce WH, Yao JST, et al: The use of prebypass arteriography and Doppler ultrasound recordings to sort patients for extended femoral distal bypass. Ann Surg 198:78, 1983.
12. King TA, Yao JST, Flynn WR, et al: Extending operability by prebypass intraoperative arteriography. In Bergan JJ, Yao JST (eds): Evaluation and Treatment

of Upper and Lower Extremity Circulatory Disorders, Grune & Stratton, Orlando, Florida, pp. 61, 1984.
13. Fedde CW, James EC, Antico DA: Techniques for intraoperative arteriography
    after arterial reconstruction of the lower extremity. Surg Gynecol Obstet 145:
    427, 1977.
14. Sigel B, Tortoriello T, Jacovitch J, et al: Sterile, portable radiation shield for
    the operating room. Arch Surg 115:347, 1980.

12

Intraoperative Carotid Monitoring

JAMES J. SCHULER
University of Illinois
College of Medicine at Chicago
Chicago, Illinois

Prior to 1950 there existed a widely held clinical belief that the majority of cerebrovascular accidents were caused by hemorrhage from the middle cerebral artery or its branches. In 1951 Fisher and Adams (1) reported the results of the examination of the brains of 373 patients who had died shortly after sustaining a cerebrovascular accident and found hemorrhagic infarction in only 66 (18%). They concluded that the majority of cerebrovascular accidents were caused by emboli or occlusion and that many of the transient cerebral symptoms that frequently preceded the cerebrovascular accident were embolic in nature. Fisher and Adams further state that "no case of vascular disease of the brain is completely investigated if the carotid arteries have not been examined" (1). This report in conjunction with the ability to safely perform arterial anastomoses led to the operation of May 19, 1954, in which Eastcott resected the diseased proximal internal carotid artery of a 66-year-old woman who had been having transient ischemic attacks and restored arterial continuity with an end-to-end anastomosis of the distal internal carotid to the common carotid artery (2). Even though a previous carotid artery reconstruction for completed stroke had been performed by Carrea, Molins, and Murphy of Buenos Aires in 1951 and reported in 1955 (3), it was the widely publicized report of Eastcott, Pickering, and Rob (2), which appeared in *Lancet*, that gave the greatest impetus to and laid the foundation for all subsequent carotid surgery. At present it is estimated that approximately 50,000 carotid endarterectomies are performed annually in the United States alone (4) and that carotid endarterectomy is the second most common vascular surgical procedure performed, exceeded only by aortocoronary bypass.

The first true carotid endarterectomy performed by techniques remarkably similar to those still in use today was reported by Cooley et al. in 1956 (5). This operation was performed using both a carotid shunt and systemic hypothermia, both of which were considered to be essential to prevent cerebral ischemia during carotid clamping. It is likely that the emphasis placed upon the presumed need for some form of "cerebral protection" in their report tended to focus the attention of subsequent investigations on this aspect of carotid surgery and divert attention away from other equally and possibly more important factors such as proper patient selection, appropriate timing of surgery relative to resolved stroke, anesthetic technique, and technical perfection during the procedure.

In the ensuing 30 years since the report of Cooley et al. (5), surgeons who perform carotid endarterectomy have adopted one of three approaches to the use of a temporary indwelling shunt. There are those who always shunt, those who never shunt, and those who shunt selectively on the basis of some form of monitoring to assess cerebral perfusion. Those who shunt routinely are of the opinion that patients who will experience irreversible cerebral ischemia during carotid clamping and, therefore, require a shunt cannot be accurately selected by any of the current methods of carotid monitoring and, therefore, even though many patients may not require a shunt, all patients should be shunted. Those who never shunt feel that the number of patients who will experience irreversible cerebral ischemia during carotid clamping without a shunt in place is lower than the number of patients in whom a neurologic deficit will be caused by the routine insertion of a shunt because of the disadvantages inherent in the use of the shunt. Such disadvantages include embolization of air, atheromatous debris, or thrombus through the shunt; distal intimal injury or disruption, which later causes internal carotid occlusion or becomes a source of embolization; and difficulty in obtaining a technically perfect distal end point of the endarterectomy while the shunt is in place. Those who shunt selectively believe that the majority of patients do not require a shunt and those who do can be identified accurately by one of the methods of monitoring cerebral perfusion described below. This chapter will describe and discuss those various methods of intraoperative carotid monitoring used to determine the need for a temporary shunt during carotid endarterectomy and analyze the results of carotid endarterectomy in those series in which shunts were always used versus those in which shunts were never used, versus those series in which shunts were used selectively on the basis of some type of intraoperative monitoring.

LOCAL-REGIONAL VERSUS GENERAL ANESTHESIA

Historically, many of the early carotid endarterectomies were performed under local or regional (cervical block) anesthesia. This provided the surgeon with the

first type of intraoperative carotid monitoring in that it allowed the assessment of
the patients cerebral tolerance to trial carotid clamping. The technique consisted
of temporarily applying a clamp to the common carotid artery with the patient
awake and responding and then having the patient speak and move the extremities
on the contralateral side for a period of 3-5 min of carotid clamp time. If there was
no change in the patient's level of consciousness and no decrease in contralateral
motor function, the assumption was made that collateral cerebral circulation was
adequate and the carotid endarterectomy was completed. If there occurred a change
in sensation or a decrease in motor function, the clamp was removed thus restor-
ing cerebral flow. After a period of 5-10 min of restored cerebral perfusion, the
carotid clamps were reapplied, the arteriotomy performed, and a shunt inserted
to maintain cerebral perfusion during the carotid endarterectomy. At first glance
this approach would appear to be ideal. However, local-regional anesthesia has a
number of significant disadvantages: (a) it may produce anxiety and lead to hyper-
ventilation that causes hypocapnia, which has been shown to increase cerebral vascular resistance and decrease cerebral blood flow (6); (b) the patient may become
agitated, uncooperative, or experience changes in their level of consciousness mid-
way through the endarterectomy thus indicating the need for a shunt at a point in
time when it is most difficult to insert a shunt; (c) if the patient becomes restless
or agitated, this may distract the attention of the surgical team from the performance of a technically perfect endarterectomy. In spite of these disadvantages, certain surgical groups continue to use local-regional anesthesia and obtain acceptable
intraoperative and perioperative stroke rates (7,8) while others (9-12) report stroke
rates higher than the presently acceptable perioperative stroke rate of approximately 2% (4) (Table 1). Some authors (13,14) who have performed a large number of
carotid endarterectomies under both local-regional and general anesthesia report
an improvement in postoperative morbidity and mortality rates that they attribute
to the use of general anesthesia.

At present the vast majority of carotid endarterectomies are performed under
general anesthesia. This has a number of distinct advantages. Under general anesthesia, the anesthetist has complete control of the airway and thus can prevent
hyper- or hypoventilation, which can lead to hypocarbia or hypercarbia, respectively, neither of which is desirable if normal cerebral perfusion is to be maintained.
Hypocarbia causes intense cerebral vasconstriction and a decrease in cerebral blood
flow (6,14) while hypercarbia, even though it causes an overall decrease in cerebral
vascular resistance and an increase in overall cerebral blood flow (6,15,16), causes
a further reduction in cerebral blood flow to ischemic areas of the brain shown to
be already hypoperfused under normocarbic conditions (17). It is felt that this occurs secondary to a "cerebral vasomotor paralysis" in which the vessels in an ischemic area of the brain do not respond to changes in arterial CO_2. Under such circumstances an increase in arterial CO_2 will lower cerebral vascular resistance in
nonischemic areas of brain and cause a "steal" from already ischemic areas of brain

Table 1 Results of Carotid Endarterectomy Using the Response to Temporary Carotid Clamping Under Local-Regional Anesthesia to Determine the Need for a Shunt

Author (Ref.)	Number of Endarterectomies Performed	RND[a]		PND[b]		TND[c]	
		N	%	N	%	N	%
Peitzman et al. (7)	314	3	0.9	7	2.2	10	3.1
Rich and Hobson (8)	209	7	3.0	5	2.2	12	5.2
Hobson et al. (9)	50	4	8.0	1	2.0	5	10.0
Gabelman et al. (10)	54	1	2.0	2	4.0	3	6.0
Erwin et al. (11)	21	2	11.1	1	5.5	3	16.6
Bosiljevac and Farha (12)	165	6	3.6	6	3.6	12	7.2
Kwaan et al. (38)	125	3	2.4	0	0	3	2.4
Average	134	3.7	2.8	3.1	2.3	6.8	5.1

[a]Reversible Neurologic Deficit Rate includes TIAs, RINDS, and strokes that resolved completely.
[b]Permanent Neurologic Deficit Rate.
[c]Total Neurologic Deficit Rate.

rendered unresponsive to changes in arterial CO_2 (18). Even though the above sequence of events has been shown to occur in areas of significant ischemia in response to hypercapnia, Nakagawa et al. (19) have recently demonstrated that mild hypercapnia (pCO_2 43-55 mmHg) increased cerebral perfusion in mildly ischemic areas of brain as assessed by a return to normal of previously suppressed somatosensory-evoked potentials from the ischemic area of brain.

In addition to allowing for complete and continuous control of arterial CO_2, general anesthesia has a further beneficial effect on cerebral circulation. The inhalation anesthetic agents halothane, enflurane, and closely related agents cause a generalized cerebral vasodilatation (20-22) and an increase in cerebral blood flow, in addition to which halothane has been shown to decrease significantly the cerebral metabolic rate as measured by a decrease in cerebral oxygen consumption (20). A further advantage of general anesthesia is that is allows the surgeon to perform an unhurried endarterectomy on a quiet sleeping patient and thus concentrate all his attention on the one factor that all authors agree is essential to the safe conduct of carotid surgery, i.e., a technically perfect and complete endarterectomy.

CURRENT ANESTHETIC PRACTICES
AND ROUTINE MONITORING

At present there are two types of parameters that are commonly monitored during carotid surgery. The first includes the monitoring of those parameters that influence cerebral blood flow regardless of whether a shunt is used selectively, always, or never. These are arterial PO_2, PCO_2, and systolic blood pressure. The monitoring of all of these parameters can be greatly facilitated by the insertion of an intra-arterial cannula, usually a radial artery line, connected to a continuous display blood pressure monitor. The insertion of an inline, three-way stopcock in the above system allows for the frequent withdrawal of arterial blood gases to assess PO_2 and CO_2 and thus continually adjust ventilation to maintain PO_2 within the normal range and PCO_2 at normal to high normal levels. Continuous monitoring of systolic blood pressure is performed so that intraoperative and postoperative hypertension and hypotension can be immediately detected and treated since numerous reports have shown that sustained hypertension or hypotension increases the perioperative stroke rate (23-25). The second type of monitoring consists of the various methods of directly or indirectly evaluating the adequacy of cerebral blood flow during carotid clamping to assess the need for a temporary shunt.

MONITORING TO ASSESS THE NEED
FOR A SHUNT

Measurements of Jugular Venous Oxygen Content

One of the earliest types of monitoring of cerebral perfusion to assess the need for a shunt was the continuous measurement of jugular venous oxygen saturation ipsilateral to the side of carotid endarterectomy. This technique was an application of the Fick principle to the cerebral circulation. It assumes that if arterial blood is fully saturated with oxygen and cerebral oxygen consumption is constant, then cerebral blood flow will be directly proportional to internal jugular blood oxygen saturation. Based upon the original work of Kety and Schmidt (26) and early experience with the clinical application of jugular venous oxygen measurements during carotid endarterectomy by Lyons et al. (27) and Clauss and co-workers (28), it was felt that the minimal jugular venous oxygen saturation below which adequate cerebral perfusion could be assumed was 50-60%. The technique consisted of inserting a flexible cannula into the ipsilateral jugular vein and advancing it into the lateral sinus. Blood samples were withdrawn periodically through the cannula and jugular venous oxygen saturation was measured with an oxygen electrode. If jugular venous oxygen saturation fell below 50% mild hypertension and/or hypercarbia was induced to increase cerebral perfusion and if this failed to elevate jugular venous oxygen saturation above 50% a shunt was inserted.

Although the above mentioned previous reports (27,28) indicated that this was a reliable method for assessing decreased cerebral perfusion and thus indicating the need for either changes in anesthetic technique (hypertension or hypercarbia) or a temporary shunt, Larson et al. (29) found no relationship between the jugular venous blood oxygen saturation and loss of consciousness during trial carotid occlusion in patients undergoing endarterectomy under local anesthesia or the development of postoperative neurologic deficits in patients operated upon under general anesthesia. They conclude that although jugular venous oxygen saturation may accurately reflect total cerebral flow it cannot identify patients with areas of focal cerebral ischemia who may require a shunt. The fallibility of jugular venous oxygen saturation as an indicator of ipsilateral cerebral ischemia is due to the fact that internal jugular vein blood is derived from the venous outflow of *both* cerebral hemispheres due to the mixing that occurs in the various cerebral venous sinuses and that this degree of mixing is quite variable between patients. Because of this jugular venous oxygen saturation cannot reasonably be expected to accurately reflect ipsilateral hemispheric flow only, and will certainly not reflect small areas of focal ischemia within an otherwise normally perfused hemisphere. Because of this the measurement of jugular venous oxygen saturation never came into widespread use as a method of carotid monitoring and today it is of historical interest only.

Carotid Artery Stump Pressures

In 1969 Moore and associates (30) observed that awake patients under local-regional anesthesia who tolerated temporary carotid cross-clamping had qualitatively "brisk" backbleeding from the internal carotid artery, whereas those who did not tolerate temporary cross-clamping had "sparse" backbleeding. From this observation they surmised that the degree of cerebral collateral circulation could be quantitated by measuring the internal carotid artery back pressure distal to a proximal occluding clamp. In their first report of 48 carotid endarterectomies, 43 patients had carotid stump pressures of >25 mmHg and all tolerated cross-clamping well whereas the five patients with stump pressures <25 mmHg did not tolerate cross-clamping and required a shunt. Other reports corroborating the clinical utility of the method soon followed (31-34); however some reports indicated that a stump pressure <50 mmHg was a better indicator of the need for a shunt (32,34).

The technique of measuring carotid artery back pressure as described by Moore and co-workers (30-33) is as follows. After the carotid artery system is dissected, the patient is systemically anticoagulated with heparin and a 22-gauge needle connected to a pressure monitor with rigid tubing is inserted into the common carotid artery and systemic pressure is noted. Then the common carotid artery proximal to the needle and the external carotid are clamped, leaving the internal carotid artery unclamped so that the system measures collateral pressure through the circle of Willis. When the common and external carotid arteries are clamped, flow in the ipsilateral carotid system is stopped and the pressure measured is an "end pressure" in a closed system and therefore not dependent upon the degree of stenosis of the lesion distal to the needle but only on the functional integrity of the circle of Willis.

The measurement of carotid stump pressure as an indicator of the need for a shunt has become quite popular not only because of the inherent ease and simplicity of the technique itself but also because of the overall good results regarding a decrease in perioperative neurologic deficits reported by the various surgical groups that utilize the technique (30-34). However the measurement of carotid stump pressure has a number of real as well as theoretical drawbacks that detract from its ability to accurately determine cerebral perfusion and predict the need for a shunt. Among the real disadvantages are the fact that the measurement of carotid stump pressure as described above provides information relative to cerebral perfusion at only one point in time. Changes in mean arterial pressure during the time the carotid artery is clamped may cause the measured carotid stump pressure to vary as pointed out by Gee et al. (35). Additionally, Archie and Feldtman (36) have pointed out that carotid stump pressure alone is an inherently inaccurate predictor of cerebral perfusion pressure since jugular venous pressure may be quite variable and cerebral perfusion pressure is dependent on the *magnitude of the difference* between arterial pressure (carotid stump pressure) and venous pressure (jugular venous pressure). Since changes in PCO_2, PO_2, and the depth of anesthesia also influence cerebral perfusion and since changes in these parameters obviously cannot be detected by a technique that provides information at only one point in time, it is not surprising to note that a number of investigators have questioned the validity of the technique (35,36) as well as its clinical utility in being a reliable predictor of which patients require a shunt (37-41).

The theoretical disadvantages of using carotid stump pressure to predict the need for a shunt are similar to the disadvantages of using jugular venous oxygen saturation in that, although carotid back pressure may give a fairly accurate indication of overall cerebral perfusion, it cannot identify small focal areas of relative ischemia that may, during carotid clamping, be rendered sufficiently ischemic to undergo actual infarction. As Moore points out (42), these focal areas of ischemia exist primarily in patients with previous cerebral infarction and because of this he has expanded his criteria for use of a shunt to include any patient with a previous cerebral infarction regardless of a stump pressure as well as all patients with a carotid stump pressure <25 mmHg. The results relative to perioperative stroke rate of monitoring carotid stump pressure to determine the need for a shunt are listed in Table 2.

Continuous EEG Monitoring

The use of continuous EEG monitoring during carotid artery surgery was first introduced in the mid-1960s (13,43) and since then numerous reports (44-53) have described further refinements or adjuncts to the technique as well as attesting to

Table 2 The Results of Carotid Endarterectomy Using Carotid Stump Pressure
Measurements to Determine the Need for a Shunt

Author (Ref.)	Number of Endarterectomies Performed	RND[a]		PND[b]		TND[c]	
		N	%	N	%	N	%
Hobson et al. (9)	50	4	8.0	1	2.0	5	10.0
Erwin et al. (11)	18	2	11.1	1	5.6	3	16.7
Moore et al. (31)	107	3	2.8	2	1.8	5	4.6
Archie and Feldtman (36)	100	2	2.0	2	2.0	4	4.0
Smith et al. (37)	159	0	0.0	4	2.5	4	2.5
Average	86.8	2.2	2.5	2	2.3	4.2	4.8

[a]Reversible Neurologic Deficit Rate includes TIAs, RINDS, and strokes that resolved completely.
[b]Permanent Neurologic Deficit Rate.
[c]Total Neurologic Deficit Rate.

the clinical utility of this method of monitoring cerebral function to assess the need
for a shunt during carotid endarterectomy. The use of continuous EEG as a monitoring technique is based upon the logical supposition that EEG changes indicative of neuronal dysfunction are secondary to neuronal ischemia induced by carotid cross-clamping and, therefore, the insertion of a shunt should reverse neuronal
ischemia and dysfunction and should cause the EEG to return to baseline. The direct relationship between regional cerebral ischemia and regional neuronal dysfunction has been adequately demonstrated (54-56) and it is now fairly well accepted
that the primary determinant of neuronal dysfunction is a decreased pO_2 caused
by decreased regional cerebral blood flow (56).

The technique of continuous EEG monitoring has been best described by Callow and O'Donnell (57). Twenty standard scalp electrodes and two ear electrodes
are applied as prescribed by the 10-20 International Montage of EEG Electrode
placement and connected to a 16-channel continuous EEG recorder. A baseline
EEG tracing is obtained prior to the induction of anesthesia. Following the induction of anesthesia, those EEG changes produced by the anesthetic are allowed to
"stabilize" so that a new baseline EEG tracing under general anesthesia is recorded.
Following this, the EEG is continuously recorded and a record of all medications
administered, as well as the depth of anesthesia, is recorded to enable the interpret-

ing encephalographer to discern the difference between anesthetic- or medication-induced changes in the EEG as compared with ischemia-induced changes. Significant EEG changes indicative of neuronal ischemia consist of the appearance or increase in theta- or delta-wave activity, and/or the suppression of alpha- or beta-wave activity of greater than 50% (58). These changes usually occur ipsilateral to the side of carotid clamping, however, they may rarely occur bilaterally. These changes are usually evident within 1 min of carotid clamping and when they appear are assumed to indicate the need for a shunt that in almost all instances causes a return of the EEG to postanesthetic baseline levels. The percentage of patients who require a shunt on the basis of the above criteria has varied between 7% (51) and 29% (54) and averages approximately 20% (59). This variability in the reported need for a shunt based on EEG monitoring is probably accounted for by differences in the interpretation of the EEG regarding what constitutes a major change (58).

The use of continuous EEG monitoring to determine the need for a shunt has several attractive advantages. The first is that it is completely safe. However, the main advantage is that it provides a *continuous* method of monitoring neuronal *function* from various areas of the brain rather than providing only one measurement of cerebral perfusion from the entire cerebral hemisphere as does carotid stump pressure measurement. In addition since the EEG has been reported to change quickly (within 1 min) of the onset of neuronal ischemia, abrupt major changes in the EEG following removal of the shunt and closure of the carotid arteriotomy are indicative of thrombosis and/or embolization from the site of endarterectomy and allow the surgeon immediately to reopen the artery and remove the thrombus or correct the problem causing the embolization, thus minimizing the duration and extent of cerebral ischemia.

There are a number of real as well as theoretical disadvantages to the use of continuous EEG monitoring. The EEG recording apparatus is large and tends to make for a "crowded" operating area unless the machinery is housed in an adjacent room as described by Sundt et al. (60). Although some authors have claimed (57,58) that the EEG changes induced by ischemia are fairly characteristic and can be interpreted accurately by a surgeon familiar with a normal tracing, most groups who employ EEG monitoring require a neurologist trained in encephalography to be present during the carotid endarterectomy, thus adding to the overall cost of the procedure. In this latter regard, the computer-assisted interpretation of the EEG as described by either Chiappa et al. (59) or Cucchiara et al. (61) may eliminate the need for an encephalographer to be present. A further disadvantage of EEG monitoring, pointed out by Sundt et al. (54), is the inability of the EEG to detect cerebral ischemia in "deep" areas of the brain such as the internal capsule where relatively small areas of infarction can lead to large clinical deficits.

In addition to the above mentioned disadvantages, EEG monitoring has one more significant shortcoming. The EEG cannot distinguish between temporary and

Table 3 The Results of Carotid Endarterectomy Using EEG Monitoring to Determine the Need for a Shunt

Author (Ref.)	Number of Endarterectomies Performed	RND[a]		PND[b]		TND[c]	
		N	%	N	%	N	%
Beebe et al. (39)	50	0	0.0	2	4.0	2	4.0
Whittemore et al. (44)	150	1	0.7	1	0.7	2	1.3
Ricotta et al. (45)	100	0	0.0	0	0.0	0	0.0
Baker et al.	213	3	1.4	1	0.5	4	1.8
Hansebout et al. (48)	42	1	2.4	2	4.8	3	7.0
Phillips et al. (50)	37	0	0.0	0	0.0	0	0.0
Matsumoto et al. (51)	130	0	0.0	0	0.0	0	0.0
Chiappa et al. (59)	367	2	0.5	7	1.9	9	2.4
Sundt et al. (60)	1352	14	1.0	12	0.9	26	1.9
Byer et al. (67)	47	2	4.2	3	6.4	5	10.6
Average	248.8	2.3	0.9	2.8	1.1	5.1	2.0

[a]Reversible Neurologic Deficit Rate includes TIAs, RINDS, and strokes that resolved completely.
[b]Permanent Neurologic Deficit Rate.
[c]Total Neurologic Deficit Rate.

permanent neuronal dysfunction. It is quite likely but unprovable that in many instances the EEG changes induced by carotid clamping are no different than those that would be recorded during a transient ischemic attack and would return to normal following completion of the endarterectomy and restoration of flow without a shunt having been placed, just as a patient's clinical status returns to normal following the resolution of a TIA. It is quite likely that the inability of the EEG to discriminate temporary (reversible) neuronal dysfunction from permanent neuronal dysfunction leads to the use of a shunt much more frequently than is really required to prevent a permanent neurologic deficit. This is supported by the fact that on the average 20% of patients who undergo EEG monitoring during carotid surgery will be judged to require a shunt (59); however, in large series of patients undergoing carotid endarterectomy in whom shunts were never used, the neurologic deficit rate is certainly not 20%, but rather approximately 2% (62-65). From this it can only be concluded that the majority of the EEG changes detected during cross-clamping are indicative of temporary neuronal dysfunction, at least within the time frame during which carotid endarterectomy is usually performed, and, therefore, a shunt is not really required. Further support for the above comes from the recent report by Ferguson (66), in which all patients undergoing carotid endarterectomy had continuous EEG monitoring; however no shunts were used regardless of the EEG changes. In this series of 102 patients only one of the 35 patients in whom a "major" EEG change was noted sustained a neurologic deficit whereas three patients in whom no EEG changes occurred sustained a neurologic deficit.

Although the report of Ferguson (66) as well as others (67) indicates that EEG monitoring is not completely accurate as a predictor of the need for a shunt, it is probably safe to state that at present EEG monitoring is the most widely employed method used to determine the need for a shunt. The results of this method of monitoring are outlined in Table 3.

Measurement of Regional Cerebral Blood Flow (rCBF)

In spite of the fact that the measurement of cerebral blood flow in various regions of the brain would seem to be the ideal method of monitoring to determine the need for a shunt, the measurement of regional cerebral blood flow (rCBF) has not been widely utilized in this regard. Boysen in 1971 (68) was the first to evaluate rCBF as an indicator of the need for a shunt and in this initial report indicated that a flow of 30 ml/100 g per min was the minimum rCBF below which a shunt was required. Other reports regarding both the clinical utility of rCBF, as well as the correlation between rCBF and other monitoring techniques such as EEG and carotid stump pressure measurements, soon followed (55,66,69-72).

The technique consists of rapidly injecting 200-400 μCi of Xenon-133 dissolved in saline either into the internal carotid artery above the stenosis or into the common carotid artery with the external carotid artery occluded. The clearance of the Xenon-133 is measured by anywhere from one to as many as 16 scintillation detectors located over the ipsilateral hemisphere. Regional cerebral blood flow values are then calculated by either a 2-min clearance using the initial slope technique (68,71) or the complete 10-min clearance method as described by Hoedt-Rassmussen et al. (73).

The measurement of rCBF as described above has not achieved widespread clinical application, primarily because the equipment is bulky, expensive, and requires the presence and interpretative skills of nuclear medicine personnel. However, a number of groups have used rCBF measurements in conjunction with other types of carotid monitoring, primarily EEG, in an attempt to quantitate the actual cerebral blood flow level at which neuronal ischemia occurs and hopefully improve the accuracy and increase the clinical utility of these other methods. Normal cerebral blood flow is approximately 50-55 ml/100 g per min (20,26,68,74). Sharbrough et al. (55) reported a good correlation between rCBF measurements and

EEG changes during carotid clamping. Above mean CBF flow levels of 30 ml/100 g per min, no EEG changes occurred. Minor EEG changes begin to appear in most patients at flow levels between 18 and 30 ml/100 g per min and so-called "major" EEG changes are seen in most patients whose CBF decreases below 18 g/100 ml per min. Sharbrough et al. (55) further state that the "severity" of the EEG changes roughly parallels the decrease in clamped CBF at flow levels less than 18 ml/100 g per min and that these changes revert to normal following the insertion of a shunt. Because of this as well as an extensive clinical experience with monitoring both rCBF and EEG as a means of determining the need for a shunt Sundt et al. (60) recommend the use of a shunt if rCBF falls below 18-20 ml/100 g per min.

At present rCBF measurement has a limited clinical role because of its complexity and expense but it has served and will continue to serve as an accurate and reproducible "standard" against which both existing monitoring techniques as well as new technologies (75-77) that may become applicable in the area of carotid monitoring can be evaluated and compared.

Miscellaneous Carotid Monitoring Techniques

Falor and Housel (78) have reported the use of superior thyroid artery cannulation and continuous pressure monitoring to determine the need for a shunt. This method assumes that the collateral "back pressure" in the superior thyroid artery approximates the internal carotid artery stump pressure and, therefore, at pressures less than 50 mmHg a shunt should be employed. Although this technique has the obvious advantage of continuous measurement of pressure, it appears to be a very indirect way of assessing hemispheric perfusion pressure and, other than the fact that it is continuous, does not provide any real advantage over conventional methods of monitoring carotid stump pressures.

In those patients in whom a shunt is used, continuous oculoplethysmographic (OPG) monitoring (79) as well as supraorbital photoplethysmographic (PPG) monitoring (80) during the time that the shunt is in place have been used to insure that the shunt is actually functioning as intended. According to these reports, a change in the OPG or supraorbital PPG while the shunt is in place alerts the surgeon to the possibility of a malfunction within the shunt such as a kink, thrombosis, or shunt occlusion from Rummel tourniquets or clamps used to secure the shunt. Both of these techniques are simple and continuous and for those surgeons who elect to use a shunt they appear to offer an added dimension of safety.

The Results of Carotid Endarterectomy Relative to the Use of a Shunt

The results of carotid endarterectomy relative to perioperative reversible neurologic deficit (RND), permanent neurologic deficit (PND), and total neurologic deficit (TND) rates in those reported series in which shunts were always used, selectively used based on either measurement of carotid stump pressure or EEG monitoring, or never used are depicted in Table 4. The reports referenced in Table 4 do not represent an all-inclusive review of the literature nor have they been selected because of exceptionally "good" or "bad" results, or exceptionally large series but rather represent only those reports that were encountered in the course of writing

Table 4 The Results of Carotid Endarterectomy Relative to Whether a Shunt Was Always Used, Used Selectively Based on Some Type of Carotid Monitoring, or Never Used

Author (Ref.)	Number of Endarterectomies Performed	RND[a] N	RND[a] %	PND[b] N	PND[b] %	TND[c] N	TND[c] %
Always Shunt							
Thompson and Talkington (83)	1140	10	0.9	8	0.7	18	1.6
White et al. (23)	252	5	2.0	5	2.0	10	4.0
Towne and Bernhard (24)	253	5	2.0	9	3.6	14	5.5
Giannotta et al. (81)	152	4	2.5	4	2.5	8	5.3
Average	449.3	6.0	1.3	6.5	1.4	12.5	2.8
Selectively Shunt							
Hobson et al. (9)[d]	50	4	8.0	1	2.0	5	10.0
Erwin et al. (11)[d]	18	2	11.1	1	5.6	3	16.6
Moore et al. (31)[d]	107	3	2.8	2	1.8	5	4.6
Archie and Feldtman (36)[d]	100	2	2.0	2	2.0	4	4.0
Smith et al. (37)[d]	159	0	0.0	4	2.5	4	2.5
Beebe et al. (39)[e]	50	0	0.0	2	4.0	2	4.0
Whittemore et al. (44)[e]	150	1	0.7	1	0.7	2	1.3
Ricotta et al. (45)[e]	100	0	0.0	0	0.0	0	0.0
Baker et al. (46)[e]	213	3	1.4	1	0.5	4	1.8
Hansebout et al. (48)[e]	42	1	2.4	2	4.8	3	7.0
Phillips et al. (50)[e]	37	0	0.0	0	0.0	0	0.0
Matsumoto et al. (51)[e]	130	0	0.0	0	0.0	0	0.0

Table 4 (Continued)

Author (Ref.)	Number of Endarterectomies Performed	RND[a]		PND[b]		TND[c]	
		N	%	N	%	N	%
Chiappa et al. (59)[e]	367	2	0.5	7	1.9	9	2.4
Sundt et al. (60)[e]	1352	14	1.0	12	0.9	26	1.9
Byer et al. (67)[e]	47	2	4.2	3	6.4	5	10.6
Average	194.8	2.3	1.2	2.5	1.3	4.8	2.5
Never Shunt							
Wells et al. (13)	66	0	0.0	1	1.5	1	1.5
Baker et al. (18)	100	2	2.0	2	2.0	4	4.0
Baker et al. (41)	304	9	3.0	5	1.6	14	4.6
Carmichael (62)	440	4	0.9	7	1.6	11	2.5
Whitney et al. (63)	1637	17	1.0	37	2.2	54	3.2
Ott et al. (64)	309	6	1.9	4	1.3	10	3.2
Bland and Lazar (65)	280	2	0.7	3	1.1	3	1.1
Allen and Preziosi (82)	154	4	2.6	1	0.6	5	3.2
Average	411.3	5.5	1.3	7.5	1.8	13.0	3.2

[a]Reversible Neurologic Deficit Rate includes TIAs, RINDS, and strokes that resolved completely.
[b]Permanent Neurologic Deficit Rate.
[c]Total Neurologic Deficit Rate.
[d]Shunt insertion was based on measurement of carotid stump pressures.
[e]Shunt insertion was based on continuous EEG monitoring.

this chapter and that contained sufficient information to identify accurately perioperative neurologic deficit rates. As such no conscious selection process was at work and, hopefully, the various series in the three groups (always shunt, selectively shunt, never shunt) are included with as little bias as possible under the circumstances. In light of this, it is remarkable to note the similarity in the average RND, PND, and TND rates among the three groups. It is also quite interesting to note that in all three groups the average RND, PND, and TND rates fall within the 2-4% range of perioperative neurologic deficits, which is considered "acceptable" by prominent surgeons with a large experience in performing carotid endarterectomy (4,41,60,83).

A number of inferences could be drawn from an examination of Table 4. These include: (a) acceptable results can be achieved by following *any* of the three policies, i.e., always shunt, selectively shunt, or never shunt; (b) results may not be so much dependent upon one's policy regarding the use of a shunt as they are upon other important factors such as appropriate patient selection, quality of perioperative anesthetic management, and overall technical excellence; (c) that the number of strokes in the group that never shunts, in whom most strokes are presumed to be on the basis of ischemia during carotid clamping, is approximately equal to the number of strokes caused by technical misadventures in the group that always shunts, in whom most strokes are presumed to be technical in nature, and at least some of these are secondary to the use of the shunt; (d) that the two most commonly employed monitoring techniques used to determine the need for a shunt (EEG monitoring and measurement of carotid stump pressure) are not sufficiently accurate to identify all patients who will experience an ischemic infarction if a shunt is not used or conversely these methods are not sufficiently accurate to identify all patients who do not require a shunt and thus, remove them from the risk of a shunt-induced technical problem, which may cause a stroke. From the information presently available in the literature, it is impossible to conclude which, if any, of the above inferences are legitimate. It is not the intent of this chapter to attempt to demonstrate an optimal type of carotid monitoring to determine the need for a shunt or to endorse any one policy relative to the use of a shunt as being better than any other; but rather to describe the various methods of carotid monitoring commonly available in such a way as to allow the reader to make meaningful decisions as to what approach is most beneficial in light of his own personal results and experience in performing carotid endarterectomy.

REFERENCES

1. Fisher M, Adams RD: Observations on brain embolism with special reference to the mechanism of hemorrhagic infarction. J Neuropath Exp Neurol 10:92, 1951.
2. Eastcott HHG, Pickering GW, Rob CG: Reconstruction of internal carotid artery in a patient with intermittent attacks of hemiplegia. Lancet 2:994, 1954.
3. Carrea R, Molins M, Murphy G: Surgical treatment of spontaneous thrombosis of the internal carotid artery in the neck. Carotid-Carotideal Anastomosis: Report of a Case. Acta Neurol Lat Am 1:71, 1955.
4. Thompson JE: Carotid endarterectomy, 1982–The state of the art. Br J Surg 70:371, 1983.
5. Cooley DA, Al-Namaan YD, Carton CA: Surgical treatment of arteriosclerotic occlusion of common carotid artery. J Neurosurg 13:500, 1956.
6. Lassen NA: Control of cerebral circulation in health and disease. Circ Res 34: 749, 1974.

7. Peitzman AB, Webster MW, Loubeau J-M, Grundy BL, Bahnson HT: Carotid endarterectomy under regional (conductive) anesthesia. Ann Surg 196:59, 1982.

8. Rich NM, Hobson RW: Carotid endarterectomy under regional anesthesia. Am Surg 41:253, 1975.

9. Hobson RW, Wright CB, Sublett JW, Fedde CW, Rich NM: Carotid artery back pressure and endarterectomy under regional anesthesia. Arch Surg 109: 682, 1974.

10. Gabelman CG, Gann DS, Ashworth CJ, Carney WI: One hundred consecutive carotid reconstructions: Local versus general anesthesia. Am J Surg 145:477, 1983.

11. Erwin D, Pick MJ, Taylor GW: Anaesthesia for carotid artery surgery. Anaesthesia 35:246, 1980.

12. Bosiljevac JE, Farha SJ: Carotid endarterectomy: Results using regional anesthesia. Am Surg 46:403, 1980.

13. Wells BA, Keats AS, Cooley DA: Increased tolerance to cerebral ischemia produced by general anesthesia during temporary carotid occlusion. Surgery 54: 216, 1963.

14. Larson CP: Anesthesia and control of the cerebral circulation. In Wylie EJ and Ehrenfeld WK (eds): Extracranial Cerebrovascular Occlusive Disease: Diagnosis and Management, WB Saunders, Philadelphia, p. 152, 1970.

15. Kety SS, Schmidt CF: The effects of altered arterial tensions of carbon dioxide and oxygen on cerebral blood flow and cerebral oxygen consumption of normal young men. J Clin Invest 27:484, 1948.

16. Patterson JL Jr, Heyman A, Battey LL, Ferguson RW: Threshold of response of the cerebral vessels of man to increase in blood carbon dioxide. J Clin Invest 34:1857, 1955.

17. Boysen G, Ladegaard-Pedersen HJ, Henriksen H, Olesen J, Paulson OB, Engell HC: The effects of Pa CO_2 on regional cerebral blood flow and internal carotid arterial pressure during carotid clamping. Anesthesiology 35:286, 1971.

18. Baker WH, Rodman JA, Barnes RW, Hoyt JL: An evaluation of hypocarbia and hypercarbia during carotid endarterectomy. Stroke 7:451, 1976.

19. Nakagawa Y, Ohtsuka K, Tsuru M, Nakamura N: Effects of mild hypercapnia on somatosensory evoked potentials in experimental cerebral ischemia. Stroke 15:275, 1984.

20. Christensen MS, Hoedt-Rasmussen K, Lassen NA: Cerebral vasodilatation by halothane anaesthesia in man and its potentiation by hypotension and hypercapnia. Br J Anaesth 39:927, 1967.

21. McKay RD, Sundt TM, Michenfelder JD, Gronert GA, Messick JM, Sharbrough FW, Piepgras DG: Internal carotid artery stump pressure and cerebral blood flow during carotid endarterectomy: Modification by halothane, enflurane, and innovar. Anesthesiology 45:390, 1976.

22. McDowall DG: The effects of general anaesthetics on cerebral bloodflow and cerebral metabolism. Br J Anaesth 37:236, 1965.

23. White JS, Sirinek KR, Root HD, Rogers W: Morbidity and mortality of carotid endarterectomy: Rates of occurrence in asymptomatic and symptomatic patients. Arch Surg 116:409, 1981.

24. Towne JB, Bernhard VM: The relationship of postoperative hypertension to complications following carotid endarterectomy. Surgery 88:575, 1980.

25. Bove EL, Fry WJ, Gross WS, Stanley JC: Hypotension and hypertension as consequences of baroreceptor dysfunction following carotid endarterectomy. Surgery 85:633, 1979.

26. Kety S and Schmidt F: The nitrous oxide method for the quantitative determination of cerebral blood flow in man: Theory, procedure and normal values. J Clin Invest 27:476, 1948.

27. Lyons C, Clark LC, McDowell H, McArthur K: Cerebral venous oxygen content during carotid throbintimectomy. Ann Surg 160:561, 1964.

28. Clauss RH, Hass WK, Ransohoff J: Simplified method for monitoring adequacy of brain oxygenation during carotid surgery. New Engl J Med 273: 1127, 1965.

29. Larson CP, Ehrenfeld WK, Wade JG, Wylie EJ: Jugular venous oxygen saturation as an index of adequacy of cerebral oxygenation. Surgery 62:31, 1967.

30. Moore WS, Hall AD: Carotid artery back pressure: A test of cerebral tolerance to temporary carotid occlusion. Arch Surg 99:702, 1969.

31. Moore WS, Yee JM, Hall AD: Collateral cerebral blood pressure: An index of tolerance to temporary carotid occlusion. Arch Surg 106:520, 1973.

32. Hays RJ, Levinson SA, Wylie EJ: Intraoperative measurement of carotid back pressure as a guide to operative management for carotid endarterectomy. Surgery 72:953, 1972.

33. Hunter GC, Sieffert G, Malone JM, Moore WS: The accuracy of carotid back pressure as an index for shunt requirements: A reappraisal. Stroke 13:319, 1982.

34. Hughes RK, Bustos M, Byrne JP: Internal carotid artery pressures: A guide for use of shunt during carotid repair. Arch Surg 109:494, 1974.

35. Gee W, Kaupp HA, McDonald KM, Goodreau JJ, Lerner SM: The collateral hemispheric systolic pressure. Arch Surg 118:908, 1983.

36. Archie JP, Feldtman RW: Determinants of cerebral perfusion pressure during carotid endarterectomy. Arch Surg 117:319, 1982.

37. Smith LL, Jacobson JG, Hinshaw DB: Correlation of neurologic complications and pressure measurements during carotid endarterectomy. Surg Gynecol Obstet 143:233, 1976.

38. Kwaan JHM, Peterson GJ, Connolly JE: Stump pressure: An unreliable guide for shunting during carotid endarterectomy. Arch Surg 115:1083, 1980.

39. Beebe HG, Pearson JM, Coatsworth JJ: Comparison of carotid artery stump pressure and EEG monitoring in carotid endarterectomy. Am Surg 44:655, 1978.

40. Sublett JW, Seidenberg AB, Hobson RW: Internal carotid artery stump pressures during regional anesthesia. Anesthesiology 41:505, 1974.

41. Baker WH, Dorner DB, Barnes RW: Carotid endarterectomy: Is an indwelling shunt necessary? Surgery 82:321, 1977.

42. Moore WS: Operative technique. In Rutherford RB (ed): Vascular Surgery, WB Saunders, Philadelphia, pp 1248, 1984.

43. Perez-Borja C, Meyer JS: Electroencephalographic monitoring during reconstructive surgery of the neck vessels. Electroenceph Clin Neurophysiol 18: 162, 1965.

44. Whittemore AD, Kauffman JL, Kohler TR, Mannick JA: Routine electroencephalographic (EEG) monitoring during carotid endarterectomy. Ann Surg 197:707, 1983.

45. Ricotta JJ, Charlton MH, DeWeese JA: Determining criteria for shunt placement during carotid endarterectomy: EEG versus back pressure. Ann Surg 198:642, 1983.

46. Baker JD, Gluecklich B, Watson CW, Marcus E, Kamat V, Callow AD: An evaluation of electroencephalographic monitoring for carotid study. Surgery 78:787, 1975.

47. Callow AD, Matsumoto G, Baker D, Cossman D, Watson W: Protection of the high risk carotid endarterectomy patient by continuous electroencephalography. Cardiovas Surg 19:55, 1978.

48. Hansebout RR, Blomquist G, Gloor P, Thompson C, Trop D: Use of hypertension and electroencephalographic monitoring during carotid endarterectomy. Can J Surg 24:304, 1981.

49. Marshall BM, Lougheed WM: The use of electroencephalographic monitoring during carotid endarterectomy, as an indicator for the application of a temporary by-pass. Can Anaes Soc J 16:331, 1969.

50. Phillips MR, Johnson WC, Scott RM, Vollman RW, Levine H, Nabseth DC: Carotid endarterectomy in the presence of contralateral carotid occlusion: The role of EEG and intraluminal shunting. Arch Surg 114:1232, 1979.

51. Matsumoto GH, Baker JD, Watson CW, Gleucklich B, Callow AD: EEG surveillance as a means of extending operability in high risk carotid endarterectomy. Stroke 7:554, 1976.

52. Trojaborg W, Boysen G: Relation between EEG, regional cerebral blood flow and internal carotid artery pressure during carotid endarterectomy. Electroenceph Clin Neurophys 34:61, 1973.

53. Harris EJ, Brown WH, Pavy RN, Anderson WW, Stone DW: Continuous electroencephalogic monitoring during carotid artery endarterectomy. Surgery 62:441, 1967.

54. Sundt TM, Sharbrough FW, Anderson RE, Michenfelder JD: Cerebral blood flow measurements and electroencephalograms during carotid endarterectomy. J Neurosurg 41:310, 1974.

55. Sharbrough FW, Messick JM, Sundt TM: Correlation of continuous electroencephalograms with cerebral blood flow measurements during carotid endarterectomy. Stroke 4:674, 1973.

56. Paulson OB, Sharbrough FW: Physiologic and pathophysiologic relationship between the electroencephalogram and the regional cerebral blood flow. Acta Neurol Scand 50:194,1 974.

57. Callow AD, O'donnell TF: EEG monitoring in cerebrovascular surgery. In Bergan JJ and Yao JST (eds): Cerebrovascular Insufficiency, Grune & Stratton, New York, pp. 327, 1983.

58. Ferguson GG, Gamache FW: Cerebral protection during carotid endarterectomy: Intraoperative monitoring, anesthetic techniques, and temporary

shunts. In Smith RR (ed): Stroke and the Extracranial Vessels, Raven Press, New York, pp. 187, 1984.

59. Chiappa KH, Burke ST, Young RR; Results of electroencephalographic monitoring during 367 carotid endarterectomies: Use of a dedicated minicomputer. Stroke 10:381, 1979.

60. Sundt TM, Sharbrough FW, Piepgras DG: The significance of cerebral blood flow measurements during carotid endarterectomy. In Bergan JJ and Yao JST (eds): Cerebrovascular Insufficiency. Grune & Stratton, New York, pp. 287, 1983.

61. Cucchiara RF, Sharbrough FW, Messick JM, Tinker JH: An electroencephalographic filter-processor as an indicator of cerebral ischemia during carotid endarterectomy. Anesthesiology 51:77, 1979.

62. Carmichael JD: Carotid surgery in the community hospital: 467 consecutive operations. Arch Surg 115:937, 1980.

63. Whitney DG, Kahn EM, Estes JW, Jones CE: Carotid artery surgery without a temporary indwelling shunt: 1,917 consecutive procedures. Arch Surg 115: 1393, 1980.

64. Ott DA, Cooley DA, Chapa L, Coelho A: Carotid endarterectomy without temporary intraluminal shunt: Study of 309 consecutive operations. Ann Surg 191:708, 1980.

65. Bland JE, Lazar ML: Carotid endarterectomy without shunt. Neurosurgery 8:153, 1981.

66. Ferguson GG: Intraoperative monitoring and internal shunts: Are they necessary in carotid endarterectomy? Stroke 13:287, 1982.

67. Byer JA, Henzel JH, Dexter JD: Correlation of intraoperative electroencephalography with neurologic deficit after carotid endarterectomy. Southern Med J 72:956, 1979.

68. Boysen G: Cerebral blood flow measurement as a safeguard during carotid endarterectomy. Stroke 2:1, 1971.

69. Boysen G, Engell HC, Pistolese GR, Fiorani P, Agnoli A, Lassen NA: On the critical lower level of cerebral blood flow in man with particular reference to carotid surgery. Circulation 49:1023, 1974.

70. Vorstrup S, Hemmingsen R, Henriksen L, Lindewald H, Engell HC, Lassen NA: Regional cerebral blood flow in patients with transient ischemic attacks studied by Xenon-133 inhalation and emission tomography. Stroke 14:903, 1983.

71. Waltz AG, Sundt TM, Michenfelder JD: Cerebral blood flow during carotid endarterectomy. Circulation 45:1091, 1972.

72. Rowed DW, Vilaghy MI: Intraoperative regional cerebral blood flow during carotid endarterectomy. Can J Neurol Sci 8:235, 1981.

73. Hoedt-Rassmussen K, Sveinsdottir E, Lassen NA: Regional cerebral blood flow in man determined by intra-arterial injection of radioactive inert gas. Circ Res 18:237, 1966.

74. Bloor BM, Glista GG: Observations on simultaneous internal carotid artery and total cerebral blood flow measurements in man. Neurosurgery 2:249, 1977.

75. Ogawa A, Sakurai Y, Suzuki J: Continuous measurements of regional cerebral blood flow using krypton-81m. Stroke 14:623, 1983.

76. Uematsu S, Yang A, Preziosi TJ, Kouba R, Toung TJK: Measurement of carotid blood flow in man and its clinical application. Stroke 14:256, 1983.

77. Hill TC, Magistretti PL, Holman BL, Lee RGL, O'Leary DH, Uren RF, Royal HD, Mayman CI, Kolodny GM, Clouse ME: Assessment of regional cerebral blood flow (rCBF) in stroke using SPECT and N-isopropyl-(I-123)-p-iodamphetamine (IMP). Stroke 15:40, 1984.

78. Falor WH, Hansel JR: Superior thyroid artery cannulation for monitoring carotid artery operation. Arch Surg 111:1036, 1976.

79. Pearce HJ, Lowell J, Tubb DW, Brown HJ: Continuous oculoplethysmographic monitoring during carotid endarterectomy. Am J Surg 138:733, 1979.

80. Pearce HJ, Becchetti JJ, Brown HJ: Supraorbital photoplethysmographic monitoring during carotid endarterectomy with the use of an internal shunt: An added dimension of safety. Surgery 87:339, 1980.

81. Giannotta SL, Dicks RE, Kindt GW: Carotid endarterectomy: Technical improvements. Neurosurgery 7:309, 1980.

82. Allen GS, Preziosi TJ: Carotid endarterectomy: A prospective study of its efficacy and safety. Medicine 60:298, 1981.

83. Thompson JE, Talkington CM: Carotid endarterectomy. Ann Surg 184:1, 1976.

13

Intraoperative Hemodynamic Assessment of the Adequacy of Extremity and Portal Vascular Reconstruction

LARRY R. WILLIAMS
University of South Florida
Tampa, Florida

Veterans Administration
 Medical Center
Bay Pines, Florida

Obtaining a successful result in any vascular reconstruction requires appropriate preoperative diagnosis of the hemodynamic abnormality responsible for symptoms, flawless technical performance of an appropriately chosen procedure, and attentive follow-up to insure a continued satisfactory result. Since the actual operative technique plays a major role in most vascular procedures, the intraoperative assessment of the completed reconstruction must be an integral part of each operation. This chapter will address methods of intraoperative hemodynamic assessment of procedures for lower extremity revascularization and for portal decompression.

LOWER EXTREMITY REVASCULARIZATION

A variety of methods for assessing the adequacy of lower extremity arterial reconstructive procedures have been utilized with varying success. Many different clinical parameters are estimated by most vascular surgeons. In addition, completion arteriography has been well documented as a useful tool in detecting technical errors at operation (1,2). Arteriography is, however, an anatomic assessment and does not provide information relative to the hemodynamic adequacy of the bypass.

Quantitative hemodynamic assessments have been investigated by various authors in an attempt to document the functional status of arterial bypass grafts. These have included determination of graft flow rates, segmental pressure measurements, and plethysmographic assessments. Thus, clinical evaluation, anatomic documentation with completion arteriography, and functional hemodynamic analysis are complementary in the overall assessment of the adequacy of lower extremity revascularization.

Clinical Assessment

The most common method for assessing a completed bypass is by palpation of the pulse in the graft or distal to the distal anastomosis. In many instances, this provides adequate documentation that the graft is functioning well. However, an "easily detectable" pulse can be totally misleading. The appreciation of a pulse is very subjective, and even experienced examiners may incorrectly perceive distal pulses when none are in fact present. The transmission of a palpable pulse via stenosed vessels or by a totally thrombosed graft is a common phenomenon. This may occur even when the vessel is accessible for direct palpation. The detection of a thrill over the anastomosis, likewise, is not reliable. A thrill may be caused by a stenotic area with increased flow velocity or nonlaminar flow. On the other hand, the altered geometry caused by the anastomosis itself may produce a palpable thrill.

Some authors have attempted to assess the adequacy of infrainguinal revascularization by examining the foot following completion of the bypass. This can be done by including the prepped foot within the operating field. Alternatively, the foot can be enclosed within a clear bag so that it can be visualized throughout the operation. Estimation of skin color, capillary refill, and temperature are extremely variable in the immediate reperfusion state. General or regional anesthesia, ambient and patient temperature, cardiac output, and collateral circulation may have a marked effect on regional blood flow and skin microcirculation. Obesity, pedal edema, and skin pigmentation also make examination of the foot highly subjective. Thus, assessment of lower extremity bypass results based on examination of the foot is unreliable.

Graft Flow Measurements

Direct measurement of the blood flow through vein grafts is a means by which some authors have attempted to quantitate the results of lower extremity bypass. A square wave electromagnetic flow probe, placed snugly around the vessel, measures the voltage induced by the flow of blood (electrolyte) at right angles to the probe's magnetic field. Amplification and electronic subtraction of artifact yield a signal that can be displayed on a strip chart recorder.

Flow measurements can be taken directly over vein grafts or distal to the bypassed segment over the native artery. Measurement of blood flow in PTFE grafts is unreliable due to an unacceptable amount of interference with the electrical fields. It must be remembered that one of the major industrial uses of PTFE is in electrical insulation.

Dean et al. (3) measured blood flow rates in 98 patients with reversed autogenous saphenous vein femoropopliteal bypass grafts and found that the intraoperative flow rates were an excellent predictor of early graft failures. Vein grafts with basal graft flows of less than 70 cc/min universally thrombosed in the early postoperative period. Graft flow rates correlated well with preoperative ankle/ brachial blood pressure indices and with the angiographic patency of outflow vessels (Fig. 1). Therefore, distal occlusive disease and outflow resistance may have been responsible for the lower graft flow rates. Thus, it appeared that any vein graft with a flow rate of less than 70 cc/min was inadequate and either revision or more distal bypass would be necessary. Higher flow rates, however, did not insure success of the graft. Four patients in whom early graft failure was attributed to technical errors at operation had graft flow rates greater than 100 cc/min.

Similar studies likewise have documented that graft flow rates are related to the hemodynamic success of the grafts (4-7). The minimum acceptable flow rate

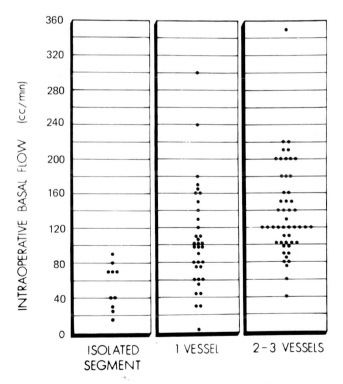

Figure 1 Intraoperative basal graft flow rates with respect to angiographic patency of outflow vessels. (From Dean et al., Br J Surg 55:134, 1968, with permission.)

is difficult to determine. In general, however, grafts with low flow rates are less likely to remain patent postoperatively. Little et al. (4) reported that 80% of grafts with intraoperative flow rates of 60 cc/min or less, failed. Terry et al. (5) reported a 54% early graft thrombosis rate when flow rates were less than 100 cc/min. However, in two of four patients with flow rates less than 50 cc/min, grafts remained patent.

Mannick and Jackson (6) studied 14 patients with femoropopliteal vein grafts and found that the intraoperative graft flow rates correlated very well with the angiographic estimation of outflow. The flow rates did not, however, predict which grafts were not adequate due to technical errors or which grafts would fail in the early postoperative period. In three patients flow rates of less than 25 cc/min and in one patient a flow rate of only 15 cc/min were recorded. Despite these extremely low flow rates, no technical errors could be detected and these grafts remained patent postoperatively.

Thus, in contrast to Dean's findings, even grafts with very low flow rates may be successful. The flow rates ultimately obtained in femoropopliteal vein grafts do not necessarily correlate with the technical adequacy of the procedure, but are a result of multiple factors. Inokuchi et al. (12) were unable to correlate intraoperative graft flow rates and subsequent outcome (Fig. 2). Barner et al. (7) likewise found no correlation between early graft failure and intraoperative flow measurements in 29 lower extremity vein grafts. Barner et al. stressed that long procedures on exposed limbs in cool rooms, under general anesthesia, resulted in significant vasoconstriction. Dean et al. (3) and Mannick et al. (6) also felt that increased outflow resistance, whether due to vasoconstriction or arterial occlusive disease, was responsible for low graft flow rates in many cases.

Some investigators have attempted to gain more information from intraoperative flow measurements by pharmacologic vasodilatation of the distal arterial bed (3,8). Papaverine is commonly used for this purpose. Intraarterial injection of 15-40 mg (usually 30 mg) of papaverine ordinarily results in at least a doubling in the arterial flow rate. Despite the theoretic advantage, results of graft flow rates following pharmacologic vasodilatation have been extremely variable and not predictive of the presence of correctible technical errors or early graft failure (3,8).

Renwick et al. (9) attempted to solve the problem of variability in intraoperative vein graft flow rates by implanting electromagnetic flow probes to remain in place postoperatively. They found that average flow rates rose from 50 to 100 cc/min in the operating room to over 250 cc/min 8-12 hr postoperatively (Fig. 3). In one patient early graft occlusion was detected by a drop in the postoperative flow to zero. Multiple mechanical difficulties, problems with calibration, and the need to remove the probes has limited acceptance of this technique.

Kouchoukous (10) studied the pulsatile blood flow patterns in 12 reversed saphenous vein grafts in an attempt to enhance the usefulness of intraoperative flow measurements. Although still quite subjective, patients with rapid deceleration of

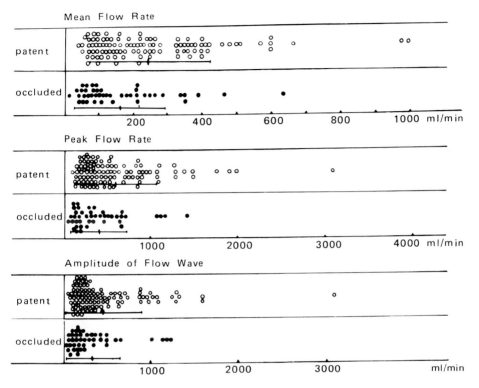

Figure 2 Comparison of outcome of revascularization and intraoperative flow measurements illustrating inability to predict graft patency based on flow rates. (From Inokuchi et al., Am J Surg 138:219, 1979, with permission.)

the pulse contours had better outflow tracts and better graft patency rates than patients with slow rates of deceleration (less than 15 cc/sec/sec).

More in-depth analysis of the postreconstruction arterial waveform has been performed by Lee et al. (11). By breaking the waveform down into 13 separate measurable components, quantitative analyses were possible (Fig. 4). Calculation of the ratio of deceleration duration to pulse duration was the only waveform characteristic that seemed to have value. High ratios, supposedly due to poor run-off with inelastic distal vessels implied a poor prognosis. Specific results of these waveform analyses in patients undergoing lower extremity bypass were not reported by Lee, however, similar measurements by Inokuchi et al. (12) failed to show a correlation between any specific waveform parameters and early graft thrombosis. Inokuchi et al. felt that subjective categorization of the waveforms into general groups based on inspection of the contours was simpler and seemed to supply more information relative to graft patency.

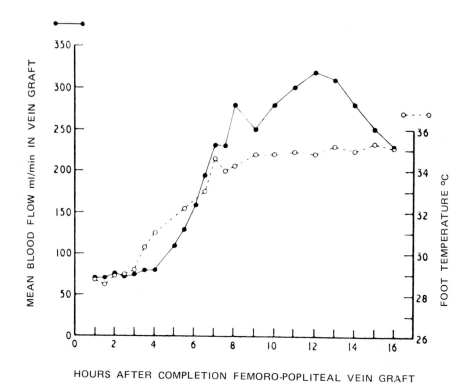

Figure 3 Serial blood flow measured with a probe implanted at the time of femoropopliteal bypass. (From Renwick et al., Surgery 64:544, 1968, with permission.)

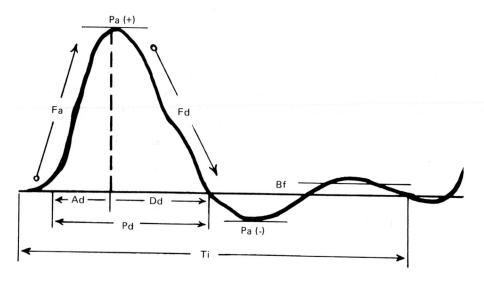

Ascer et al. (13) used an analog computer to integrate the pressure generated during injection of a given volume of saline through the completed distal anastomosis. Although several assumptions are necessary to allow calculations that conform to the physical laws of fluid dynamics, relative outflow resistances can be estimated. The outflow resistances following femoropopliteal bypass ranged from 0.08 to 1.38 units and following femorodistal bypass ranged from 0.18 to 2.34 units. In 13 grafts with outflow resistances of 1.2 units or more, occlusion occurred within the first postoperative month. The ouflow resistance as calculated by Ascer et al. did not correlate well with preoperative estimates of outflow resistance such as distal occlusive disease on arteriography, ankle brachial pressure index, or pulse volume recordings of ankle waveforms. The exact role of this sophisticated technique in assessing the adequacy of lower extremity revascularization has yet to be determined.

Pressure Measurements

Intraoperative measurement of the blood pressure distal to a vascular reconstruction is a relatively simple means of evaluating the functional status of the procedure (14,15). Doppler-derived pressures are easily performed and calculation of the extremity/systemic index helps to standardize the measurements. Variations in the extremity pressure due to systemic pressure and cardiac output changes are thus minimized. Comparisons to preoperative values, at different times during the procedure and from patient to patient are, therefore, more meaningful when the blood pressure index is used.

Equipment required for Doppler blood pressure measurements is readily available in most operating suites (Fig. 5). The technique involves prepping and draping the foot into the operative field. Ankle and thigh blood pressure cuffs and a Doppler pencil probe, which have been previously gas sterilized, can then be used by the surgeon without the need for a break in sterile technique. A nearby sphygmomanometer and portable Doppler flow detector with speaker output are connected by passing the appropriate lines off the sterile field. Following completion of the bypass, but prior to closure of the wounds, Doppler blood pressure is determined at the ankle. For suprainguinal procedures, pressures are measured at the thigh level. Systemic pressure is simultaneously recorded by the

---

Figure 4 Multiple parameters used to quantitate the pulsatile arterial waveform. Parameters: Fa = acceleration; Ad = acceleration duration; Pa(+) = peak amplitude; Dd = deceleration duration; Fd = deceleration; Pd = pulse duration; Pa(-) = peak amplitude; Bf = base line flow; Pf = positive flow/cardiac cycle; Nf = negative flow/cardiac cycle; Ef = effective flow/cardiac cycle; Ti = time interval between cycles; Mf = mean flow. (From Lee et al., Surg Gynecol Obstet 132:803, 1971, with permission.)

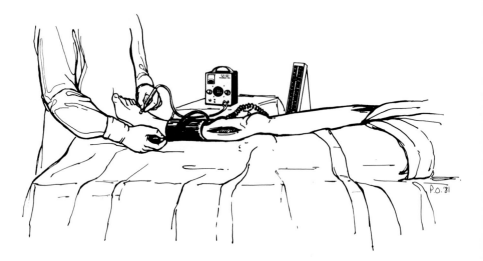

Figure 5 Technique for intraoperative blood pressure measurement using the sterile cuff and Doppler flow detector. (From Williams et al., Am J Surg 144:578, 1982, with permission.)

anesthesiologist with either a previously standardized radial arterial line or brachial cuff. The extremity/systemic blood pressure index can then be easily calculated and compared with the preoperative value.

Since the equipment and entire lower extremity are sterile and easily accessible, complete hemodynamic evaluation of the infrainguinal arterial system and bypass is possible. There is no limitation by incisions or nonsterile portions of the leg. Moving the cuff along the extremity to the level of interest allows the measurement of pressures in a segmental fashion over the graft, at the distal anastomosis or at the ankle.

It may be difficult to apply a cuff in certain situations. For example, the proximal-most thigh is somewhat inaccessible for placement of an appropriately fitting cuff. Direct intraarterial pressure measurements can be performed to supplement the Doppler-derived cuff pressures (16).

The technique for intraoperative pressure measurements is straightforward. A 19-gauge needle attached to a three-way stopcock is connected to arterial pressure tubing, which is passed off the sterile field to an anesthesiologist. This tubing can be connected either to a radial arterial line with a second three-way stopcock or directly to a pressure transducer and monitor. Puncture of the exposed artery or graft in question is performed and extremity/systemic indices can be calculated. If there is concern that a proximal subcritical stenosis is present, papaverine may be injected through the three-way stopcock. A 15% or greater fall in pressure at the common femoral level during increased flow delineates a proximal subcritical stenosis.

Just as preoperative Doppler pressure indices require correlation with the clinical situation, so do intraoperative measurements. There are no specific parameters that have been established with regard to the interpretation of intraoperative measurements. Although each patient must be assessed individually, the information obtained ordinarily provides a straightforward estimation of the functional status of the reconstruction.

The finding of a low pressure index at the ankle should prompt a search for a critical stenosis at some proximal level. If there is any question that the inflow to the graft is inadequate, measurement of the pressure with the cuff over the proximal graft will resolve it. If the pressure index at the proximal graft level is less than 0.9, an inflow problem is likely and investigation of the proximal anastomosis and/ or inflow to the graft should be undertaken. This may require direct pressure measurement above and below the proximal anastomosis. Detection of low pressure above the anastomosis incriminates the aortoiliac system. Diagnosis of a gradient across the proximal anastomosis identifies the anastomosis as the critical area.

If the pressure at the proximal graft level is equal to systemic pressure, the cuff is moved down the leg and serial pressures are determined to find the level at which the pressure fails. If the pressure index with the cuff at the distal end of the graft is unity, but falls with the cuff over the proximal-most runoff vessels, the distal anastomosis should be suspect. While imaging techniques (completion arteriography or real-time B-mode imaging) are useful adjuncts in this area, direct pressures can help to pinpoint the hemodynamic problem (17).

When the pressure at the ankle is low in the face of a normal pressure distal to the distal anastomosis, intervening arterial occlusive disease is most often responsible. In this situation one cannot expect the distal pressure to reflect accurately the functional status of the graft unless there is some means of predicting how much the distal pressure index should be increased following appropriate proximal bypass. A separate chapter in this volume describes a simple, accurate means for predicting the minimum amount of increase in ankle/brachial index that should be expected following lower extremity bypass (18). Since this calculation very seldom overestimates the post bypass ankle/brachial index, any intraoperative index that is less than predicted should prompt a search for a proximal hemodynamic problem.

In patients undergoing suprainguinal bypasses, the thigh/systemic index supplies a more consistent reflection of satisfactory reconstruction. Systemic hemodynamic changes due to hypovolemia, low cardiac output, hypothermia, and peripheral vasoconstriction cause a significant variability in ankle pressures.

Plethysmography

Various forms of plethysmography have been used to evaluate vascular procedures in the operating room. Creech et al. (19) first suggested intraoperative monitoring of digital blood flow with plethysmography in 1957. Griffen et al. (20) employed

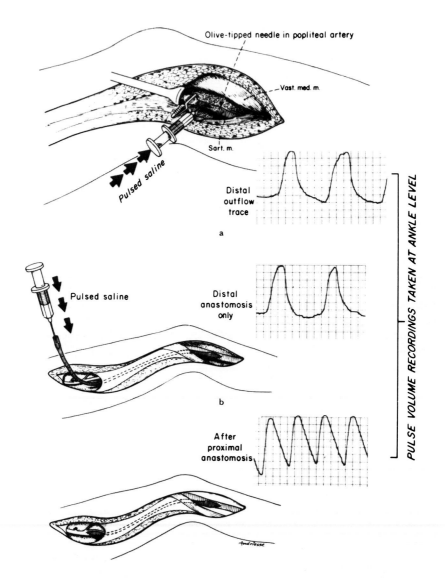

Figure 6 Technique for intraoperative pulse volume recordings with pulsed injection of saline into the distal arterial system (a) through the graft following the distal anastomosis (b), and upon restoration of circulation (c). (From O'Donnell et al., Surg Gynecol Obstet 145:252, 1977, with permission.)

segmental strain gauge plethysmography in 135 patients undergoing lower extremity revascularization. They found that intraoperative assessment of the bypass detected a significant number of correctable technical errors (7/135). Reoperation rates were significantly lower in patients who had intraoperative plethysmographic assessment when compared with a control group in which no assessment was made. Strain gauge plethysmographic measurements offer no specific advantage over previously mentioned techniques.

O'Donnell et al. (21,22) have used the pulse volume recorder, a form of air plethysmography, for intraoperative assessment. This procedure involves the placement of monitoring cuffs about the ankles or calves distal to the operative field. Baseline pulse wave contours and amplitudes are recorded after the induction of anesthesia when the patient is hemodynamically stable. Following completion of the reconstruction, repeat pulse volume recordings are obtained and compared with the baseline waveforms. Alternatively, an artificial pulse waveform can be generated by injection of saline through the distal arterial system or through the graft in a pulsed manner (Fig. 6). Thus, the patency of the arterial system between the injection site and the monitoring cuff can be assessed before the reestablishment of blood flow. Just prior to wound closure, repeat tracings can insure graft patency and good distal flow.

Although the pulse volume recorded method is quite similar to methods utilizing the Doppler, the addition of segmental systolic blood pressures offers a significant quantitative advantage. Reliance on intraoperative distal waveforms and simulated waveforms is somewhat qualitative and may lead to subjective error.

PORTAL HYPERTENSION

Preoperative Measurements

In patients considered for surgical treatment of portal hypertension, hemodynamic assessment plays a large role. Several techniques are available for the preoperative documentation of elevated portal pressure. Transcutaneous splenic pulp pressure reflects portal pressure but is seldom utilized at present because of significant variations in both normal and cirrhotic patients (23). More direct measurements can be made by exposure and recanalization of the umbilical vein or by percutaneous transhepatic portal vein puncture (24).

The most frequently used method for determination of portal pressure is wedged hepatic vein pressure (WHVP) obtained by advancement of a catheter into the hepatic vein at the time of panhepatic angiography (25-27). Subtraction of the inferior vena cava (IVC) pressure from the WHVP (corrected WHVP) gives an accurate estimation of the free portal pressure (FPP) (28). In normal patients the corrected WHVP varies from 3 to 10 mmHg. In patients with sinusoidal or postsinusoidal block, the degree of portal hypertension is accurately reflected by the corrected WHVP and is characteristically 15 mmHg or more. With presinusoidal block, on the other hand, the WHVP is low or normal and direct portal pressure measurements need to be performed if determination of actual free portal pressure is desired.

Measurement of right atrial pressure as well as IVC pressure will diagnose any pressure gradient within the IVC. Elevated IVC pressure due to an enlarged caudate lobe of the liver causing extrinsic compression is not ordinarily a contraindication to portacaval shunt. Turcotte cautions, however, that if chronic intrinsic caval stenosis with a resultant pressure gradient is identified, mesoatrial shunt should be considered instead of routine portacaval shunt (29).

Numerous complex techniques for the preoperative estimation of hepatic blood flow have been investigated. These include use of the Fick principle, indicator dilution techniques, and peripheral blood clearance of radioactive gold and phosphate (30). While theoretically appealing, their clinical utility in the selection of patients for portal decompression or in prediction of postshunt survival or encephalopathy has yet to be determined.

Intraoperative Measurements

Once a patient has been selected for portasystemic shunting, intraoperative pressure determinations can provide additional useful information. Cannulation of an enlarged omental vein and direct measurement of portal pressure not only confirms the diagnosis, but allows for comparison after completion of the shunt (Fig. 7). Alternatively, pressures can be measured following dissection of the portal or superior mesenteric vein and on both sides of an occluding clamp (hepatic occluded portal pressure) (HOPP) and splanchnic occluded portal pressure (MPP) and may reflect the magnitude of prograde portal blood flow (31). The corrected free portal pressure is determined by subtracting the IVC pressure from the measured portal pressure.

In Orloff's series of 180 emergency portacaval shunts, the average FPP was 267 mm saline. This correlated well with preoperative corrected WHVP (29 mm saline) (31). Drapanas likewise documented the consistency of preoperative corrected WHVP (329 mm water) and intraoperative FFP (342 mm water) in 35 patients undergoing mesocaval shunts (32). There is no firm evidence to suggest that selection of the type of shunt to be performed should be based on any specific pressure measurements at operation.

An adequate shunt should provide for at least a 50% reduction in portal pressure. If less of a reduction is realized, or if there is a pressure gradient across the anastomosis, careful inspection of the shunt for technical errors or thrombosis, both directly and by ultrasound or angiography, are in order. If no obvious cause can be identified and corrected to bring about the appropriate reduction in portal pressure, the shunt must be redone or another type of shunt created. Left untreated, shunts that have not reduced FPP very often thrombose in the early postoperative period.

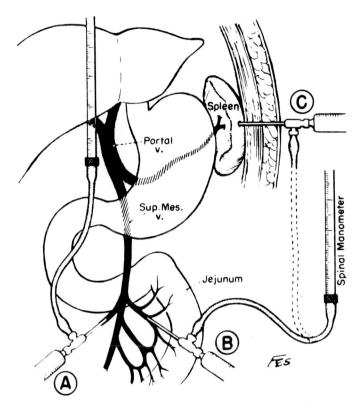

Figure 7 Methods for measuring portal venous pressure (A and B); mesenteric vein cannulation (C) splenic pulp pressure. (From Sedgwick et al., with permission.)

Warren has emphasized that decompression following selective distal spleno-renal shunt may not be total, and interpretation of intraoperative pressure measurements must take this into account. Nevertheless, any pressure gradient that exists directly across the splenorenal anastomosis is indicative of some technical difficulty at the anastomosis and should prompt investigation. Following adequate distal splenorenal shunting, there may be a progressive loss of portal perfusion as flow from high to low pressure increases collateral venous channels. Warren has studied multiple metabolic parameters in these patients and has found that these gradual circulatory changes are not associated with profound metabolic deterioration.

Although encephalopathy remains a complex entity related to blood ammonia levels, hepatic reserve, and central nervous system neurotransmitters, all agree that diversion of blood flow from the liver results in an increased incidence of encephalopathy as well as gradual deterioration of remaining liver function. Drapanas (32)

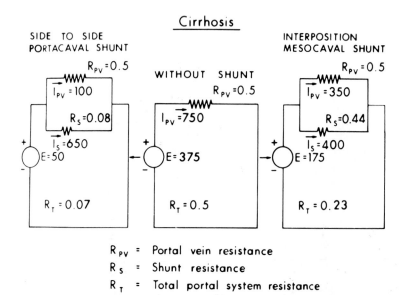

Figure 8   Example of an electrical analogue of the portal system based on pressure and flow measurements in a small group of patients. (From Drapanas et al., Ann Surg 181:523, 1975, with permission.)

and McDermott (30) have both shown that preshunt hepatic blood flow does not correlate with ultimate survival or encephalopathy. However, a drop in the hepatic occluded portal pressure (HOPP) of 100 ml of saline or more results in an increased incidence of encephalopathy following portacaval shunt. This is a reflection of the rather abrupt diversion of prograde portal flow. In contradiction, Orloff, in a similar series, found that patients with high mean portal pressures (MPP) (who suffer the greatest reduction in FPP postshunt) actually fared better with regard to survival and encephalopathy when compared to patients with low MPP.

Further prospective analysis is necessary before the exact relationship between portal pressures, flow, and specific postoperative results can be stated firmly. To that end, Drapanas has suggested an electrical analogue of the portal hemodynamic system (Fig. 8). On the basis of direct measurements in 80 patients undergoing mesocaval shunts, the system involves calculation of intrahepatic sinusoidal resistance and prediction of portal flow changes after various types of shunts. Although basic assumptions are necessary, the system may be helpful in elucidating complex portal system hemodynamics.

REFERENCES

1. Renwick S, Royle JP, Martin P: Operative angiography after femoropopliteal arterial reconstruction: Its influence on failure rate. Br J Surg 55:134, 1968.
2. Crowley JG: Intraoperative angiography. Am Surg 46:328, 1980.
3. Dean RH, Yao JST, Stanton PE, Bergan JJ: Prognostic indicators in femoropopliteal reconstructions. Arch Surg 110:1287, 1975.
4. Little JM, Sheil AGR, Lowenthal J: Prognostic value of intraoperative blood flow measurements in femoropopliteal bypass vein grafts. Lancet 2:648, 1968.
5. Terry HJ, Allen JS, Taylor GW: The relationship between blood flow and failure of femoropopliteal reconstructive arterial surgery. Br J Surg 59:549, 1972.
6. Mannick JA, Jackson BT: Hemodynamics of arterial surgery in atherosclerotic limbs direct measurement of blood flow before and after vein grafts. Surgery 59:713, 1966.
7. Barner HB, Judd DR, Kaiser GC, Willman VL, Hanlon CR: Blood flow in femoropopliteal bypass vein grafts. Arch Surg 96:619, 1968.
8. Flanigan DP, Williams LR, Schwartz JA, Schuler JJ, Gray B: Hemodynamic evaluation of the aortoiliac system using pharmacologic vasodilatation. Surgery 93:709, 1983.
9. Renwick S, Gabe IT, Shillingford JP, Martin P: Blood flow after reconstructive arterial surgery measured by implanted electromagnetic flow probes. Surgery 64:544, 1968.
10. Kouchoukous NT: Pulsatile blood flow patterns in femoropopliteal venous bypass grafts. Surg Forum 18:192, 1967.
11. Lee BY, Trainor FS, Madden JL: Significance of arterial blood flow in reconstructive arterial procedure. Surg Gynecol Obstet 132:803, 1971.
12. Inokuchi K, Kusaba A, Kiyose T: Flow waveform analysis in vascular surgery. Am J Surg 138:219, 1979.
13. Ascer E, Veith FJ, Morin L, White-Flores SA, Scher LA, Samson RH, Weiser RK, Rivers S, Gupta SK: Quantitative assessment of outflow resistance in lower extremity arterial reconstructions. J Surg Res 37:8, 1984.
14. Yao JST, Bergan JJ: Application of ultrasound to arterial and venous diagnosis. Surg Clin North Am 54:23, 1974.
15. Williams LR, Flanigan DP, Schuler JJ, Lim LT: Intraoperative assessment of limb revascularization by Doppler derived segmental blood pressure measurements. Am J Surg 144:578, 1982.
16. Schwartz JA, Flanigan DP, Williams LR, Schuler JJ, Gray B: Preoperative hemodynamic evaluation of aortoiliac occlusive disease: Correlation with intraoperative measurements. Cur Surg 40:278, 1983.
17. Flanigan DP, Williams LR, Schuler JJ: Perioperative and intraoperative assessment in limb revascularization. In Bergan JJ and Yao JST (eds): Evaluation and Treatment of Upper and Lower Extremity Circulatory Disorders, Grune & Stratton, Orlando, 1984.
18. Williams LR, Flanigan DP, Schuler JJ, O'Connor RJA, Castronuovo JJ: Prediction of improvement in ankle blood pressure following arterial bypass. J Surg Res 37:175, 1984.

19. Creech O, DeBakey MD, Culotta R: Digital blood flow following reconstructive arterial surgery. Arch Surg 74:5, 1957.
20. Griffin LH, Wary CH, Vaughan BL, Moretz WH: Detection of vascular occlusions during operation by segmental plethysmography and skin thermometry. Ann Surg 173:389, 1971.
21. O'Donnell TF, Cossman D, Callow AD: Noninvasive intraoperative monitoring: A prospective study comparing Doppler systolic occlusion pressure and segmental plethysmography. Am J Surg 135:539, 1978.
22. O'Donnell TF, Raines JK, Darling RC: Intraoperative monitoring using the pulse volume recorder. Surg Gynecol Obstet 145:252, 1977.
23. Green L, Weisberg H, Rosenthal WS, Douvies PA, Katz D: Evaluation of esophageal varices in liver disease by splenic-pulp manometry, splenoportography and esophagastroscopy: Diagnostic discrepancies. Am J Dig Dis 10:284, 1965.
24. Piccone VA, LeVeen HH, White JJ, Skinner GB, MacLean LD: Transumbilical portal hepatography, a significant adjunct in the investigation of liver disease. Surgery 61:333, 1967.
25. Paton A, Reynolds TB, Sherlock S: Assessment of portal venous hypertension by catheterization of hepatic vein. Lancet 1:918, 1953.
26. Taylor WJ, Myers JD: Occlusive hepatic venous catheterization in the study of the normal liver, cirrhosis of the liver and non-cirrhotic portal hypertension. Circulation 13:368, 1956.
27. Fomon JJ, Warren WD: Hemodynamic studies in portal hypertension. In Annu Rev Med 20:277, 1969.
28. Smith G: An assessment of the validity of preoperative hemodynamic studies in portal hypertension. Surgery 74:130, 1973.
29. Warren WD, Restrepo JE, Respess JC, Muller WH: The importance of hemodynamic studies in management of portal hypertension. Ann Surg 158:387, 1963.
30. McDermott WV: Evaluation of the hemodynamics of portal hypertension in the selection of patients for shunt surgery. Ann Surg 176:449, 1972.
31. Orloff MJ, Bell RH, Hyde PV, Skivolocki WP: Long-term results of emergency portacaval shunt for bleeding esophageal varices in unselected patients with alcoholic cirrhosis. Ann Surg 192:325, 1980.
32. Drapanas T, LoCicero J, Dowling JB: Hemodynamics of the interposition mesocaval shunt. Ann Surg 181:523, 1975.

14

Intraoperative Arteriography

ALLAN R. PASCH and JAMES J. SCHULER
University of Illinois
College of Medicine at Chicago
Chicago, Illinois

INTRODUCTION

Despite advance in the noninvasive assessment of peripheral vascular disease, arteriography has remained an essential tool in the evaluation of the vascular system. Arteriography provides anatomic information not always available from other diagnostic modalities, and complements data obtained from physical examination and noninvasive studies. In Chapter 11, the use of arteriography in the operating room prior to revascularization to delineate patency of distal vessels not visualized on preoperative conventional arteriography and to assess the optimal site of the distal anastomoses was discussed. Another use of intraoperative arteriography is in the assessment of the technical result of revascularization at the completion of vascular reconstruction or bypass. Completion intraoperative arteriography allows the opportunity to detect technical defects that, if uncorrected, may compromise the ultimate success of the procedure. In this chapter, we will discuss this particular application of arteriography and assess its overall role in the modern perioperative assessment of the vascular patient.

GENERAL CONSIDERATIONS

The same contraindications and precautions regarding conventional arteriography apply to the use of arteriography in the operating suite. Of prime consideration is the risk of allergic reactions to contrast media. In general, arteriography is safer than other radiologic procedures involving the use of contrast media. In a review of over 300,000 cases, arteriography had a 2% incidence of adverse reactions, versus 4% and 8% for excretory urography and intravenous cholangiography, respectively (1). More importantly, only two patients experienced fatal anaphylactic reactions after more than 40,000 arteriographic procedures. Though no specific data regarding the safety of operative angiography is available, the operating room represents an ideal location for the controlled treatment of serious reactions should they occur, and it is unlikely that operative angiography contributes significantly to operative morbidity or mortality.

Again referring to data obtained from patients undergoing preoperative angiography, it has been shown that patients with a history of a major anaphylactic reaction to contrast material are not at an increased risk for future major reactions (2). Despite this seemingly reassuring data, it would seem prudent to avoid intraoperative angiography in these individuals. Atopic individuals and patients with a history of a mild reaction to contrast media (nausea, urticaria, pruritus) are two to three times more likely to have subsequent mild reactions than normal individuals. However, the clinical significance of these mild symptoms in patients under regional or general anesthesia is probably small.

Almost all of the currently used contrast agents consist of iodine coupled to an anion (diatrizoate or iothalamate) plus a cation (sodium or methylglucamine). For cerebral angiography, sodium salts appear to be more toxic, and should be avoided (3). The major physiologic effect of contrast material is arterial vasodilatation and a resultant temporary decrease in systolic blood pressure. Thus, adequate volume status is necessary prior to arteriography to avoid precipitous drops in blood pressure. Contrast medium is excreted by glomerular filtration in the kidney and will cause an osmotic diuresis, again requiring careful attention to fluid management. In the presence of renal dysfunction, hepatic excretion becomes important.

The most commonly seen nonallergic complication of arteriography is renal failure, due to a combination of a decrease in renal blood flow and a direct toxic effect of contrast media on the kidney. Diabetes mellitus, preexistent azotemia, impaired liver function, dehydration, and the use of large amounts of contrast material have been incriminated as risk factors for the development of renal failure after angiography, with the degree of risk increasing in patients with multiple predisposing conditions (4-6). Even in the absence of overt renal failure, a mild reduction in creatinine clearance is common, occurring in up to 31% of patients after conventional angiography performed preoperatively (7).

No specific study of changes in renal function after intraoperative arteriography has been performed. Since the dye load during intraoperative angiography is considerably less than that used in conventional angiography, the contribution of intraoperative angiography to postoperative acute renal failure is probably small.

COMPLETION ANGIOGRAPHY

Infrainguinal and Aortoiliac Revascularization

Early graft failure rates of 2-22% have been reported after femoropopliteal bypass and up to 32% following femorotibial bypass, mainly due to technical errors at the time of surgery (8-11). Graft patency cannot always be restored, and even if early reoperation is successful long-term graft patency may be affected adversely (12). Early reoperation also results in higher mortality and increases the risk of wound complications (13,14). Intraoperative completion angiography offers the opportunity to minimize the need for early reoperation by detecting technical flaws which, even though they may be hemodynamically insignificant, may yet lead to early graft occlusion.

In 1924, Brooks first described direct operative angiography (15). Since then, numerous techniques for performing arteriography after femoropopliteal bypass have been described, including cannulation of a tributary of the saphenous vein or direct cannulation of the proximal saphenous vein with performance of the angiogram prior to completing the proximal anastomosis (16-18). Our preferred method is similar to prebypass intraoperative arteriography as described elsewhere in this book. A 19-gauge scalp needle is placed in the proximal graft. The proximal graft is clamped, and is connected by tubing to a three-way stopcock. The surgeon stands behind a Mayo stand draped with lead protection. The radiograph is taken after hand injection of 20-30 cc of undiluted Renografin 60, with no time delay required. If an in situ bypass was performed, radiopaque markers (i.e., 21-gauge needles) should be inserted in the skin perpendicular to the graft at regular intervals to help localize any abnormalities seen during angiography. As illustrated in Figure 1, technical flaws that may be detected by completion angiography include graft twisting, graft thrombus, arterial thrombus, and anastomatic narrowing. After in situ saphenous vein bypass, additional information, such as the presence of intact valve cusps and arteriovenous fistulae, may be detected.

The rationale for completion angiography following aortofemoral bypass is not as strong. The incidence of early graft failure is only 1-3% (20,21), and the potential benefits of completion angiography are therefore proportionately lower than after infrainguinal bypass. When performing intraoperative aortography, inflow occlusion is mandatory. Despite this, poor visualization due to dilution of dye with blood has been reported after simple hand injection (22), and a pressure injection with serial angiography may be needed for optimal visualization. This technique is cumbersome and not readily available in most operating rooms.

However, completion angiography of femoral and distal vessels is often helpful following aortofemoral bypass, since up to 10% of patients will experience distal emboli or thrombus formation during aortic surgery (23,24). Also, a significant number of patients without distal thrombus/embolus fail to have pedal pulses after

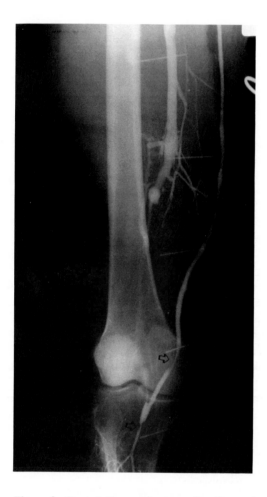

Figure 1 Completion angiogram after femoralpopliteal bypass with in situ saphenous vein, demonstrating arteriovenous fistulae, external compression of the
distal graft by the gastrocremius muscle, and thrombus in the popliteal artery.

surgery due to intense vasoconstriction. Intraoperative completion femoral angiography can identify both spasm and thrombus in these patients. Another use of
distal arteriography after aortofemoral bypass is in patients with known multisegmental occlusive disease, 9-19% of whom may eventually require infrainguinal
vascular reconstruction after aortofemoral bypass (25,26). In this group of patients in whom it is difficult to predict who will require subsequent infrainguinal
bypass for complete relief of symptoms, the distal angiogram obtained at the time

Table 1   Results of Completion Angiography after Infrainguinal
and Aortic Revascularization

Series	Patients	Positive Angiograms
Renwick et al. (27)	55	15 (27%)
Plecha and Pories (30)	183	43 (24%)
Courbier et al. (28)	1810	82 (5%)
Dardik et al. (33)	391	34 (9%)
Bowald et al. (22)	136	39 (29%)
Crowley (31)	131	23 (18%)
Liebman et al. (29)	171	10 (5%)
Hackler and Bunt (34)	35	6 (17%)
Total	2912	252 (9%)

of aortofemoral bypass will allow one to perform the infrainguinal bypass, if it is
required, without need for repeat angiography.

The results of completion intraoperative angiography following aortic and infrainguinal reconstruction are summarized in Table 1 (22,27-34). Of 2912 completion angiograms reported in the literature, 252 (9%) were abnormal. The results
of completion angiography differ when grouped according to the type of reconstruction, i.e., endarterectomy versus bypass, and when grouped according to the
location of the reconstructed segment. One hundred thirteen of 1596 angiograms
(7%) following infrainguinal revascularization were abnormal, compared with 44
of 872 (5%) after aortofemoral reconstruction. In both locations, the incidence
of defects was higher (18% and 14%, respectively) following endarterectomy. Excluding the endarterectomy data, the incidence of positive angiograms was 5.6%
for infrainguinal bypass and 3.9% after aortoiliac or aortofemoral bypass.

The above retrospective data clearly demonstrate the ability of completion
angiography to detect technical errors after vascular reconstruction. However, does
revision of these angiographic defects result in improved graft patency, i.e., are these
defects clinically significant? Furthermore, how accurate is arteriography compared
with noninvasive modalities of intraoperative evaluation?

To address the first question, Renwick obtained completion angiograms in 55
of 110 consecutive femoropopliteal bypasses and revised 15 defects (27%) seen on
angiography (27). The early reoperative rate in the 55 patients with completion
angiography was zero, compared with 18% in the group without angiography. In
a less controlled study, Bowald observed 90% early patency after revision of 20

angiographic abnormalities, versus a 20% patency in 19 grafts with angiographic defects that were not revised (22). Thus, the intraoperative correction of defects seen on completion angiography appears to affect the outcome favorably after infrainguinal bypass.

Surprisingly little data is available regarding the accuracy of intraoperative angiography. In an experimental study comparing uniplanar completion angiography to serial biplane arteriography and to ultrasonography, specificity was over 90% for all three modalities (35). However, single-plane completion angiography was quite insensitive (50% overall) compared with 70% for biplanar angiography and 92% for ultrasonography. In a subsequent clinical study of 67 vascular repairs evaluated intraoperatively by uniplanar completion angiography and ultrasonography, the accuracy of the former was only 85% compared with 96% for ultrasonography, due to several falsely positive angiographic results (36). Our most recent experience with 239 direct comparisons of operative angiography and operative ultrasonography is summarized in Chapter 15; accuracy of ultrasound (97%) remained higher than angiography (93%) due to the false positive results of the latter. In other clinical series employing angiography alone, both false negative and false positive results have been reported (28-30).

When is completion angiography worthwhile? Both the rate of early graft failure and the incidence of angiographic abnormalities are low following aortofemoral bypass, and the X-ray image following hand-injected aortography is often unsatisfactory. For these reasons, we do not routinely perform completion aortography in this setting, though it or completion femoral angiography may prove useful in selected difficult cases. In contrast, we recommend that completion angiography be routinely obtained following femoropopliteal and femorotibial bypass grafts. High-quality films are easily and rapidly obtained with equipment that is universally present in most hospitals. Though preliminary data indicate a higher accuracy of operative ultrasonography, this technology is not consistently available in many operating rooms. In addition, arteriography provides information regarding the distal runoff and presence of distal thrombi or emboli that is not available with ultrasonic imaging of the anastomosis.

Miscellaneous Indications

In addition to being useful following infrainguinal bypass, intraoperative completion angiography is useful in a variety of other settings in vascular surgery. After femoral or popliteal embolectomy, assessment of the distal circulation is often difficult. Residual distal emboli or thrombus may be present despite the return of pedal pulses or an improvement in ankle Doppler indices. Conversely, it is difficult to know if the failure to restore distal pulses (which occurs in up to 36% of patients) reflects residual emboli or preexistent atherosclerotic disease (37-38). In these patients, completion angiography can define the problem and prevent needless catheter manipulation of atherosclerotic tibial vessels.

We have also found completion angiography to be beneficial following the repair of injured arteries. Since the vast majority of injured vessels are treated by short segment interposition grafts of reversed saphenous vein, arteriography allows assessment of the proximal and distal anastomoses and also detects the presence of distal thrombus or spasm. In this predominantly young population, intense spasm of tibial vessels is often seen after a proximal arterial injury. Completion intraoperative arteriography can document this spasm and obviate needless exploration. In a recent series of 139 arterial injuries at our institutions, completion angiography detected five anastomotic defects and six instances of distal thrombus (39). We feel that detection and intraoperative correction of these technical errors contributed to the 4% rate of early graft thrombosis and the 1% incidence of limb loss in the series.

Another application of completion angiography is after repair of renal vessels. Acute occlusion of aortorenal bypass grafts may occur in up to 14% of patients and nephrectomy is required in over one-third of patients undergoing reoperation (40-42). Whereas progression of disease may be responsible for late graft failure, technical errors account for most early problems and early reoperation can often be avoided by the use of completion angiography. After renal revascularization, postoperative urograms and nuclear scans are of limited value in determining graft or arterial patency; despite acute arterial occlusion such diagnostic tests may be normal due to preexistent collateral circulation. Also, signs of graft failure such as hypertension and renal dysfunction may not become immediately apparent.

After transaortic renal endarterectomy, Stoney et al. routinely obtain intraoperative completion angiography by clamping aortic inflow and outflow and injecting dye directly into the aortic segment containing the orifices of the renal arteries (43). In an early series of 84 patients without operative angiograms, three cases of unrecognized occlusion led to eventual nephrectomies. In a more recent experience with 99 patients with routine angiography, two patients required revision of technical defects seen at completion angiography. Certainly the impact of completion angiography on the success of renal artery reconstruction is difficult to assess, and treatment failures occur in some patients due to problems in patient selection rather than graft occlusion. Nonetheless, arteriography can minimize those failures due to technical errors and early thrombosis.

Surgery of the venous system remains a frontier in vascular surgery, and is infrequently performed. However, intraoperative angiography of the venous system can be useful in procedures such as portal vein decompression, creation of arteriovenous fistulae for hemodialysis, or femoral vein thrombectomy.

Classic intraoperative assessment of the various shunts performed to decompress the portal vein and its tributaries involves measurement of the decrease in mesenteric venous pressure compared with preoperative levels. Though angiography and venography are important to determine shunt patency, they have usually been applied postoperatively. However, intraoperative venography has been reported to assess distal splenorenal shunts, since division of connections between the mesenteric and splenic venous systems is crucial to achieve selective shunting. Nagasue et al. (44) performed direct intraoperative portography in 13 patients before and after creation of a Warren shunt. Thirty cc of 60% meglumine sodium amidotrizoate is injected into a catheter in the superior mesenteric vein while an equal volume of dye is simultaneously injected through a needle placed directly in the splenic pulp. In four patients, unsuspected and undivided veins between the portal and splenic systems were demonstrated by direct intraoperative portography.

Another application of intraoperative venography is during creation of arteriovenous fistulae for hemodialysis. Since an inadequate cephalic vein is the most common reason for failure of radiocephalic fistulae, Hertzer (45) has described intraoperative venography to delineate the cephalic vein. In this technique, a 21-gauge scalp vein needle is inserted into a vein on the dorsum of the hand. A radiograph of the forearm is obtained after injection of 15 cc of contrast material. Completion intraoperative venography can also be used to assess the anastomoses after arteriovenous fistula or shunt creation and is easily performed by occluding arterial inflow and directly injecting the venous outflow or the shunt.

A final application of intraoperative venous angiography is after femoral vein thrombectomy. Though anticoagulation remains the standard treatment of acute deep venous thrombosis, there are numerous reports on the role of thrombectomy for acute ileofemoral venous thrombosis. Plate et al. (46) have described insertion of a 5.0 French feeding tube into a venous tributary for intraoperative completion venography after femoral venous thrombectomy, which can also be utilized for postoperative phlebograms.

Carotid Endarterectomy

The most controversial aspect of completion arteriography is its application and utility following carotid endarterectomy. The 1% incidence of neurologic complications seen after preoperative carotid arteriography (47-48) has led to reluctance on the part of some surgeons to employ intraoperative carotid angiography, where the additional dangers of emboli from air or fresh platelet aggregates are possible and neurologic complications as high as 2% have been reported (49). However, other surgeons routinely employ arteriography after endarterectomy, feeling that the benefits gained outweigh the risk of the procedure (50).

Technique is crucial to minimize the incidence of complications associated with intraoperative carotid arteriography. A 10-cc syringe with attached tubing and scalp vein needle is filled with heparinized saline. After meticulously removing all air bubbles, the needle is inserted in the common carotid artery proximal to the arteriotomy and its position verified by a return of arterial blood. The apparatus is flushed and clamped, and the syringe filled with 10 cc of undiluted Conray 60 (60% methylglucamine iothalamate). Since dyes containing sodium salts have been shown to be more toxic, these should be avoided for cerebral angiograpy (3).

Table 2 Results of Completion Angiography Following Carotid
Endarterectomy

Series	Patients	Positive Angiograms
Blaisdell (51)	100	26 (26%)
Anderson et al. (49)	131	7 (5%)
Scott et al. (56)	107	56 (52%)[a]
Lye et al. (57)	230	24 (10%)[b]
Gaspar (52,53)	813	66 (8%)[c]
Jernigan et al. (54)	603	15 (3%)
Alpert et al. (58)	40	2 (5%)
Zierler et al. (59)	150	23 (15%)[d]
Courbier et al. (55)	100	5 (5%)
Total	2274	224 (10%)

ECA = External carotid artery; ICA = internal carotid artery; CCA
= common carotid artery.
[a]Includes 27 ECA defects (six revised) and 29 ICA defects (12
revised).
[b]All cases represent ICA spasm.
[c]Includes 30 ECA revisions.
[d]Includes five ECA and eight ICA defects, not revised.

After occluding the proximal common carotid artery, the entire 10 cc is injected
rapidly and the film exposed with no delay.

In 1967, Blaisdell performed 100 angiograms following carotid endarterectomy
and detected defects in 26, including intracerebral thrombus in one patient (51).
Morbidity included hemiplegia in a single patient after normal arteriography. Since
then, numerous other centers (Table 2) have reported their experience with intraoperative completion carotid angiography (49,51-59). Gaspar et al. have a large
experience with over 800 completion intraoperative carotid angiograms (52,53).
In their series over 8% were abnormal, including lesions of the internal carotid (4%),
external carotid (3%), and common carotid arteries (1%). Examining their most
recent 457 angiograms in greater detail, they reported 11 patients with intracerebral thrombus. Two angiograms were falsely positive. After 18 revisions, four patients developed complications, including one death and three strokes.

Jernigan et al. documented angiographic abnormalities requiring revision in
15 of 603 (2.5%) consecutive carotid endarterectomies (54). In another study,
Courbier reexplored five of 100 patients with defects on completion angiography,

and noted a 2% stroke rate in this group compared with an 8.2% incidence of stroke in 206 historical controls at his institution (55). Courbier also obtained repeat carotid angiograms at a mean postoperative interval of 19.2 months. Of 60 minor abnormalities of the internal or common carotid artery noted at completion angiography but not revised, only 14 (23%) progressed to significant stenosis or occlusion.

In a similar study, Scott noted a 3.6% stroke rate in a group of 107 patients with completion angiograms, versus a 6.8% rate in 146 historical controls at the same hospital (56). Anderson observed defects in 5.3% of 131 completion angiograms, but accrued a 2.3% rate of complications associated with angiography, including two neurologic events (49). Using a method of completion contact angiography, Alpert discovered technical errors in two of 40 (5%) internal carotid arteries (58). In this method using portable dental X-ray equipment, the small film is placed directly in the operative field. The major advantage is reduced radiation scatter compared with conventional angiography.

Despite extensive published experience on completion angiography after carotid endarterectomy, there is no consensus regarding the indications for its use. There is agreement that completion angiograms will detect technical defects in a substantial number of patients. However, several major issues remain. First, what is the risk of obtaining this information, and can this information be obtained more safely by other modalities. Second, the ultimate issue is whether the detection and correction of angiographic defects results in a lower incidence of neurologic morbidity, i.e., do the detected defects have clinical significance and what type of defects require corrections.

The major disadvantage of completion arteriography is the risk of angiograph-induced neurologic complications. The rarity of these complications, plus the inability to segregate completion angiography and the operative procedure itself as causative factors, makes it difficult to estimate the risk of stroke from intraoperative angiography. However, in the literature there appears to be a 1-2% incidence of stroke related to completion angiography (49,51,54). Regardless of the absolute risk of angiography, it is clear that noninvasive modalities lessen or eliminate this consideration.

As discussed in Chapter 15, in addition to being safe, ultrasound is highly sensitive in detecting technical flaws after carotid endarterectomy (60). In a study directly comparing both intraoperative completion angiography and intraoperative Doppler spectral analysis, the latter exhibited 100% sensitivity though overall accuracy was reduced by a 10% rate of falsely positive results (59). Thus, it appears that noninvasive modalities can accurately detect technical errors after carotid endarterectomy, without the potential morbidity inherent in angiography.

The issue of the role of completion angiography in reducing stroke is not clear. Numerous events may account for perioperative stroke, including cerebral ischemia during clamping, embolization, thrombosis of the internal carotid artery, and intracerebral bleeding secondary to uncontrolled hypertension. Due to this multiplicity of factors affecting the incidence of stroke, prevention of technical errors will reduce but not eliminate perioperative stroke. For example, in Hertzer's series of 255 patients with digital subtraction angiography performed a few days after carotid endarterectomy, four patients with perioperative stroke had normal angiograms, and presumably did not have a stroke due to a technical error (61).

A further problem applicable both to arteriography and ultrasound is that these tests may detect defects of questionable clinical significance. Again looking at Hertzer's series, he found angiographic defects in 16 patients (6%), but only two had sustained perioperative neurologic complications. Courbier's longer follow-up of untreated defects seen on completion angiography also suggests a benign natural history for minor defects (55). Correction of these defects by unnecessary revision may not lessen perioperative stroke, and may even increase the risk of complications.

The decision routinely to employ intraoperative carotid angiography is a delicate tradeoff between the potential risks and benefits of this procedure. For the surgeon with an excessive perioperative stroke rate (i.e., 5-10%), technical flaws leading to thrombosis or embolization are likely to be implicated in a sizable number of strokes, and angiography can be reasonably expected to reduce the incidence of perioperative stroke. However, these technical errors can also be detected with less morbidity by ultrasound. For the surgeon with a stroke rate of 1-2%, the benefits from angiography may be more difficult to demonstrate. In such a case, if other modalities for the detection of technical defects (i.e., ultrasound) are available, we do not feel routine completion angiography following carotid endarterectomy is of benefit. Rather, selective utilization in difficult cases (high bifurcation, distal extension of plaque, inavailability of ultrasound) is more likely to yield benefits.

SUMMARY AND CONCLUSIONS

Intraoperative completion angiography is a very useful adjunct to the vascular surgeon after arterial reconstruction. Following elective lower extremity bypass, femoral embolectomy, and interposition grafting for trauma, completion arteriography should be employed routinely due to its ability to detect technical errors that may otherwise result in early graft failure. Following aortofemoral bypass, the yield from arteriography is considerably lower and benefits from routine use are unlikely. In contrast, the occult but serious nature of renal artery graft thrombosis makes the use of completion angiography rewarding in this setting. Following carotid endarterectomy, completion angiography may also yield useful information. However, the morbidity of carotid angiography and the accuracy of alternate methods such as ultrasound leads us to recommend selective application of angiography following carotid surgery.

REFERENCES

1. Shehadi WH, Toniolo G: Adverse reactions to contrast media. Radiology 137: 299, 1980.
2. Shehadi WH: Contrast media adverse reactions: Occurrence, recurrence, and distribution patterns. Radiology 143:11, 1982.
3. Rose, Jeffrey S: Contrast media, complications, and preparation of the patient. In Rutherford RB (ed): Vascular Surgery, WB Saunders, Philadelphia, pp. 244-252, 1984.
4. Swartz RD, Rubin JE, Leeming BW, Silva P: Renal failure following angiography. Am J Med 65:31, 1978.
5. D'Elia JA, Gleason RE, Alday M, Malarick C, Godley K, Warram J, Kaldany A, Weinrauch LA: Nephrotoxicity from angiographic contrast material. Am J Med 72:719, 1982.
6. Lang EK, Foreman J, Schlegel JU, Leslie C, List A, McCormick P: The incidence of contrast medium induced acute tubular necrosis following arteriography. Radiology 138:203, 1981.
7. Mason RA, Arbeit La, Giron F; Renal dysfunction after arteriography. J Am Med Assoc 253:1001, 1985.
8. Brewster DC, LaSalle AJ, Robison JG, Strayhorn EC, Darling RC: Femoropopliteal graft failures. Arch Surg 118:1043, 1983.
9. Cranley JJ, Hafner CD: Revascularization of the femoropopliteal arteries using saphenous vein, polytetrafluoroethylene and umbilical vein grafts. Arch Surg 17:1543, 1982.
10. Reichle FA, Rankin KP, Tyson RR, Finestone AJ, Sherman C: Long-term results of 474 arterial reconstructions for severely ischemic limbs. Surgery 85:93, 1979.
11. Reichle FA, Martinson MW, Rankin KP: Infrapopliteal arterial reconstruction in the severely ischemic lower extremity. Ann Surg 191:59, 1980.
12. Craver JM, Ottinger LW, Darling RC, Austen WG, Linton RR: Hemorrhage and thrombosis as early complications of femoropopliteal bypass grafts. Surgery 74:839, 1973.
13. Flinn WR, Harris JP, Rudo ND, Bergan JJ, Yao JST: Results of repetitive distal revascularization. Surgery 91:566, 1982.
14. Sproul G, Pinto JM, Trummer MJ, Stevens DM: Reoperation for early complications of arterial surgery. Arch Surg 104:814, 1972.
15. Brooks B: Intra-arterial injection of sodium iodide. J Am Med Assoc 82: 1016, 1924.
16. Liddicoat JE, Bekassy SM, DeBakey ME: Intraoperative arteriography during femoral-popliteal bypass. Arch Surg 110:839, 1975.
17. Johnson WC: Operative angiography for femoro-popliteal vein bypass reconstruction. Am J Surg 126:120, 1973.
18. Pinkerton JA Jr: Operative arteriography. Arch Surg 110:841, 1975.
19. Flanigan DP, Williams LR, Keifer T, Schuler JJ, Behrend AJ: Prebypass operative arteriography. Surgery 92:627, 1982.

20. Malone JM, Moore WS, Goldstone J: The natural history of bilateral aorto-femoral bypass grafts for ischemia of the lower extremities. Arch Surg 110: 1300, 1975.

21. Crawford ES, Bomberger RA, Glaeser DH, Saleh SA, Russell WL: Aortoiliac occlusive disease: Factors influencing survival and function following reconstructive operation over a twenty-five year period. Surgery 90:1055, 1981.

22. Bowald S, Eriksson I, Fagerberg S: Intraoperative angiography in arterial surgery. Acta Chir Scand 144:463, 1978.

23. Tchirkow G, Beven EG; Leg ischemia following surgery for abdominal aortic aneurysm. Ann Surg 188:166, 1978.

24. Strom JA, Bernhard VM, Towne JB: Acute limb ischemia following aortic reconstruction. Arch Surg 119:470, 1984.

25. Martinez BD, Hertzer NR, Beven EG: Influence of distal arterial occlusive disease on prognosis following aortobifemoral bypass. Surgery 88:795, 1980.

26. Jones AF, Kempczinski RF: Aortofemoral bypass grafting. Arch Surg 116: 301, 1981.

27. Renwick S, Royle JP, Martin P: Operative angiography after femoropopliteal arterial reconstruction—its influence on early failure rate. Br J Surg 55:134, 1968.

28. Courbier R, Jausseran JM, Reggi M: Detecting complications of direct arterial surgery. Arch Surg 112:1115, 1977.

29. Liebman PR, Menzoian JO, Mannick JA, Lowney BW, LoGerfo FW: Intraoperative arteriography in femoropopliteal and femorotibial bypass grafts. Arch Surg 116:1019, 1981.

30. Plecha FR, Pories WJ: Intraoperative angiography in the immediate assessment of arterial reconstruction. Arch Surg 105:902, 1972.

31. Crowley JG: Intraoperative angiography. Am Surg 46:328, 1980.

32. Dardik II, Ibrahim IM, Sprayregen S, Veith F, Dardik H: Routine intraoperative angiography. An essential adjunct in vascular surgery. Arch Surg 110: 184, 1975.

33. Dardik H, Ibrahim IM, Koslow A, Dardik II: Evaluation of intraoperative arteriography as a routine for vascular reconstructions. Surg Gynecol Obstet 147:853, 1978.

34. Hackler MT, Bunt TJ: Negative impact of routine postreconstructive intraoperative angiography in lower extremity revascularization. Am Surg 49:15, 1983.

35. Coelho JCU, Sigel B, Flanigan DP, Schuler JJ, Spigos DG, Tan WS, Justin J: An experimental evaluation of arteriography and imaging ultrasonography in detecting arterial defects at operation. J Surg Res 32:130, 1982.

36. Sigel B, Coelho JCU, Flanigan DP, Schuler JJ, Machi J, Beitler JC: Detection of vascular defects during operation by imaging ultrasound. Ann Surg 196: 473, 1982.

37. Green RM, DeWeese JA, Rob CG: Arterial embolectomy before and after the Fogarty catheter. Surgery 77:24, 1975.

38. Elliott JP Jr, Hazeman JH, Szilagyi DE, Ramakrishnan V, Bravo JJ, Smith RF: Arterial embolization: Problems of source, multiplicity, recurrence and delayed treatment. Surgery 88:833, 1980.

39. Pasch AR, Bishara RA, Lim LT, Meyer JP, Schuler JJ, Flanigan DP: Optimal limb salvage in penetrating civilian vascular trauma. J Vasc Surg 3:189, 1986.

40. Dean RH, Wilson JP, Burko H, Foster JH: Saphenous vein aortorenal bypass grafts. Ann Surg 180:469, 1974.

41. Stanley JC, Whitehouse WM, Zelenock GB, Graham LM, cronenwett JL, Lindenauer SM: Reoperation for complications of renal artery reconstructive surgery undertaken for treatment of renovascular hypertension. J Vasc Surg 2: 133, 1985.

42. Stanley JC, Ernst CB, Fry WJ: Fate of 100 aortorenal vein grafts. Surgery 74: 931, 1973.

43. Stoney RJ: Transaortic renal endarterectomy. In Rutherford RB (ed): Vascular Surgery, WB Saunders, Philadelphia, pp. 1130-1135, 1984.

44. Nagasue N, Ogawa Y, Yukawa H, Hirose S: Intraoperative direct portography to achieve selective distal splenorenal shunt. Surg Gynecol Obstet 161:52, 1985.

45. Hertzer NR: Circulatory access for hemodialysis. In Rutherford RB (ed): Vascular Surgery, WB Saunders, Philadelphia, pp. 244-252, 1984.

46. Plate G, Einarsson E, Ohlia P, Jensen R, QvarFordt P, Eklof B: Thrombectomy with temporary arteriovenous fistula: The treatment of choice in acute iliofemoral venous thrombosis. J Vasc Surg 1:867, 1984.

47. Kerber CW, Cromwell LD, Drayer P, Bank WO: Cerebral ischemia. I. Current angiographic techniques, complications and safety. Am J Roentgenol 130: 1097, 1978.

48. Mani RL, Eisenberg RL, McDonald EJ Jr, Pollock JA, Mani JR: Complications of catheter crebral arteriography: Analysis of 5000 procedures. I. Criteria and incidence. Am J Roentgenol 131:864, 1978.

49. Andersen CA, Collins GJ Jr, Rich NM: Routine operative arteriography during carotid endarterectomy: A reassessment. Surgery 83:67, 1978.

50. Moore WS: Operative technique. In Rutherford RB (ed): Vascular Surgery, WB Saunders, Philadelphia, pp. 1248-1266, 1984.

51. Blaisdell FW, Lim R Jr, Hall AD: Technical results of carotid endarterectomy: Arteriographic assessment. Am J Surg 114:239, 1967.

52. Rosental JJ, Gaspar MR, Movius HJ: Intraoperative arteriography in carotid thromboendarterectomy. Arch Surg 106:806, 1973.

53. Larson SR, Gaspar MR, Movius HJ, Rosental JJ, Bell DD, Lemire GG: Intraoperative arteriography in cerebrovascular surgery. In Bergan JJ and Yao JST (eds): Cerebrovascular Insufficiency, Grune & Stratton, New York, pp. 353-365, 1983.

54. Jernigan WR, Fulton RL, Hamman JL, Miller FB, Mani SS: The efficacy of routine completion operative angiography in reducing the incidence of perioperative stroke associated with carotid endarterectomy. Surgery 96:831, 1984.

55. Courbier R, Jausseran JM, Bergeron P, Reggi M, Formichi M, Ferdani M: Routine intra-operative carotid angiography: Its impact on operative morbidity and carotid restenosis. J Vasc Surg (in press).

56. Scott SM, Sethi GK, Bridgman AH: Perioperative stroke during carotid endarterectomy: The value of intraoperative angiography. J Cardiovasc Surg 23: 353, 1982.

57. Lye CR, Morrow IM, Downs AR: Carotid artery spasm. Arch surg 117:1531, 1982.

58. Alpert J, Brener BJ, Parsonnet V, Meisner K, Sadow S, Brief DK, Goldenkranz RJ: Carotid endarterectomy and completion contact arteriography. J Vasc Surg 1:548, 1984.

59. Zierler RE, Bandyk DF, Thiele BL: Intraoperative assessment of carotid endarterectomy. J Vasc Surg 1:74, 1984.

60. Douglas DJ, Flanigan DP, Schuler JJ, Buchbinder D: Intraoperative ultrasound imaging of the carotid artery during carotid endarterectomy. J Vasc Surg (in press).

61. Hertzer NR, Beven EG, Modic MT, O'Hara PJ, Vogt DP, Weinstein MA: Early patency of the carotid artery after endarterectomy: Digital subtraction angiography after two hundred sixty-four operations. Surgery 92:1049, 1982.

15

Intraoperative Ultrasound Assessment of Vascular Reconstructions

DANIEL J. DOUGLAS and D. PRESTON FLANIGAN
University of Illinois College of Medicine at Chicago
Chicago, Illinois

Technical errors and intraluminal defects resulting from the performance of a vascular anatomosis can lead to early graft thrombosis and occlusion (1). Also, technical defects created during the performance of a carotid endarterectomy can lead to carotid artery thrombosis or act as a source of embolism, both of which may cause a subsequent hemispheric stroke.

The technical defects that can lead to subsequent graft failure or stroke include intimal flaps, anastomotic or endarterectomy suture line strictures, and intraluminal thrombi. These defects have been shown by intraoperative arteriography to occur as often as 24% of the time at anastomotic sites (2) and as often as 26% of the time at the site of carotid endarterectomy (3).

The detection and correction of these defects prior to the termination of the operation should lead to improved early graft patency for vascular bypass procedures and a decreased incidence of perioperative stroke for carotid endarterectomies. This would in turn lead to fewer early reoperations, which have been shown to increase patient mortality (1,4).

Inspection and palpation are not reliable methods of detecting these defects (3,5). In addition, many of these defects are not hemodynamically significant, and therefore, may not be detected by electromagnetic flowmeter determination (6) or segmental Doppler examination. The use of pulsed Doppler and spectrum analysis has been shown to be a sensitive method of detecting intraluminal defects, but requires an arteriogram to provide an image of the defect that is creating the flow disturbance in order to decide if the defect is significant enough to warrant reentry into the artery (7).

255

Routine use of intraoperative completion arteriography has been advocated by many as a means of assessing the technical adequacy of a vascular reconstruction (2,3,5,6,8-10). Even though arteriography provides an image of the endarterectomy site or anastomosis, it is an invasive procedure with complications, which include the creation of intraluminal defects (11), radiation exposure to both the surgeon and patient, contrast medium toxicity (12), and stroke when used to assess the results of carotid endarterectomy (13). Also, the image that arteriography provides is uniplanar (usually the anterior to posterior projection) and static. Although the incidence of complications resulting from the use of intraoperative arteriography is relatively low, it seems desirable to have a noninvasive method for evaluating the technical adequacy of an anastomosis or endarterectomy, especially when evaluating the extracranial carotid bifurcation.

Intraoperative high-resolution, real-time, B-mode ultrasonography is a noninvasive method of evaluating the technical adequacy of a vascular reconstruction that offers several advantages over arteriography. It is a safe procedure without the complications that can occur with arteriography. It provides a dynamic image in several planes, thereby detecting defects that might otherwise be missed with a uniplanar image. In addition, it may be repeated as often as is necessary to ensure an adequate technical result without concern over dye load or radiation exposure.

Prior to using intraoperative ultrasound routinely in clinical practice, both the ability of ultrasound to detect technical defects and the relative accuracy of ultrasound as compared with arteriography in detecting these defects were evaluated experimentally in our laboratory.

EXPERIMENTAL RESULTS

Intraoperative ultrasound was evaluated in two separate animal experiments. In the first experiment (14) the accuracy of ultrasound in detecting surgically created vascular defects was assessed. A series of defects, including intimal flaps, strictures, intraluminal thrombi, and subintimal hematomas, were surgically created in canine aortas and femoral arteries. All of the strictures, intraluminal thrombi, and subintimal hematomas were correctly identified by ultrasound. Intimal flaps that were 2 mm or larger were identified 100% of the time and intimal flaps measuring 1 mm were identified 68% of the time. In 89.7% of the instances, the ultrasound measurement of flap size was within 1 mm of the actual measured size, for a correlation coefficient of 0.84.

In the second experimental study (15) intraoperative ultrasound was compared to both portable and serial biplane arteriography in their ability to detect vascular defects that were surgically created in canine aortas. All three methods of intraoperative assessment were equally accurate in detecting strictures, however, ultrasound was more accurate and sensitive than both portable and serial biplane arteriography in detecting 2-mm and 5-mm intimal flaps and intraluminal thrombi.

Since intraoperative ultrasound proved to be a reliable method for detecting technical defects and because it was found to be as accurate as intraoperative arteriography and is without the complications of arteriography, it was used clinically to assess the technical adequacy of vascular reconstructions.

MATERIALS AND METHODS

Over the past 5.5 years, during which time intraoperative ultrasound has been used at our institution, a variety of small parts, high-resolution, real-time, B-mode scanners have been utilized. The machine is positioned near the operating table in clear view of the operator. Either a 7.5-MHz or 10-MHz probe is used. This frequency usually offers adequate tissue penetration for vascular reconstructions and provides a high-resolution image that will detect defects as small as 1 mm. The probe and cord are either gas-sterilized or, more commonly, covered by a sterile disposable plastic sleeve that has been filled at one end with acoustic gel. The probe is hand-held by the operator and positioned in the wound directly over the site to be examined without coming into contact with the vessel. Sterile saline is then instilled into the wound to assure acoustic coupling between the probe and vessel. This will allow visualization of the entire vessel as well as the anterior vessel wall without compression. For peripheral vascular sites, the wound edges are retracted upward to ensure that the saline will remain in the wound.

Longitudinal scans in several different planes are made to ensure complete visualization of the vessel lumen. Transverse scans are then performed to offer three-dimensional information. The entire operative site including the anastomosis, clamp sites, suture line, or entire extent of an endarterectomy are scanned. The ultrasound is performed just after completion of an anastomosis or endarterectomy and release of all clamps. Permanent records are kept on video cassette or Polaroid prints.

When a defect is found, the decision to reenter the vessel and correct the defect is based upon the type, size, and location of the defect. Defects that are corrected are those that, in the judgment of the surgeon, may lead to early graft failure or may be a potential cause of perioperative stroke if left uncorrected in the carotid artery position.

CLINICAL RESULTS

Between October 1979 and March 1985, intraoperative ultrasound was used at our institution to evaluate the technical results of 998 anastomotic or endarterectomy sites in 550 vascular reconstructions. The various types and relative frequencies of vascular reconstructions evaluated are represented in Table 1. Over one-fourth of the operations in which intraoperative ultrasound was used were carotid endarterectomies.

Table 1 Type and Number of Vascular Reconstructions
Evaluated with Intraoperative Ultrasound

Operation		N
Infrainguinal bypass		204
Femoropopliteal	(93)	
Femorotibial	(67)	
Femoropopliteal-tibial	(21)	
Popliteal-tibial	(19)	
Iliopopliteal	(2)	
Iliopopliteal-tibial	(1)	
Axillopopliteal	(1)	
Carotid endarterectomy		155
Suprainguinal bypass		142
Aortofemoral (bifemoral)		
Aorotioliac (biiliac)	(83)	
Femorofemoral	(40)	
Axillofemoral (bifemoral)	(14)	
Aortoaorta	(5)	
Portal decompression shunts		11
Splenorenal	(7)	
Mesocaval	(2)	
Porotcaval	(2)	
Carotid subclavian bypass		6
Miscellaneous		32
Total		550

Technical defects were detected using intraoperative ultrasound in 199 of the
998 (20%) anastomotic or endarterectomy sites that were examined. Of the total
number of operations in which intraoperative ultrasound was used, technical defects were present in 36%. The relative frequencies of technical defects detected
by ultrasound are represented in Table 2. Intimal flaps were the most common defects found, representing nearly two-thirds of all defects. Anastomotic or endarterectomy suture line strictures, intraluminal thrombi, residual plaque, and kinking
were somewhat less frequent, collectively comprising the remaining one-third of
the defects. Representative ultrasound images of an intimal flap, stricture, and intraluminal thrombus are illustrated in Figures 1, 2, and 3, respectively.

Sixty-two (31%) of the 199 defects found were corrected by reentering the
anastomotic or endarterectomy site. This represented 6% of all sites evaluated with

Table 2 Type and Frequency of Technical Defects Detected with Intraoperative Ultrasound

Type of Defect	N	%
Intimal flaps	130	65
Strictures	32	16
Intraluminal thrombi	24	12
Residual plaque	11	6
Kink	2	1
Total	199	100

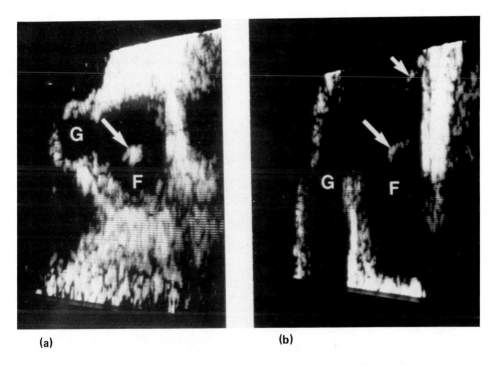

(a)   (b)

Figure 1 Intraoperative ultrasound image of a 2-mm intimal flap at the femoral to graft anastomosis of a femoropopliteal bypass. (a) Transverse plane; (b) longitudinal view.

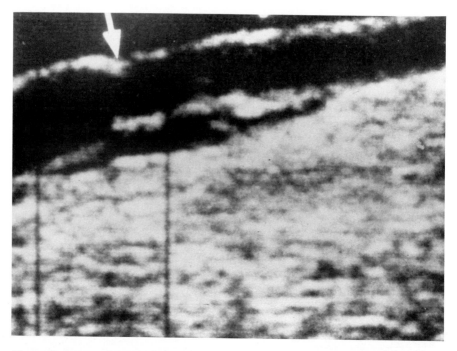

Figure 2 Intraoperative ultrasound image of a 40% stricture involving the suture line of a saphenous vein composite graft.

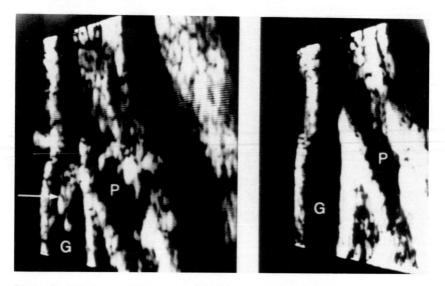

Figure 3 (Left) Intraoperative ultrasound image of a 5-mm intraluminal thrombus at a graft to popliteal anastomosis. (Right) Ultrasound image of the same segment of artery after surgical correction of the defect.

Table 3 Type, Size, and Location of Technical Defects
Corrected

Type of Defect	Number and Location
Intimal flap	24 (39%)
1 mm	1 Fem
2 mm	3 Tib, 1 Pop
3 mm	3 ECA, 3 Fem, 1 ICA, 1 Tib
4 mm	2 Fem, 1 Iliac
5 mm	3 Fem, 1 Pop, 1 ICA
7 mm	1 ICA, 1 Aorta, 1 Fem
Stricture	19 (30%)
20%	1 Pop, 1 Tib
30%	1 ICA, 1 B, 1 Tib, 1 Fem
40%	1 ASVG, 1 PC, 1 Fem
50%	3 ICA, 2 Fem, 1 Tib
60%	1 Tib
90%	1 Iliac
Thrombus	16 (26%)
1 mm	2 Tib, 2 Fem, 1 SR
2 mm	2 Tib, 1 CCA, 1 PC
3 mm	1 Fem
5 mm	1 Pop, 1 Fem
Occluded	2 Tib, 1 ASVG, 1 SR
Plaque	2 (3%)
3 mm	1 ICA
10 mm	1 Tib
Kink	1 (2%) Tib

Abbreviations: Fem = Femoral artery; Tib = tibial artery;
Pop = popliteal artery; ECA = external carotid artery; ICA
= internal carotid artery; CCA = common carotid artery;
B = brachial artery; ASVG = autogenous saphenous vein
graft; PC = portacaval shunt; SR = splenorenal shunt.

intraoperative ultrasound. The type and location of defects that were repaired are
represented in Table 3. The majority of these defects were intimal flaps 3 mm or
larger, strictures 30% or greater, and intraluminal thrombi. The intraoperative ultrasound image and corresponding arteriogram of a 5-mm intimal flap found in a popliteal artery at the site of a vascular clamp is illustrated in Figure 4 and represents a
defect that was repaired.

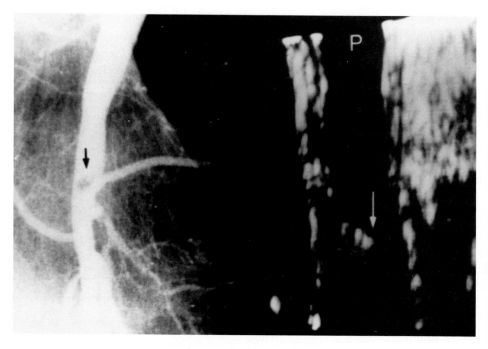

Figure 4 Intraoperative ultrasound image and corresponding arteriogram of a 5-mm intimal flap in a popliteal artery resulting from the application of a vascular clamp.

Sixty-seven percent of the defects detected were thought to be insignificant in size or location and were not repaired. The majority of these defects were small intimal flaps or strictures that were located in relatively large-diameter vessels such as the 2-mm intimal flap found at the proximal extent of a carotid endarterectomy that is illustrated in Figure 5.

COMPARISON BETWEEN ARTERIOGRAPHY AND ULTRASOUND

Of the 998 anastomotic or endarterectomy sites evaluated by intraoperative ultra-sound, intraoperative arteriography was also performed in 211. These 211 sites examined by both methods of intraoperative assessment allowed an excellent opportunity to compare the two methods. When both the ultrasound and arteriogram were negative for technical defects, this was considered a true negative examination.

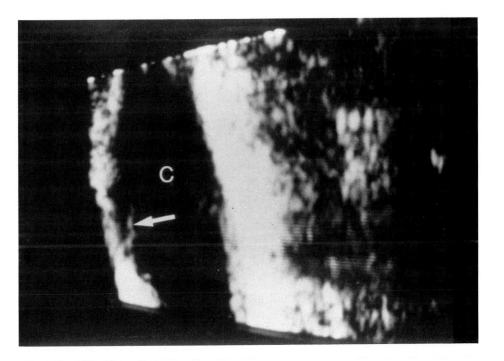

Figure 5 Intraoperative ultrasound image of a 2-mm intimal flap at the proximal extent of an endarterectomy in the common carotid artery.

When either method detected a defect and this was substantiated by reexploration and confirmation, this was considered a true positive examination. False negative and false positive examinations were determined by reexploration.

The true positive, true negative, false positive, and false negative examinations of each method of intraoperative assessment are represented in Table 4. The sensitivity, specificity, accuracy, and positive and negative predictive values of each method were then calculated. The results are illustrated in Table 5.

As can be seen from Table 5, the sensitivity, specificity, accuracy, and negative predictive value of both methods of assessment are comparable. However, intraoperative ultrasound is clearly superior to intraoperative arteriography with regard to the positive predictive value of the test. This reflects the higher number of false-positive arteriograms relative to the number of false-positive ultrasound examinations. Therefore, the number of negative reexplorations would be less if intraoperative ultrasound were used as a guide to reexploration of a vessel.

Table 4 Comparison between Ultrasound and Arteriography

Ultrasound			Arteriography		
	N	%		N	%
TP	27	13	TP	27	13
TN	178	84	TN	170	80
FP	4	2	FP	12	6
FN	2	1	FN	2	1
Total	211	100	Total	211	100

Abbreviations: TP = true positive; TN = true negative; FP = false positive; FN = false negative.

Table 5 Comparative Accuracy of Ultrasound and Arteriography

	Ultrasound (%)	Arteriography (%)
Sensitivity	93.1	93.1
Specificity	97.8	93.4
Accuracy	97.2	93.4
Positive predictive value	87.1	69.2
Negative predictive value	98.9	98.8

INTRAOPERATIVE ULTRASOUND IN CAROTID SURGERY

The use of intraoperative ultrasound in the evaluation of carotid endarterectomy deserves special mention, as it is probably in this location that ultrasound imaging in vascular surgery has its greatest utility. Because the limits of endarterectomy and clamp sites are within the confines of the wound, the entire area of concern can be evaluated with ultrasound. Also, because intraoperative arteriography carries with it the risk of stroke and the possibility of producing intraluminal defects that may subsequently lead to stroke, and because the run-off vessels need not be visualized, intraoperative ultrasonography is preferred to intraoperative arteriography for routine assessment of the technical adequacy of carotid endarterectomy.

Our experience with intraoperative ultrasound imaging of the carotid artery was analyzed separately from the rest of the vascular reconstructions. Technical defects were detected in 43 (28%) of the 155 endarterectomy sites evaluated and included intimal flaps (73%); strictures (18%); and kinks, residual plaque, and intraluminal thrombi (9% collectively). Seven percent of the endarterectomy sites were reentered to correct a defect. Defects that were corrected were again largely intimal flaps 3-mm or larger, strictures 30% or greater, intraluminal thrombi, and kinks.

In follow-up averaging 13 months, there was no statistically significant difference in ipsilateral hemispheric stroke between those patients with a normal intraoperative ultrasound, those patients who had a defect detected and corrected, and those patients with insignificant defects that were not repaired. This suggested that reentering and correcting a defect, which was judged by the surgeon as being significant by virtue of its type, size, and location, did not, in and of itself, lead to a higher incidence of perioperative stroke. Also, the decision not to correct smaller or less significant defects was correct since leaving these defects uncorrected again did not lead to a higher incidence of perioperative stroke.

SUMMARY

In our experience with the use of intraoperative ultrasound, technical defects have been detected in over one-third of the vascular reconstructions in which it has been used. Since many of these defects may lead to early graft failure or potentiate perioperative strokes when in the carotid position, it is probably reasonable to evaluate the technical adequacy of all vascular reconstructions.

For this purpose, intraoperative ultrasound offers several advantages over intraoperative arteriography. The safety of ultrasound is supported by the fact that there have been no complications attributable to its use since we began using it in the evaluation of vascular reconstructions. Arteriography, on the other hand, is an invasive procedure with the potential of producing complications of its own. Intraoperative ultrasound provides images in several different planes at several different points in time as opposed to the static image in only one plane offered by arteriography. Also, ultrasound may be repeated as often as is necessary to ensure an adequate technical reconstruction.

Although the sensitivity, specificity, accuracy, and negative predictive value of the two tests are comparable, the positive predictive value of intraoperative ultrasound is higher and, will therefore, lead to fewer negative reexplorations.

Even though intraoperative ultrasound is superior to arteriography in several respects, it does have certain limitations. Ultrasound has a high resolution and is able to detect defects that may be insignificant and thus can be safely left uncorrected. However, it is not entirely clear exactly which defects can be safely left uncorrected and which defects may jeopardize a vascular reconstruction. To this point this decision has been based upon the size, type, and location of the defect. Undoubtably a more exact definition of insignificant defects will be provided with further experience with intraoperative ultrasound and patient follow-up.

Another limitation of intraoperative ultrasound is its inability to visualize vessels beyond the confines of the surgical wound. This is not an important consideration in assessing the technical results of carotid endarterectomy. Further, since arteriography can cause stroke when used to assess the results of this procedure, we prefer to use intraoperative ultrasound as a sole means of assessing carotid endarterectomy. Also, because of the technical limitations of arteriography in abdominal vascular procedures and femoral anatomoses, we also use only ultrasound to evaluate the results of these reconstructions. However, with more peripheral vascular reconstructions, we feel it is important to visualize the run-off vessels, and therefore, use both methods of assessment in these procedures.

In conclusion, both intraoperative ultrasound and intraoperative arteriography each have their own advantages and limitations. Many vascular reconstructions require the use of both tests in a complementary fashion. On the other hand, vascular reconstructions such as abdominal procedures and carotid endarterectomies can be assessed exclusively with intraoperative ultrasound. Intraoperative ultrasound is an important, safe, and accurate method of assessing the technical adequacy of vascular reconstructions and will likely prove to be a valuable means of decreasing the incidence of early bypass graft failure and perioperative stroke when used routinely.

REFERENCES

1. Craver JM, Ottinger LW, Darling RC, Austen WG, Linton RR: Hemorrhage and thrombosis as early complications of femoropopliteal bypass grafts: Causes, treatment, and prognostic implications. Surgery 6:839, 1973.
2. Plecha FR, Pories WJ: Intraoperative angiography in the immediate assessment of arterial reconstruction. Arch Surg 105:902, 1972.
3. Blaisdell FW, Lim R, Hall AD: Technical result of carotid endarterectomy. Arteriographic assessment. Am J Surg 114:239, 1967.
4. Sprone G, Pinto JM, Trummer MJ, Stevens DM: Reoperation for early complications of arterial surgery. Arch Surg 104:814, 1972.
5. Rosental JJ, Gaspar MR, Movius HJ: Intraoperative arteriography in carotid thromboendarterectomy. Arch Surg 106:806, 1973.
6. Bowald S, Eriksson I, Fagerberg S: Intraoperative angiography in arterial surgery. Acta Chir Scand 144:463, 1978.
7. Zierler RE, Bandyk DF, Thiele BL: Intraoperative assessment of carotid endarterectomy. J Vasc Surg 1:73, 1984.
8. Courbier R, Jausseran JM, Reggi M: Detecting complications of direct arterial surgery: The role of intraoperative arteriography. Arch Surg 112:1115, 1977.

9. Dardik II, Ibrahim IM, Sprayregen S, Veith F, Dardik H: Routine intraoperative angiography: An essential adjunct in vascular surgery. Arch Surg 110: 184, 1975.
10. Crowley JG: Intraoperative angiography. Am Surg 46:328, 1980.
11. Pories WJ, Plecha FR, Castele TJ, Strain WH: Complications of arteriography and phlebography. In: GH Beebe (ed), Complications in Vascular Surgery, JB Lippincott, Philadelphia, 1973, p. 1.
12. Ansell G: Adverse reactions to contrast agents: Scope of problem. Invest Radiol 5:373, 1970.
13. Anderson CA, Collins GJ, Rich NM: Routine operative arteriography during carotid endarterectomy: A reassessment. Surg 83:67, 1978.
14. Coelho JCU, Sigel B, Flanigan DP, Schuler JJ, Spigos DG, Nyhus LM: Detection of arterial defects by real-time ultrasound scanning during vascular surgery: An experimental study. J Surg Research 30:535, 1981.
15. Coelho JCU, Sigel B, Flanigan DP, Schuler JJ, Spigos DG, Tan WS, Justin J: An experimental evaluation of arteriography and imaging ultrasonography in detecting arterial defects at operation. J Surg Research 32:130, 1982.

16

Detection of Vascular Defects Utilizing Intraoperative Spectral Analysis

BRIAN L. THIELE
The Milton S. Hershey Medical Center,
The Pennsylvania State University
  College of Medicine
Hershey, Pennsylvania

INTRODUCTION

Objective intraoperative assessment of arterial reconstruction is a widely accepted principle and practice in vascular surgery, and it is essential if optimal results are to be obtained by excluding technical error as a cause of early failure. In recent years there has been a proliferation of techniques for this purpose, each of which has its own advantages and disadvantages. Although arteriography has been the technique most commonly used, ultrasound technology in particular has been used increasingly because of its dual capability of providing morphologic and physiologic information. The use of pulsed Doppler ultrasound with real-time spectral analysis for assessing the technical adequacy of arterial reconstruction in multiple locations is reviewed here.

THE RATIONALE

The major goal of any intraoperative method of assessing the technical adequacy of arterial reconstruction is to identify problems likely to predispose to immediate or premature failure. The types of procedures in which intraoperative evaluation is likely to be of greatest value include those that are technically demanding because of the small size of the anastomoses involved, such as femorotibial bypass grafts, or those in which failure is likely to be associated with catastrophic sequelae, such as carotid endarterectomy. Additionally, renal and visceral artery reconstruction

269

create circumstances in which postoperative assessment is extremely difficult, and the price of failed reconstruction is also catastrophic, with either renal or mesenteric infarction. The rationale for the use of intraoperative assessment in each of these procedures will be discussed separately.

CAROTID ENDARTERECTOMY

The concept of intraoperative assessment of this procedure has not been widely accepted or instituted and, when performed, has generally taken the form of operative arteriography. Much of the resistance to intraoperative assessment comes from a belief by many surgeons that it is too time-consuming and potentially hazardous, with a relatively low incidence of detected abnormalities, thereby not justifying its routine use. There is, however, compelling data from series in which operative arteriography has been used routinely for carotid endarterectomy that there is a significant incidence of unrecognized technical defects. Blaisdell et al. (1) evaluated their experience in 100 patients and identified a less than ideal technical result in 25%, with stenoses of varying degrees in 21% and complete occlusion in 4%. Early patency (10-60 days) in 95 patients was also evaluated, with 94 normal and one with complete occlusion. In this report there was a 3% perioperative neurological complication rate and a 4% mortality—excellent results for the time at which the report appeared.

Rosental et al. (2) reported the results obtained with routine operative arteriography in 260 consecutive carotid endarterectomies; significant technical defects were noted in 8%. Half of these (4%) occurred in the external carotid artery, and the other 4% were located in the common or internal carotid artery in the mainstream of the endarterectomy site. Although the authors did not report their neurological complication rate, they concluded that routine operative arteriography resulted in a more critical review of the surgical technique used and recommended its routine use.

More recently, Zierler et al. (3) reported their findings in 150 consecutive cases of carotid endarterectomy in which operative arteriography was employed routinely for assessing the technical adequacy of the procedure. In this series, defects were detected in 8% of the operative arteriograms, with 5% being in the internal carotid and 3% the external carotid. These defects were considered technically unacceptable and, in all cases in which the internal carotid was affected, were repaired, usually by patch angioplasty. In this series there were no perioperative neurological complications, a feature stressing the importance of technical factors in the development of perioperative neurological deficits.

The incidence of technical errors documented in these series is low, but had they not been identified, it is quite possible that the neurological complication rate would have been greater and likely to increase to the point of being unacceptable.

The striking similarity between the results obtained in the large series reported by Rosental et al. and that of Zierler et al. emphasizes that even when meticulous care is taken during carotid endarterectomy, technical defects can occur. In view of the potentially catastrophic sequelae, it would seem most appropriate that they be identified early.

Other approaches have been used to overcome the theoretical disadvantages of intraoperative arteriography in particular; the most common technique utilized is oculoplethysmography (4). There are, however, two major difficulties with this approach. The first of these is that it is performed in the recovery room, which for some patients will be too late to avoid the serious sequelae of technical errors during the performance of the procedure. Evaluating the adequacy of carotid endarterectomy at this time is only likely to have an impact on neurological deficits that develop in the days following surgery, which are in fact relatively uncommon. The second difficulty relates to the fact that this particular technique is sensitive only to very severe high-grade stenoses, and it is quite probable that technical defects of lesser magnitude are capable of producing serious complications and, as such, would not be identified with this approach. Clearly, if it is identified that an acceptable technical result has been obtained in the operating room, the endarterectomy site itself can virtually be excluded as a cause of subsequent neurological problems.

IN SITU DISTAL BYPASS GRAFTING

The emergence of in situ bypass grafting as the procedure of choice for distal revascularization of the lower extremity (5) provides the surgeon with a series of potential technical difficulties that lend themselves very appropriately to the need for some form of intraoperative assessment.

The first of these relates to the straightforward technical aspect of performing the distal anastomosis to very small vessels that may or may not be diseased. Although operative magnification is used routinely and contributes significantly to the avoidance of technical problems, most proponents of this procedure stress the necessity for intraoperative assessment of the distal arterial reconstruction (6). While indirect techniques such as the use of continuous-wave Doppler auscultation of the distal arteries are used by many, this really only provides relatively subjective information regarding the technical adequacy of the distal reconstruction and by no means guarantees long-term success. Operative arteriography is the most widely used method of intraoperative evaluation but provides morphological information in a single-plane view, a circumstance in which it is possible to miss problems because of the lack of three-dimensional information.

The second aspect of this procedure that requires evaluation is the completeness of valve lysis, which, again, can be assessed arteriographically but also suffers from the lack of three-dimensional information. The lack of resolution for minor defects due to varying concentrations of contrast material within the vein lumen may also contribute to difficulty identifying such problems.

Finally, optimal function of these grafts necessitates that arteriovenous fistulas be recognized and excluded, preferably avoiding circumferential mobilization of the vein. Here again, arteriographic studies are preferred, but they require that two exposures be used to encompass the full length of the graft. Arteriography in good hands may provide very good evidence of the technical adequacy of the procedure, but it does not provide any data about the functional aspects of the graft. An ideal form of intraoperative assessment of this procedure, therefore, should address this triad of issues: (a) the technical and functional characteristics of the distal reconstruction, (b) adequacy of valve lysis, and (c) exclusion of arteriovenous fistulae.

VISCERAL ARTERY RECONSTRUCTION

Visceral artery reconstruction is associated with a unique set of circumstances in which intraoperative arteriographic assessment and postoperative assessment of graft function are extremely difficult; reliance is placed on clinical assessment in the postoperative period, an approach that is relatively insensitive. In both renal and mesenteric revascularization procedures, it is almost impossible to obtain operative arteriography of good technical quality routinely because of the difficulties encountered in optimizing exposure of radiographs, in part due to the extremely high flow rates encountered in the abdominal aorta. In the case of renal revascularization, particularly when this is performed for correction of renal insufficiency, the addition of a contrast material insult to an already abnormal kidney that has also experienced varying degrees of warm ischemia is not in the best interests of optimizing postoperative renal function. In these circumstances in particular, there is a real need for an appropriate objective method for assessing the technical adequacy of the reconstruction, thus ensuring good postoperative graft function. As with carotid endarterectomy, the price of failed reconstruction is usually disastrous, with loss of the kidney due to the delay encountered in recognizing this problem. In mesenteric revascularization procedures, the patient's life may be endangered if the reconstruction fails due to the catastrophic systemic sequelae of mesenteric ischemia, and there is perhaps an even greater need to exclude the possibility of technical error.

There is no doubt that with the passage of time and increasing critical appraisal of the technical aspects of vascular reconstruction, more objective methods of intraoperative assessment of all arterial reconstructions will gradually be implemented. The overriding philosophy must be that all failures due to technical problems are potentially avoidable with meticulous initial technique and with the identification of error at the earliest possible time, which is ideally at the time of the initial procedure.

PRINCIPLES INVOLVED WITH PULSED DOPPLER
AND SPECTRAL ANALYSIS

The principle of using pulsed Doppler with spectral analysis for intraoperative assessment of arterial reconstruction rests on the understanding that minor technical abnormalities will produce a disturbance in the velocity pattern in the region of the arterial anastomosis. This disturbance is detected by identifying deviations in the Doppler spectral characteristics that differ from those seen in laminar flow conditions (7).

The second feature used with Doppler assessment of arterial reconstructions, particularly in the case of bypass grafts, is the capability of determining the maximum centerstream velocity of the graft by converting the frequency information obtained from the Doppler spectrum to velocity parameters by applying the Doppler equation (Figure 1). As will be discussed later, it is possible to correlate this

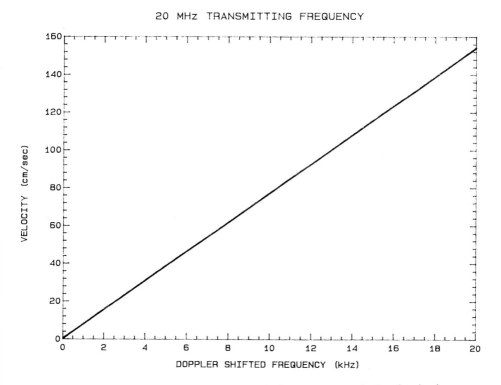

Figure 1   Relationship of centerstream peak frequency to velocity (cm/sec) as defined by the Doppler equation with a known incident angle of 60°.

particular parameter (centerstream graft velocity) with both long-term patency and the presence of technical error.

An understanding of the abnormalities seen in the presence of technical error is best appreciated by considering the velocity patterns seen in normal nonstenotic arteries, with a subsequent consideration of the patterns seen when varying degrees of stenosis similar to those produced by technical problems are present.

In the normal nondiseased state, flow in arteries is predominantly laminar throughout the cardiac cycle, although during the initial deceleration phase of systole there is a short period of instability characterized by minor deviation from the laminar flow state that is again seen during late diastole. With pulsed Doppler apparatus and spectral analysis, this is manifest by the pattern shown in Figure 2, where there is spectral broadening during the initial deceleration phase of systole and again in late diastole. With minor degrees of artificially produced stenosis in an animal model, in which the waveform shape is similar to that seen in peripheral arteries to a high-resistance vascular bed, the major change detected in the region immediately distal to the stenosis is an increase in the magnitude of spectral broadening seen during diastole, with a concomitant prolongation of this unstable period back into the deceleration phase of systole (Fig. 3). The development of a hemo-

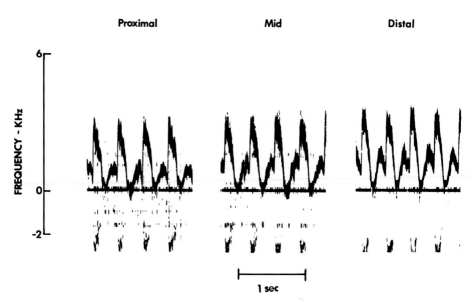

Figure 2   Spectra obtained from the centerstream of the canine distal thoracic aorta showing the mild spectral broadening in the decleration phase of systole and later in diastole as a result of transient instability in the flow pattern.

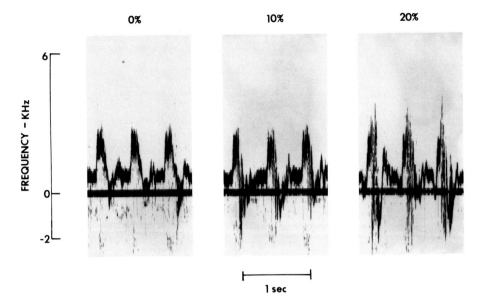

Figure 3 Spectra obtained distal to artificially created concentric stenosis in the canine thoracic aorta that did not reduce pressure or flow. The characteristic pattern is that of a progressive increase in spectral broadening as the stenosis becomes more severe without a concomitant increase in peak systolic frequency.

dynamically significant stenosis is heralded by the development of spectral broadening throughout the deceleration phase of systole associated with an increase in the peak systolic velocity (Fig. 4).

Quantitative measurement of this spectral broadening parameter and the timing relationship in the cycle is shown in Figure 5, in which the results of a number of canine experiments have been pooled. In this study (8), varying degrees of concentric stenoses were created in the thoracic aorta of dogs and centerstream velocity patterns obtained from the region immediately distal to the area of the stenosis. Maximum spectral broadening was determined by computer analysis of the spectra obtained distal to the stenosis. It can be seen that spectral broadening gradually increases in magnitude with the development of a 15% diameter-reducing stenosis, reaching a maximum with a 50% diameter-reducing stenosis. The spectra in this study were obtained with a high-frequency (20-MHz) pulsed Doppler similar to that used routinely for intraoperative assessment in the clinical situations detailed in succeeding paragraphs. This particular study provided evidence that spectral broadening was a useful parameter for identifying and differentiating between varying degrees of stenosis over a range that did not reduce pressure or flow. As such, this remains the only known parameter capable of differentiating

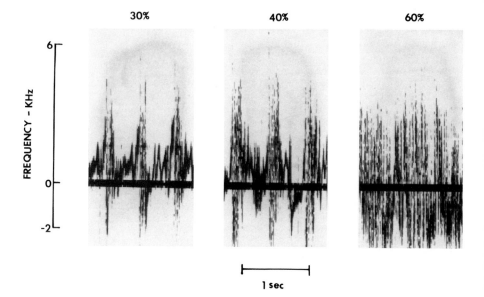

Figure 4 Spectra obtained distal to an artificially created concentric stenosis that was hemodynamically significant. The characteristic features are the presence of diffuse spectral broadening and an increase in peak systolic frequency.

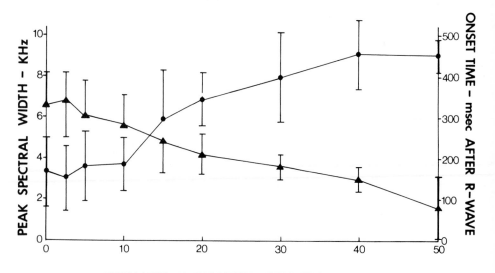

Figure 5 Relationship between maximum spectral broadening (●) and percent diameter reduction over a range of stenoses that were not hemodynamically significant. Time of maximum spectral broadening (after the "R" wave) is also depicted (▲). Spectral broadening increases with severity of stenosis and occurs earlier in the cycle, occurring 75 msec after the onset of systole with a 50% diameter-reducing stenosis (pooled data).

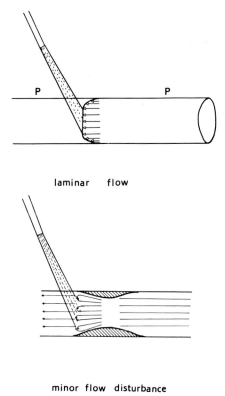

laminar flow

minor flow disturbance

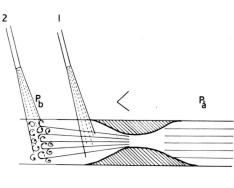

major flow disturbance

Figure 6 Schematic representation of the flow characteristics in the normal, minimally stenotic, and severely stenotic vessel.

these relatively minimal lesions. Severe stenoses (>50% diameter reduction) are associated with the production of a jet immediately beyond the area of the stenosis and, further downstream, decay of laminar flow as evidenced by the development of diffuse spectral broadening (Fig. 6).

While ideally, arterial reconstructions should manifest an absolutely normal flow distal to the region of the anastomosis, varying degrees of spectral broadening are usually present and are not indicative of major technical problems. The development of increased frequencies at peak systole in association with spectral broadening, however, are characteristic of major technical problems associated with early failure and thus necessitating immediate correction.

THE HIGH-FREQUENCY (20-MHz) PULSED DOPPLER

The concept of pulsed Doppler with spectral analysis is widely used for the non-invasive detection of disease, particularly in the carotid arteries (9). In this setting, a relatively low frequency (5 MHz) is used because of the limitations imposed by the depth of the vessel and the signal attenuation that occurs as it passes through tissues superficial to the vessel being examined. In the operative situation, the vessel under consideration is already exposed, and it is therefore possible to use a very high-frequency pulsed Doppler to evaluate the velocity characteristics of blood flow in the lumen. The specific advantage that accrues from using this higher transmitting frequency is that the sample volume within the vessel is much smaller than that which can be obtained with a lower transmitting frequency, thus increasing the sensitivity of identifying velocity pattern abnormalities. The sensing instrument used is available in two configurations, one in which the piezoelectric crystals are mounted in the head of a 16-gauge needle attached to the pulsed Doppler apparatus by long electrical leads. In the second modality, the crystals are mounted in an acrylic-cuffed probe which has similar electrical leads attached (Fig. 7). This is ideal for evaluating small grafts and is available in a variety of sizes with diameters of 4, 6, and 8 mm. Both of these probes can be gas-sterilized and attached to the Doppler instrumentation, which is mounted out of the operative field. The signal obtained is then processed using fast Fourier transform spectral analysis, which is depicted in gray scale format on a video monitor. The peak frequency can be read directly off the screen utilizing a movable cursor and converted to velocity using the table depicted in the text.

If the needle probe is used, an acrylic holder is used to insure an incident angle of 60° to the vessel being evaluated and is gently applied over the surface of the artery. If the cuff probes are used, care must be taken that a snug fit is present without producing constriction.

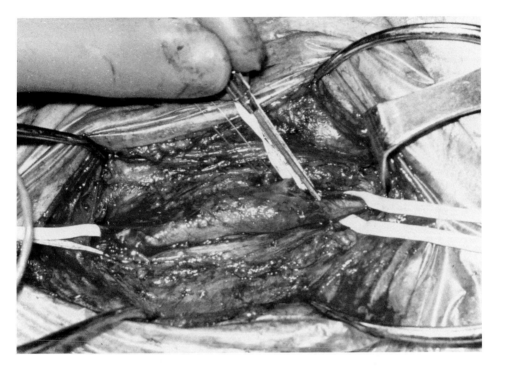

Figure 7 Photograph of high frequency (20-MHz) probe in the needle configuration being used to interrogate the carotid arteries intraoperatively.

PRACTICAL APPLICATION AND RESULTS

Carotid Endarterectomy

After complete exposure of the vessels in the operative field and prior to the application of clamps, centerstream spectra are obtained with the most appropriate probe. The vessel immediately distal to the site of the major stenosis is evaluated and the spectra obtained from this location are recorded for subsequent playback to compare with the data obtained following the endarterectomy.

Using the needle or cuffed probe, centerstream sampling is performed immediately distal to the location of the distal portion of the endarterectomy. Upon release of the clamps, it is not uncommon to observe a major flow disturbance pattern initially, which, over 4-5 min, gradually stabilizes. For this reason we obtain recordings 4-5 min after completion of the endarterectomy to assess the technical adequacy of the operation. Sampling is also performed in the common carotid in the region of the proximal endarterectomy site and also the external carotid artery.

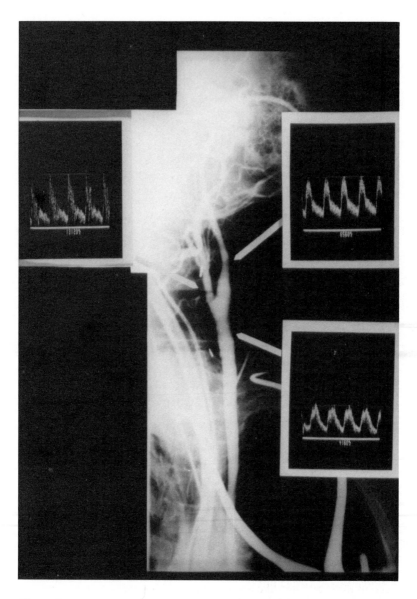

Figure 8 Intraoperative arteriogram and spectra obtained following completion of the endarterectomy with no abnormal peak frequencies or spectral broadening present at any location.

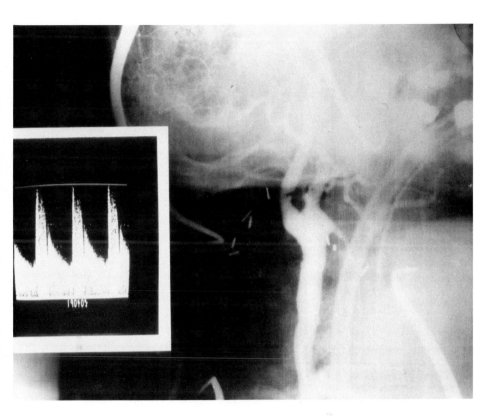

Figure 9 Operative arteriogram and spectra obtained from distal internal carotid artery in which an intimal flap is present. Note should be made of the diffuse spectral broadening indicative of a major flow disturbance.

Characteristic spectra of a technically acceptable endarterectomy are shown in Figure 8. The presence of diffuse spectral broadening in association with abnormally high peak frequencies is indicative of the presence of technical error, as shown in Figure 9, in which there is an intimal flap. Correction of the defect should be associated with production of a spectrum with relatively normal characteristics, as shown in Figure 10.

Currently in the performance of carotid endarterectomy, this procedure is used to determine when operative arteriograms should be performed. Following the endarterectomy, if normal spectra are obtained from all locations, no arteriography is subsequently performed. However, in the presence of major abnormalities in the spectra, operative arteriography is obtained to determine whether a major technical defect is present. Current experience suggests that not all the endarterectomy

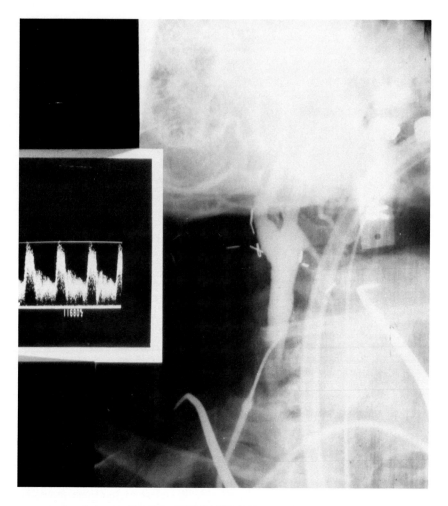

Figure 10 Arteriogram and spectra obtained from the same patient depicted in Figure 9 following correction of the defect.

segments will have absolutely normal velocity patterns immediately following endarterectomy (10), probably, in part, related to changes in configuration of the internal carotid artery associated with closure of the arteriotomy and even minor wall irregularities. As a rule these do not require correction, but in all circumstances to date there have been no false-negative studies with the pulsed Doppler apparatus, as evidenced by defects detected on routine operative arteriography initially or postoperative complications one would expect with technical problems.

Femorotibial Reconstruction

As noted earlier, intraoperative assessment should address the issues of technical adequacy of the distal reconstruction, adequacy of vein valve lysis, and, lastly, exclusion of arteriovenous fistulae.

The intraoperative assessment with the pulsed Doppler commences with an evaluation of the graft for the presence of persistent fistulae. This feature is assessed initially because the presence of such fistulae may have a significant effect

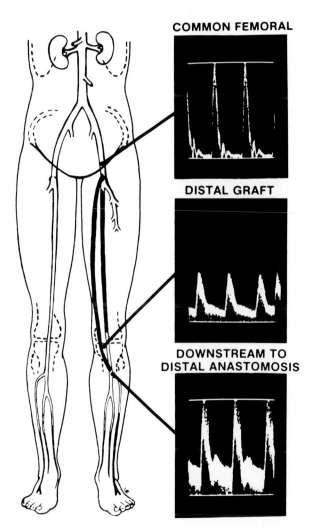

Figure 11 Vein bypass graft with characteristic spectra obtained from multiple locations showing an absence of spectral broadening and lack of high diastolic flow.

on the flow velocity characteristics of the graft and therefore needs to be excluded. The graft is assessed in segments by placing the probe over the vein graft and occluding the vein graft immediately distal with a soft clamp. The signal transmitted to the spectrum analyzer should be that of wall thump only, with no evidence of movement of red cells. If a proximal fistula exists, there will still be pulsatile flow in the graft, and the presence of such a signal warrants a careful inspection of the graft proximal to the region of occlusion for the missed branch. The author usually utilizes assessment of the vein in the thigh in two segments and the vein graft distal to the knee in two segments. Following the assessment of each of these segments for arteriovenous fistulae, an additional set of random recordings is obtained along the length of the graft to insure that there is no high diastolic flow component, which is also characteristic of residual arteriovenous fistulas (Fig. 11). Completion of the survey for missed branches is followed by a determination of the adequacy of valve lysis.

Valve Lysis Evaluation

During the actual performance of valve lysis, the location of valves is marked with a marking ink, and it is these locations that are subsequently assessed. The operator is predominantly interested in the velocity characteristics immediately distal to the area of the valve, usually for a length of 1-2 cm. The probe is positioned over the graft or, if a cuffed probe is used, encircled around the graft, and the spectra evaluated on the video screen. The presence of marked spectral broadening distal to an area of previous valve lysis suggests a residual valve leaflet or technically inadequate lysis of the valve, and the area should be reprobed with the valvulotome. The author prefers to use the needle probes for this evaluation, as they can be rapidly moved along segments of the graft without mobilization of the vein. Confirmation that all valve leaflets have been adequately lysed, as evidenced by the lack of flow disturbance patterns immediately distal to each, enables the operator to proceed to the final component of the examination—evaluation of the distal anastomosis.

Evaluation of the Distal Anastomosis

The needle probe is initially used over the hood of the graft to insure that the velocity spectra at the terminal portion of the graft are clean. The needle probe is then moved distal to the toe of the graft, approximately 5 mm, and the range selected to give the best signal. The spectrum is evaluated for the peak frequency in the presence of spectral broadening and technical defects characterized by the features already described of increased peak frequencies or diffuse spectral broadening, as depicted in Figure 12.

At the conclusion of the assessment, a cuffed probe is applied to the distal third of the graft and recordings obtained specifically to evaluate the peak frequency for conversion to peak velocity. We utilize an immediate conversion chart

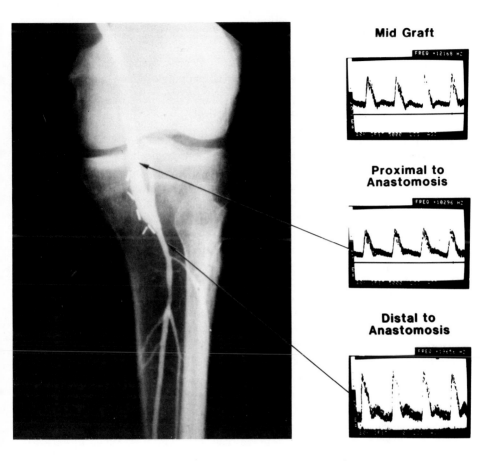

Figure 12 Detailed spectral characteristics in region of normal distal anastamosis of femoropopliteal graft. Immediately distal to the anastamosis the peak frequency increases due to a change in calibre and acceleration of blood flow.

in the operating room for this purpose, and graft velocities in excess of 65 cm/sec as noted by Bandyk et al. (11) are associated with good long-term results and an absence of technical error.

Peak velocities lower than this, and particularly those less than 40 cm/sec, are associated with early failure, and a complete reevaluation of the graft should be performed to insure that no technical defects have been missed. This usually involves a reevaluation with the pulsed Doppler apparatus and a detailed operative arteriogram. If, following these maneuvers, there is no evidence of technical error, the low flow rate is attributed to high peripheral resistance as a result of distal disease. In this setting we have on occasion used a second graft into a distal vessel in a sequential fashion to increase the centerstream velocity to values that will be associated with long-term patency.

Spectra obtained from various locations of a normal vein bypass graft without residual arteriovenous fistulae and no technical error are depicted in Figure 11.

Renal and Visceral Arterial Reconstruction

The approaches taken in renal artery revascularization consist of either using the needle probe to assess centerstream velocity in multiple locations along the graft or to apply a suitably sized cuffed probe distal to the renal anastomosis. When the original lesion is proximal in the renal artery, the latter approach is preferred because this gives an overall picture of graft function, including the technical adequacy of the distal anastomosis. In complex lesions, however, it is not uncommon for the distal anastomosis to be performed either at the bifurcation of the renal arteries or extending into the bifurcation of the renal arteries, and it is then necessary to use the needle probe placed individually over the branch vessels. In spite of the relatively small size of these arteries, the high-frequency pulsed Doppler is ideally suited for obtaining velocity spectra for evaluation.

As with the carotid arteries, it is advisable to wait approximately 5 min after clamp release to evaluate the technical adequacy of the bypass graft due to varying changes in parenchymal vascular resistance induced by the ischemia time incurred during the procedure. Here, as in other locations, the most disturbing abnormalities include very high peak frequencies at systole in association with diffuse spectral broadening. It is not uncommon to identify very high peak frequencies in cases in which renal revascularization is being performed purely for renovascular hypertension when the flow rates through the renal artery are extremely high. This is an important factor in variations in the peak frequency at systole, with the lowest peak frequencies being seen when there is severe parenchymal disease with reconstruction for renal insufficiency.

Figure 12 depicts a postoperative arterial digital arteriogram of a patient undergoing left aortorenal bypass grafting with saphenous vein with spectra obtained intraoperatively. This procedure was performed for renovascular hypertension without severe parenchymal damage and is characterized by a relatively normal waveform shape with high peak systolic frequencies and a high diastolic flow component, as is usually seen in vessels supplying a low resistance vascular bed. It should be noted that there is minimal spectral broadening in the initial deceleration phase of systole and during diastole. This approach is now used routinely for all renal artery reconstructions and is currently being evaluated with follow-up arterial digital arteriograms 3-4 days after surgery. It is hoped that if, after a suitably large series has been conducted, the intraoperative method of assessment is shown to be a highly reliable predictor of problems, it will negate the need for initial postoperative arteriography in these patients.

Visceral Artery Reconstruction

As noted earlier, the rationale for intraoperative assessment of visceral artery reconstruction is similar to that for renal arterial surgery. The procedure is similar in that either the cuffed or needle probe can be used, depending on the anatomic situation of the reconstruction. If a vein graft is used, velocity patterns immediately distal to the proximal anastomosis and distal to the distal anastomosis should be obtained, with different patterns being seen in the celiac artery compared with the superior mesenteric artery. The principles of interpretation are, however, similar in that the operator is particularly interested in identifying very high peak frequencies in association with diffuse spectral broadening. In the superior mesenteric artery, after the initial hyperemic flow phase has passed, the patterns seen by us are as shown in Figure 13, in which flow during diastole actually comes to zero. Peak frequencies are not as high as those seen in renal artery reconstruction due to

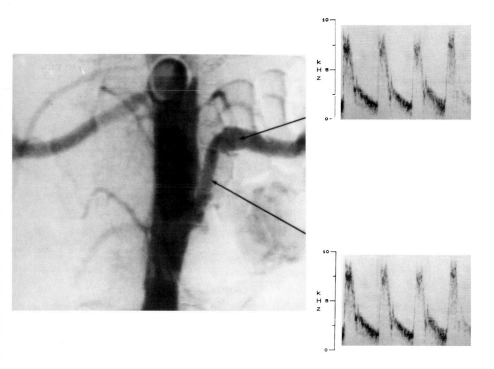

Figure 13 Arteriogram and spectra obtained following aortorenal vein bypass graft. It should be noted there is high diastolic flow, characteristic of a normal renal parenchymal revasculature. There is no abnormal spectral broadening from within the proximal or distal recording sites.

the lower overall flow rates through the superior mesenteric artery during the non-active state.

SUMMARY

The concept of intraoperative assessment of arterial reconstruction is, in this author's opinion, fundamental to minimizing failures as a result of technical error. Although arteriography is eminently suitable for a morphological evaluation in certain circumstances, it is hindered by the fact that it is not applicable under all circumstances and does not have good physician acceptance.

The use of Doppler ultrasound is a powerful tool in our current diagnostic armamentarium and is also capable of being applied to the operative situation during which the high-frequency Doppler is particularly suitable.

The suitability of this technology has been well documented by both controlled animal studies and subsequent clinical evaluation as reported by Bandyk et al. (7). In a series of controlled animal studies, major and minor defects were constructed in the abdominal aorta of dogs, and spectral broadening was shown to be an extremely sensitive indicator of the presence of even minimal wall defects produced by small intimal flaps.

Subsequent clinical evaluation of this technology with both carotid endarterectomy and femorotibial bypass grafting in which operative arteriography was used as a comparative standard demonstrated that this was an ideal surveillance method because of its 100% specificity, although it should be noted that not all cases in which the spectra were considered abnormal was a significant technical error detected (Table 1).

Table 1 Comparative Accuracy of Pulsed Doppler Spectral Analysis and Operative Arteriography in the Detection of Technical Error During Arterial Surgery[a]

Pulsed Doppler Spectral Analysis	Arteriography		
	Normal	Abnormal	Total
Normal	79	0	79
Abnormal	5	6	11
Total	84	6	90

[a]The sensitivity was 79/84 (94%); specificity, 6/6 (100%); negative predictive value, 79/79 (100%); and positive predictive value, 6/11 (54%).

The more recent applications in the field of visceral arterial surgery potentially resolve a major problem that has existed for some time. The difficulties encountered with intraoperative and early postoperative arteriographic assessment lead to a clinical setting in which the surgeon is unsure of the technical adequacy of his operative procedure, particularly in the face of alterations in function of the kidney in particular, which may or may not be related to the procedure itself.

More detailed and rigorous intraoperative assessment of all forms of arterial reconstruction is likely to become an established component of the operative aspects of vascular reconstruction, with high-frequency pulsed Doppler being particularly suited for this purpose.

REFERENCES

1. Blaisdell, FW, Lin R, Hall AD: Technical results of carotid endarterectomy—arteriographic assessment. Am J Surg 114:239-246, 1967.
2. Rosental JJ, Gaspar MR, Movius HJ: Intraoperative arteriography in carotid thromboendarterectomy. Arch Surg 106:806-808, 1973.
3. Zierler RE, Bandyk DF, Thiele BL: Intraoperative assessment of carotid endarterectomy. J Vasc Surg 1:73-84, 1984.
4. Ortega G, Gee W, Kaupp HA, McDonald KM: Postendarterectomy carotid occlusion. Surgery 90:1093-1098, 1981.
5. Leather RP, Powers SR, Karmody AM: A reappraisal of the in situ saphenous vein arterial bypass: Its use in limb salvage. Surgery 86:453-461, 1979.
6. Levine, AW, Bandyk DF, Bonier PH, Towne JB: Lessons learned in adopting the in situ saphenous vein bypass. J Vasc Surg 2:145-153, 1985.
7. Bandyk DF, Zierler RE, Thiele BL: Detection of technical error during arterial surgery by pulsed Doppler spectral analysis. Arch Surg 119:421-428, 1984.
8. Thiele, BL, Hutchison KJ, Greene FM, Forster FK, Strandness DE, Jr.: Pulsed Doppler waveform patterns produced by smooth stenosis in the dog thoracic aorta. In Taylor DEM, Steven AL (eds): Blood Flow Theory and Practice, Academic Press, Inc., New York, 1983, pp. 85-104.
9. Fell G, Phillips DJ, Chikos PM, Harley JD, Thiele BL, Strandness DE, Jr.: Ultrasonic duplex scanning for disease of the carotid artery. Circulation 64:896-900, 1978.
10. Zierler RE, Bandyk DF, Berni GA, Thiele BL: Intraoperative pulsed Doppler assessment of carotid endarterectomy. Ultrasound Med Biol 9:65-71, 1983.
11. Bandyk DF, Cato RF, Towne JB: A low flow velocity predicts failure of femoropopliteal and femorotibial bypass grafts. Surgery 98:799-809, 1985.

17

Perioperative Assessment of In Situ Bypass Graft

DALE BUCHBINDER, CAROLYN SEMROW, TIMOTHY J. RYAN, and DAVID L. ROLLINS
University of Health Sciences/The Chicago Medical School
North Chicago, Illinois

HISTORY

The concept of using the greater saphenous vein in situ as an arterial conduit to the infrainguinal arterial reconstruction has intrigued and frustrated surgeons for many decades. The course of the saphenous vein makes it anatomically accessible to all major arteries of the lower extremity for bypass surgery.

Over 20 years ago, Charles Rob created and attempted in situ saphenous vein arterial bypass (1). One of his former fellows, K.V. Hall, first reported the results of this operation in 1962 (2). Hall performed the operation by exposing the entire vein. At each valve site, the vein was opened, the valve excised, and the vein then closed (2,3). This procedure was tedious and time consuming. Connolly and others modified the procedure to render valves incompetent (valve fracture) by passing a valve stripper retrograde down the vein and rupturing each valve (4). This procedure became popular until Barner reported dismal results with the valve fracture technique, and the concept of in situ bypass was abandoned (5).

The overall concept still appealed to many surgeons. In 1972, Leather introduced the technique of valve incision, where each valve was incised by passing micro-scissors down the proximal end of the vein or through side branches (6). Leather has continued to report excellent results using this technique (7-11). These results have since been duplicated by many centers (11-14). The most impressive findings with this technique were increased operability and patency rates. Veins with distal diameter of 2 mm could be used for tibial vessel surgery. Greater than

291

90% vein utilization was achieved and 5-year patency rates of 77% were reported in the tibial positions (8,10). Buchbinder reported decreased endothelial damage and Busch reported increased endothelial prostayclin production, accounting in part for increased patency rates and decreased early failure rates (14,15).

The technique of in situ bypass has gained widespread acceptance. However, because of wide anatomical variation, double systems, and the presence of many side branches, preoperative evaluation of the saphenous vein is essential. Reliable preoperative and perioperative evaluations enable the surgeon to plan for the appropriate procedure. In the operating room, the vein must also be assessed for adequacy of valve incision, location and ligation of arterial venous connections, as well as technical adequacy of the operation. The graft also needs assessment in the postoperative period to avoid failure from valve sinus stenosis and progression of distal disease. This chapter will be devoted to the pre-, intra-, and postoperative methods of vein and bypass assessment.

PREOPERATIVE EVALUATION OF THE SAPHENOUS VEIN

The preoperative evaluation of the saphenous vein is useful for the surgeon planning in situ vein bypass. The methods of evaluation are visual inspection, vein mapping by palpation or Doppler exam, preoperative saphenous venography, operative saphenous venography, and B-mode ultrasonic imaging of the saphenous vein.

In patients with thin legs and prominent saphenous veins, the vein can be traced from its origin in the foot through the calf, and when visible a reasonable assessment can be made. However, in most patients the vein is not close enough to the surface to be evaluated adequately by inspection alone. To add to this technique, one can create a fluid wave in the vein by stroking distal to proximal over the vein, starting at the ankle. One can feel the course of the vein in the calf by palpation. A pocket Doppler can be used in addition, and a reasonable mapping of the vein can be obtained. These procedures can and should be performed at the bedside with no patient risk or discomfort. Unfortunately, these techniques give no information about to the location of side branches, double system valves, or relative size of the vein.

The gold standard for defining the anatomy of the saphenous vein is the venogram. This is not without risk. However, when done carefully, by experienced radiologists the complication rate is quite low (less than 2%) (16). Recently Shah et al. reported that of 385 preoperative venograms, 345 were performed in the angiography suite; the remaining 40 were performed in the operating room (16). Care was taken to avoid direct saphenous vein puncture. Then 2000 units of heparin were given directly into the vein on the dorsum of the foot, followed by 100 ml of radioopaque dye. Radiographs were taken in the anteroposterior plane and the

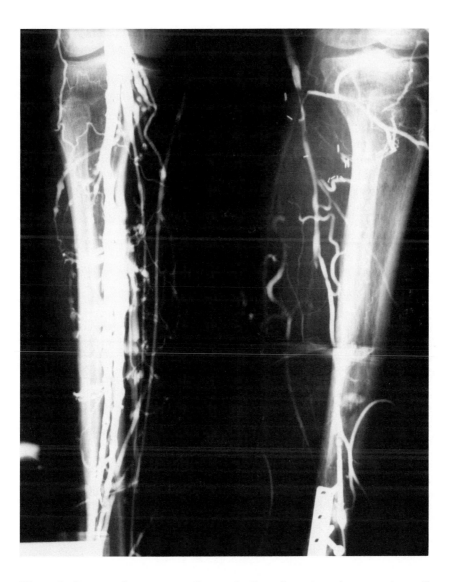

Figure 1 Preoperative venogram demonstrating adequate saphenous vein on the right and the absence of the deep system on the left.

lateral planes. A number grid was taped to the leg prior to venography; at the conclusion of the venogram, the vein was flushed with Rınger's lactate to remove the dye from the endothelial surface as soon as possible (Fig. 1).

Intraoperative venography may be performed in place of preoperative venography. Intraoperative venography is done by placing a small needle into the saphenous vein or a major tributary at the ankle when the patient is ready for surgery and propped on the operating room table. Contrast material (20-40 cc) is injected into the vein and radiographs are taken up the leg. This technique also defines the saphenous venous anatomy. The operations should proceed after the vein has been flushed with a heparinized solution, and adequately marked on the leg.

Pre-in situ assessment of the greater saphenous vein can also be performed using a high-resolution, real time, B-mode ultrasonic imager with a 7.5-MHz transducer. This procedure is performed with the patient sitting in bed with the leg extended. A small pillow or rolled towel is placed under the knee and the leg is

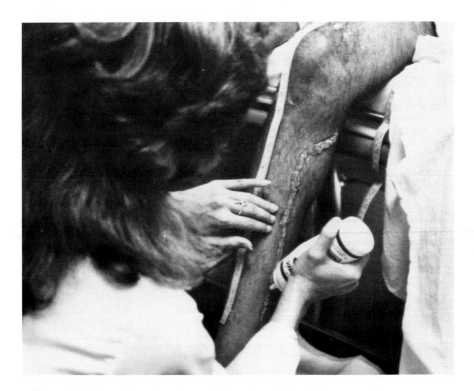

Figure 2 The position for ultrasonic imaging of the saphenous vein.

rotated laterally. The saphenous vein is then imaged starting at the ankle (Fig. 2). A waterproof pen is used to map the vein. The locations of valved and tributary vessels are marked as well. Vessel diameter is determined above the ankle. In the upper thigh it is determined by using the imager's internal calipers. The diameter marked on the leg at the site of measurement. The number and location of valves and tributary vessels as well as the diameter of the saphenous vein are recorded (Fig. 3). The authors recently have compared the results of ultrasonic venography to the operative anatomy of the saphenous vein (17). The correlation in 14 limbs was 93%. The 7% error in this technique was due to the examiners' failure to identify a triple saphenous system. All valves, tributaries, and the diameter of vessels were correctly identified.

These techniques, when used effectively, can provide information regarding the saphenous vein, its condition (usable, thrombosed, or varicose), and the location of valves and major tributaries. Ultrasonic imaging additionally can evaluate valve location and function. This data base can provide the surgeon with the knowledge needed for planning appropriate operations.

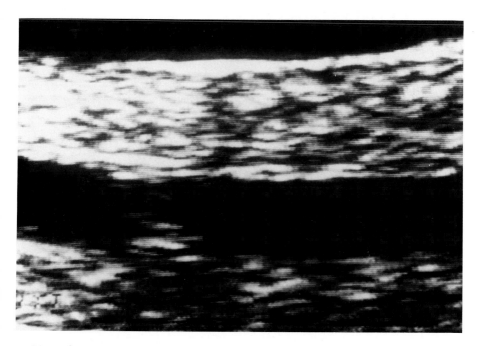

Figure 3 Ultrasonic image of the saphenous vein.

SURGICAL TECHNIQUE FOR IN SITU BYPASS

The saphenous vein and proximal arteries are exposed in the infrainguinal position. The saphenofemoral junction is dissected and the venous tributaries around the fossa ovalis are ligated and divided. The distal arteries and saphenous vein are then dissected. The saphenous vein may be exposed in its entirety through a continuous skin incision (12) or at valve sites (18). Following systemic administration of heparin, a curved vascular clamp is placed at the saphenous femoral junction and the saphenous vein is excised with a small rim of common femoral vein. The common femoral vein is closed with a running suture of 5-0 polypropylene suture. The proximal saphenous vein valve is excised under direct vision and the rest of the valves are incised using a combination of valve scissors, valvulotome, and valve cutter, as described by Leather (18).

The proximal anastomosis is usually constructed to the common femoral artery. Occasionally, it is constructed to the superficial profunda femoris arteries if the anatomy is such that the saphenous vein is more easily juxtaposed.

After the valves are incised, there should be good pulsatile flow from the distal vein end. The distal anastomosis is contructed using continuous 6-0 or 7-0 polypropylene suture. Angiography, direct pressure measurement, and noninvasive Doppler techniques are used to identify arteriovenous fistulae and to determine graft patency and arterial runoff.

INTRAOPERATIVE VEIN ASSESSMENT

There are four basic factors to be assessed when conducting a lower extremity, in situ saphenous vein bypass. These include the adequacy of valve incision, location of arteriovenous fistulas, adequacy of the distal anastomosis and runoff, and the function of the arterial graft. Completion arteriography is routinely employed to identify technical defects and arteriovenous fistulae. A 19-gauge buttergly is placed in the proximal graft and 15-20 cc of dye is injected with inflow occlusion. A series of 19-gauge needles are placed in the skin 6 cm apart to serve as a grid. Two films are usually necessary to visualize the entire graft and arterial runoff. When X-ray plates are put into a sterile bag and placed under the lower extremity, the proximal 10-15 cm of graft may not be seen and an unsuspected arteriovenous fistula or technical defect may be present (Fig. 4). However, this is an uncommon area for technical defects.

Arteriography will usually identify all arteriovenous fistulae. Fistulae greater than 1 mm should be ligated because they may decrease graft flow or cause skin necrosis. Small fistulae usually thrombose within a few days. If significant endothelial trauma has occurred, platelet thrombus will be seen as an intraluminal defect. This should be removed under direct vision via a longitudinal graftotomy, which is closed with a small vein patch. Missing valve cusps are seen as a transverse

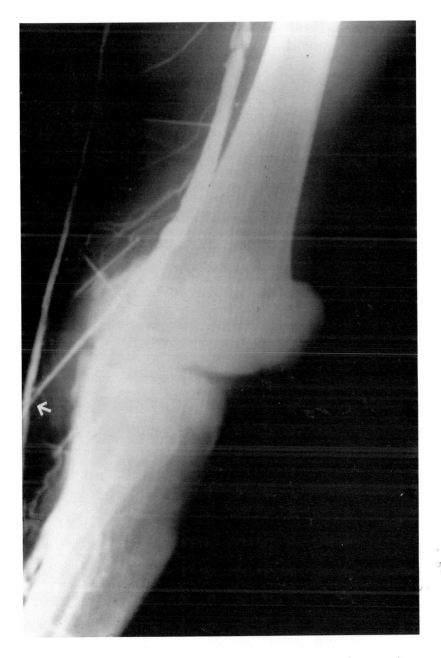

Figure 4 Completion angiogram showing needle markers and an arteriovenous connection.

linear defects across the veins. The cusps should be incised using the retrograde valvulatome or under direct vision if there is accumulated thrombus. A normal arteriogram results in a homogenous, well-defined silhouette of contrast within the vein as seen in Fig. 4 . When contrast defects are noted at the anastomosis or in the distal runoff vessels, they should be corrected.

Noninvasive techniques can be used effectively intraoperatively to assess graft function, detect anastomotic technical error, and identify arteriovenous fistulae and incompletely incised valves (19,20). A sterile Doppler probe may be placed on the vein graft and flow signals evaluated. A normal flow signal is biphasic in the graft, but may become monophasic in the distal native artery due to decreased vascular resistance from the vasodilation of ischemia. When increased pitch is heard, a technical defect or arteriovenous (AV) fistula may be present. Compression of the graft distal to the Doppler probe will differentiate the cause. Real-time spectrum analysis may be used with a continuous wave or pulsed Doppler probe to increase the accuracy of locating AV fistulae and technical error (19).

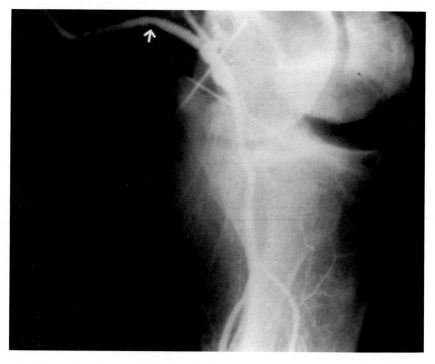

Figure 5 Completion angiogram showing a missing valve cusp.

Graft function may be determined by measuring ankle pressure using a sterile Doppler probe and blood pressure cuff. When arterial runoff is unobstructed, ankle pressure should be near systemic. Less available runoff may yield decreased ankle-brachial indices (ABI). However, when the ABI is low, a technical defect or large AV fistula should be suspected. Occasionally, a small (2.5 mm) vein or arterial spasm causes a decreased ABI and, when present, the ABI should increase within 12-24°. However, one should determine that there are no technical errors present before blame is placed on vein size or arterial spasm.

When noninvasive techniques are not available for intraoperative assessment, clinical examination for distal arterial pulses and evidence of increased pedal flow manifested by reactive hyperemia, brisk capillary, and venous filling are useful. Additionally, direct pressure measurements of graft pressures using a small needle may help to identify sites of AV fistula and technical defects.

POSTOPERATIVE TECHNIQUES FOR EVALUATION OF SAPHENOUS VEIN

The quality of the in situ saphenous vein bypass may be easily checked by pulse palpation. Because this is a surface operation, and the vein is usually directly under the skin, the presence or absence of a palpable pulse will indicate if the graft is functioning. If there is a change in pulse amplitude or a previously palpable pulse is absent, one can immediately assume that there is a problem with graft function. Our patients are followed routinely during the immediate postoperative period with segmental Doppler tracings and pressures. These are continued for the next two years at 3-month intervals. If there has been no significant change at that time, they are followed at 6-month intervals for the next 2 years, then yearly. Any degenerations in segmental pressures or wave analysis are noted and patients are returned immediately to the hospital for angiography. In the early postoperative period, a retained valve cusp or missed whole valve (>5%) may become functional causing graft stenosis or occlusion. Also an arteriovenous connection may open (>5%). Both will cause decreased distal arterial pressures, and are easily correctable with early detection (20). During late follow-ups, valve sinus stenosis and distal progression of disease have been reported. When these are diagnosed early on, they can be corrected before graft failure occurs using local anesthesia with simple vein patch or ligation procedures.

In conclusion, preoperative evaluation of the saphenous vein enables the surgeon to define anatomy, to determine location and number of valve sites, and to assess vein usability for in situ saphenous vein bypass. Intraoperative vein assessment enables the surgeon to evaluate the adequacy of valve incision, the presence or absence of unligated arteriovenous connections, and the technical adequacy of the operation. Finally, in the postoperative followup, the surgeon is able to detect early graft problems, which can be corrected before graft failure occurs.

REFERENCES

1. May AG, DeWeese JA, Rob CG: Arterialized "in-situ" saphenous vein. Arch Surg 91:43-50, 1965.
2. Hall KV: The great saphenous vein used in situ as an arterial shunt after extirpation of the vein valves. Surgery 51:492-495, 1962.
3. Hall KV, Rostad H: In situ vein bypass in the treatment of femoropopliteal atherosclerotic disease: A ten year study. Am J Surg 136:158-161, 1978.
4. Connolly JE, Stemmer GA: The non-reversed saphenous vein bypass for femoro-popliteal occlusive disease. Surgery 68:602-609, 1970.
5. Barner HB, Judd DR, Kaiser GC, et al: Late failure of arteriologic in situ saphenous vein. Arch Surg 99:781-786, 1969.
6. Leather RP, Powers SR, Karmody AM: A reappraisal of the in situ saphenous vein arterial bypass: Its use in limb salvage. Surgery 68:453-460, 1980.
7. Leather RP, Shah DM, Buchbinder D, Annest SJ, Karmody AM: Further experience with the saphenous vein used in situ for arterial bypass. Am J Surg 142:506-510, 1981.
8. Leather RP, Shah DM, Corson JD, Karmody AM: Instrumental evolution of in situ saphenous vein bypass. J Vasc Surg 1:113-123, 1984.
9. Leather RP, Shah DM, Karmody AM: Infrapopliteal arterial bypass for limb salvage. Increased patency and utilization of the saphenous vein used "in-situ." Surgery 190:1000-1008, 1981.
10. Karmody AM, Leather RP, Corson JD, Shah DM: Peroneal artery bypass for limb salvage: A reappraisal of its value in limb salvage. J Vasc Surg 1 (6):809, 1984.
11. Buchbinder D, Pasch AR, Verta MJ, Rollins DL, Ryan TJ, Schuler JJ, Flanigan DP: Ankle bypass: Should we go the distance? Am J Surg 150:216-219, 1985.
12. Levine AW, Bandyk DF, Bonier PH, Towne JB: Lessons learned in adopting the in-situ saphenous vein bypass. J Vasc Surg (in press).
13. Acher LW, Turnipseed WD: In situ distal saphenous bypass using the intraluminal valve disruption technique. Arch Surg (in press).
14. Buchbinder D, Singh JK, Karmody AM, Shah DM, Leather RP: Comparison of patency rate and structural change of "in-situ" and reversed vein arterial bypass. J. Surg Res 30:213-218, 1981.
15. Bush HL, Graber JN, Jakubowski JA, Hong SL, McCabe M, Deykin D, Nasbeth DC: Favorable balance of prostacyclin and thromboxane A-2 improves early patency of human in situ vein grafts. J Vasc Surg 1:149-159, 1984.
16. Shah DM, Chang BB, Leopold PW, Corson JD, Leather RP, Karmody AM: The anatomy of the greater saphenous venous system. J Vasc Surg (in press).
17. Buchbinder D, Semrow C, Ryan T, Calligaro K, Rollins DL: The use of B-mode ultrasonic imaging in the preoperative evaluation of the saphenous vein. Am Surg (submitted).
18. Leather RO, Karmody AM: In-situ saphenous vein arterial bypass. In Rutherford RB (ed): Vascular Surgery, W.C. Saunders Co., Philadelphia, 1984.

19. Bandyk DF, Sierler RE, Thiele BL: Detection of technical error during arterial surgery by pulsed doppler spectral analysis. Arch Surg 119:421-428, 1984.
20. Buchbinder D, Rollins DL, Verta MJ, La Rosa MD, Ryan TJ, Meyer JP, Flanigan DP: Early experience with in-situ saphenous vein bypass for distal arterial reconstruction. Surgery 99:350-356, 1986.

18

Vascular Endoscopy

JONATHAN B. TOWNE
Medical College of Wisconsin
Milwaukee, Wisconsin

Technical advances in optical instrumentation have made possible intraluminal endoscopy of the vascular system. The vascular endoscopes utilize one of three different optical principles. The most common is the fiber-optic scope, which uses multiple small fibers arranged in two bundles—one to transmit light to the tip of the scope and another to conduct the image to the eyepiece. The light bundles are combined with an irrigating channel and housed in a single plastic sheath, usually measuring 3.5-4 mm in diameter. These have the advantage of being quite flexible and are relatively small in size. The second type of scope utilizes a rod lens system and consists of glass rod lenses placed in close proximity. Light travels a greater distance in glass, which results in excellent resolution and light transmission. We have found that the image clarity and light transmission were clearly superior with the rod lens system (1). Its only drawbacks were its size, 3.5-5 mm in cross section, and its rigidity, which impeded its use in vessels. The third type of scope uses disc lenses. Since these scopes have neither the flexibility and ease of handling of the fiber-optic scopes, nor the superior optical resolution of the rod lense scope, they are less commonly used.

The most frequently reported use of vascular endoscopy is to inspect intra-operatively the arterial system following vascular reconstruction to determine the adequacy of the repair (2,3). Recently there have been reports of vascular endoscopy being used as a diagnostic modality to evaluate the venous system, cardiac chambers, and the pulmonary-arterial bed (4,5). There also have been scattered reports of endoscopy used to evaluate diagnostically the arterial tree (6,7). Vascular endoscopy must deal with certain inherent problems and limitations, the most significant of which is related to the fact that blood is an opaque medium that interferes with the visualization of the vessel wall. This can be circumvented in a variety of means. Intraoperatively one can view segments of the vascular tree isolated from the circulation by vascular clamps, which provide a bloodless field. More recently, fiber-optic scopes have been inserted into inflatable transparent balloons, which when filled with gas or saline permit viewing of the vessel wall (4,5,7). The limitation of this system is that blood flow is interrupted during visualization, resulting in temporary distal ischemia. This technique is not feasible in the ascending or arch portion of the thoracic aorta. Also, the risk of inducing atheroembolism by contact with an ulcerative lesion precludes its use in cerebral vessels. The third technique is to use a pressure irrigation system to prevent inflow of blood into the vascular segment, so that a clear medium allows visualization of the vascular wall. This technique can only be used in medium-sized vessels, has the risk of causing fluid overload, and is cumbersome to use. Unfortunately, many patients with atherosclerosis in whom endoscopy would be of value also tend to have marginal cardiac function, which would make them more prone to fluid overload. Other potential problems of endoscopy include infection either at the site of entry into the vascular system or by seeding through the arterial tree. Embolization is also of concern. Friction of the scope being passed along an arterial wall could dislodge micro- or macroaggregates of atherosclerotic debris, which could migrate distally. Likewise, in the venous system it is potentially possible to dislodge a clot resulting in a pulmonary embolis. The size of the scope has limited its usefulness in medium and small arteries. At the present time the smallest scope that is used is in the 3-4-mm range, preventing its use in visceral vessels as well as arteries in the lower extremity distal to the midsuperficial femoral artery.

DIAGNOSTIC USES

Over the past half-decade there have been several attempts to visualize the great veins, right heart, and pulmonary outflow tract in patients. Previously, the inability to see through blood has been a limiting factor to this technique. However, recently, the placing of the fiber-optic catheter in a transparent polyethylene balloon, which can be inflated when positioned in place, has revived interest in this modality. Initial work was done by Moser and colleagues, who placed a flexible latex balloon over the viewing tip of a 4-mm-diameter fiber-optic endoscope (5). Subsequent refinement of the technique has led to development of the angioscope, which is 4 mm in diameter and 80 cm long, with a central channel of 0.8 mm. This scope has 70° of flexion, a 70° angle of view, and utilizes a cold light source; it is introduced into the jugular vein after circumferential tourniquet control of the vein is obtained. The catheter is then floated to the level of interest where the balloon is inflated with carbon dioxide or a saline solution, displacing the blood and allowing visualization of the vascular wall. Their initial work was in the iliac and femoral veins. In their canine model they visualized experimentally placed emboli in the pulmonary outflow tract (8). The only untoward hemodynamic event noted in the experimental animals was transient arrhythmias induced as the endoscope traversed the tricuspid valve. Extended periods of partial obstruction of the tricuspid and pulmonary valves with the endoscope lying in the pulmonary artery did not induce any arrhythmias or alterations in the cardiac output. Tanabe and his associates developed a more refined instrument (4). This likewise was a fiber-optic instrument 4 mm in diameter and 120 cm in length. The tip of the scope was constructed so as to be rotated 120° upward and 30° downward by manipulating the knob of the handle. A polyurethane balloon expandable up to 20-50 mm in diameter was tied over the tip of the catheter. Through a small catheter built into the scope, 2-4 mm in diameter, saline or carbon dioxide gas can be injected for inflation. The scope is inserted in the saphenous vein to observe the great veins and the right side of the heart. They likewise reported visualization of the aorta by percutaneous passage through the femoral artery. When the catheter is passed to the area of interest, the balloon was inflated and gently pressed against the part to be visualized with the angulation knob. They have used this technique successfully in 45 patients, 25 of whom had cardiac pathology and 20 who had vascular disease. They reported success in visualizing the inferior and superior vena cava, the atrial septum and the orifice of the coronary sinus, the tricuspid valve, most of the ventricular septum, and the outflow tract of the right ventricle and pulmonary artery. They were able to visualize an atrial septal defect in 14 of 18 patients. Since this technology is new, its place in the evaluation and treatment of diseases of the cardiopulmonary system remains to be determined. Reported experience at this date is too small to determine morbidity and mortality rate related to this technique.

INTRAOPERATIVE EVALUATION

Vollmar and Storz first described endoscopic evaluation of aortoiliac and femoral-popliteal reconstructions (2). To obtain good visualization in an unclamped distal vessel, they infused the irrigating fluid at arterial pressure to prevent backfeeding. We have not used this technique because of the risk of washing intimal debris into the distal circulation and the poor control of the volume of irrigation infused, and have instead examined vessels isolated completely from the arterial circulation, so that the endoscopy can be done safely and expeditiously. Endoscopy is a useful technique for operative evaluation of occluded vascular grafts. At reoperation for thrombosis of femoral-tibial and femoral-popliteal bypasses in the early postoperative period, we examine the distal anastomosis through a small transverse incision in the distal graft. After performing graft thrombectomy, the anastomosis is examined for technical errors and residual thrombus. The delicate suture line need not be reopened unless a technical defect is found that requires revision of the anastomosis. Trauma to the distal vessel caused by a vascular clamp, raised intimal flaps, and stenosis of the anastomosis all can be visualized clearly with the endoscope. We have found this technique to be particularly useful in evaluating occluded limbs of aortofemoral grafts after thrombectomy. Thrombosis of a graft is most often due to outflow obstruction secondary to progression of atherosclerosis or some technical error at the distal anastomosis (9). In most instances, long-term patency of the graft can be obtained by relieving the outflow obstruction with a profundoplasty or distal bypass procedure to restore adequate blood flow to the extremity. The thrombectomy can usually be performed through an incision in the groin. When the Dacron prosthesis has been occluded for several days, the thrombus becomes organized and tightly adherent to the fabric wall, making complete removal difficult. This residual thrombus can cause continued obstruction to blood flow, resulting in rethrombosis of the graft. Previously, the only means of assessing the completeness of the thrombectomy of a graft was either to evaluate qualitatively the gush of arterial blood flow on removal of the proximal clamp following thrombectomy or to measure arterial pressure at the completion of the procedure. These methods, though generally reliable, are imprecise. In those patients who do not have a good arterial pulse following graft thrombectomy, despite repeated passage of the Fogarty balloon catheter, the only option is to perform an inflow procedure, for example, femorofemoral, axillofemoral, or replacement of the limb of the aortofemoral graft. In one patient with a tightly adherent thrombus at the bifurcation of an aortoiliac graft, we avoided inserting a new graft because we were able to extract this adherent thrombus under direct vision. In axillary-femoral graft occlusion, it is important to distinguish occlusions caused by the patient lying on the graft from those caused by stenosis at the distal anastomosis. This is done easily by opening the graft just proximal to the distal anastomosis and endoscopically examining the anastomosis. An often difficult and time-consuming dissection in a previously operated groin is avoided if the findings at endoscopy are normal.

Arterial endoscopy is useful in carotid artery surgery. During carotid endarterectomy, it is difficult to inspect the external carotid artery adequately for atheromatous debris and elevated distal intimal flaps, since the distal extent of the endarterectomy is often 2-3 cm beyond the arteriotomy in the common carotid artery. The internal carotid artery repair can be evaluated for adherence of the distal intimal flap and residual atheromatous debris. We have found atheromatous debris in the internal carotid artery of two patients that was more than 1 mm long and capable of producing a neurological deficit by embolization. The time required to perform internal carotid endoscopy did not significantly prolong cerebral ischemia time. Endoscopy generally required less than 1 min and never more than 3 min. Total carotid occlusion time never exceeded 4 min (3).

TECHNIQUE

We performed vascular endoscopy in 91 vascular reconstructions, including 42 carotid endarterectomies and 24 femoral artery reconstructions (Table 1). All

Table 1 Vascular Endoscopy Procedures Evaluated

	No.
Carotid endarterectomy	42
Femoral artery reconstructions	24
Popliteal artery anastomoses	13
Aortic and iliac procedures	7
Aortic graft after thrombectomy	3
Renal artery bypass	1
Tibial reconstructions	1
Total	91

Source: Reproduced, with permission, from Towne JB, Bernhard VM: Vascular endoscopy. Surgery 82:416, 1977.

carotid endarterectomies were done with systemic heparinization and an inlying shunt for cerebral protection. The external carotid artery was examined endoscopically prior to closure of the arteriotomy with a shunt in place and a vascular clamp placed distally to prevent backbleeding (Fig. 1). After removing visualized atheromatous debris and elevated intimal flaps, we closed the arteriotomy partially with running sutures starting distally and proximally until a 1-cm defect remained in the carotid bulb. After clamping the common carotid and distal internal arteries, the shunt was removed and the endoscope was inserted through the arteriotomy. We looked for atheromatous debris or thrombus that could embolize when flow was restored and examined the distal artery for raised intimal flaps. If there is concern about the adequacy of collateral blood supply to the brain, a partial occlusion clamp can be placed across the 1-cm defect in the carotid bulb after removing the endoscope, allowing immediate restoration of internal carotid blood flow prior to completion of the arteriotomy closure.

During profundoplasty, we visualized the femoral and profunda arteries endoscopically following endarterectomy and after completion of all but 2 cm of the patch closure (Fig. 2). After aortoiliac endarterectomy we examined portions of the repair done by the closed technique to ensure complete removal of atheromatous debris. The internal iliac artery was examined for raised distal intimal flaps following endarterectomy of the iliac bifurcation.

In difficult distal bypass procedures, the completed distal anastomosis was visualized through a small tranverse incision in the distal graft. We were able to see if the intima was secured adequately in the suture line, if the lumen was free of debris, and if the anastomosis was widely patent. We also endoscopically examined occluded limbs of aortic bifurcation grafts and axillary-femoral grafts after thrombectomy. In thrombosed axillary-femoral bypasses, the graft was opened adjacent

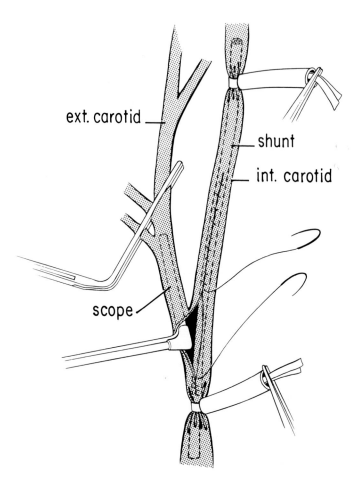

ext. carotid

shunt

int. carotid

scope

Figure 1 The choledoscoscope is inserted into the external carotid artery with the shunt in place. The vascular clamp is placed as far distally as possible on the external carotid artery to permit visualization of the distal extent of the endarterectomy. (Reprinted, with permission, from Towne JB, Bernhard VM: Vascular endoscopy. Stroke 8:569, 1977.)

to the anterior superior iliac spine, and the distal anastomosis was examined with the endoscope. Backbleeding was controlled by external pressure on the groin.

In patients with an occluded aortofemoral graft, the groin incision on the side of the occluded limb is opened and the anastomosis, common femoral, profunda femoris, and superficial femoral arteries are dissected free. Since the superficial femoral artery has usually been chronically occluded and the profunda femoral artery is the main source of blood to the lower extremity, the dissection is carried

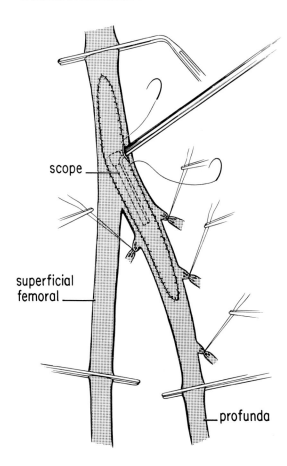

scope

superficial
femoral

profunda

Figure 2   The endoscope is inserted into the artery after completion of all but 2
cm of the patch closure on the lateral aspect of the profundaplasty. (Reprinted,
with permission, from Towne JB, Bernhard VM: Vascular endoscopy: Useful tool
or interesting toy. Surgery 82:415, 1977.)

distally in the profunda until a relatively undiseased artery is reached. The previous
anastomosis is dissected free, and a profundoplasty is performed using autogenous
vein or endarterectomized superficial femoral artery as a patch. Following completion of the outflow repair, the occluding thrombus is extracted from the graft with
Fogarty balloon catheter. A catheter with a large balloon is then passed into the
aortic portion of the bifurcation graft and inflated to prevent arterial inflow from
obscuring vision (10). The balloon is positioned so as to obstruct the aortic limb
as well as the patent contralateral limb (Fig. 3). The endoscope is passed into the
prosthesis visualizing its lumen (Fig. 4). Any residual thrombus can be readily

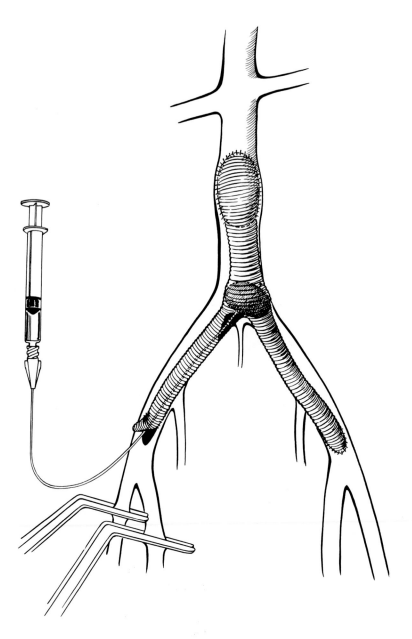

Figure 3 A balloon catheter is inserted into the aortic segment of the graft and the balloon inflated so as to occlude both the aortic flow and the backbleeding from the obstructed limb. (Reprinted, with permission, from Towne JB, Bernhard BM: Technique of intraoperative endoscopic evaluation of occluded aortofemoral grafts following thrombectomy. Surg Gynecol Obstet 148:87-89, 1979.)

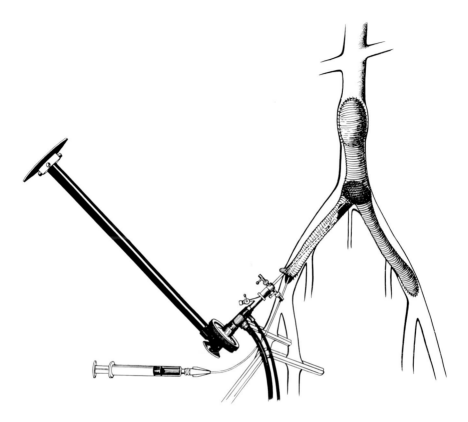

Figure 4   The endoscope is inserted into the graft and the lumen inspected for any residual adherent thrombus. Once localized, any residual debris can be easily removed with forceps. (Reprinted, with permission, from Towne JB, Bernhard VM: Technique of intraoperative endoscopic evaluation of occluded aortofemoral grafts following thrombectomy. Surg. Gynecol Obstet 148:87-89, 1979.)

localized and removed with forceps. A similar procedure is used for thrombectomy of axillofemoral, femorofemoral, and aortoiliac grafts. When inspection of the inflow tract is complete, the scope can be inserted into the outflow tract to determine that the runoff is satisfactory. The arthroscope that we use for visualization has a rod lens system with a fixed focus and a viewing angle of 90°. It is 3.5 mm in diameter and can be inserted approximately 20 cm into the lumen of the graft. A 40-cm, right-angled attachment is added to avoid contamination of the operative field during endoscopy. A standard fiber-optic light source and transmission cable are used. The graft is continuously flushed with lactated Ringer's solution which runs in by gravity flow through an irrigation channel in the scope from an intravenous bag hung 3 feet above the operative field. The endoscope, fiber-optic cable, and intravenous tubing are gas-sterilized. During endoscopy, the eyepiece is considered contaminated and not touched. When not in use, the scope is wrapped in sterile towels. Any adherent thrombus visualized with the endoscope was removed with a Randall stone forceps.

Initially, we evaluated the Hopkins choledochoscope and arthroscope, the Dyonics needlescope, and the Olympus fiber-optic bronchoscope. The image clarity and light transmission were superior in the rod lens system. These units have a fixed focus, with a significant depth of field and a viewing angle of 90°, which is much wider than in conventional endoscopy units. The choledochoscope is a rigid, right-angle instrument with a 32-cm vertical and a 5-cm horizontal limb. The horizontal limb, which measures 5 × 3.5 mm in cross section, is used for exploration. The arthroscope is a straight instrument, 23 cm long, with a cross-sectional diameter of 3.5 mm. A 40-cm, right-angle attachment can be added to the arthroscope which avoids contamination during endoscopy. A standard fiber-optic light source and transmission cable are used. The irrigation channel in the endoscope is flushed continuously with gravity flow from a bag of lactated Ringer's intravenous solution hung 3 feet above the operative field. The endoscope, fiber-optic cable, and intravenous tubing are gas-sterilized. During endoscopy the eye piece is considered to be contaminated and is not touched. When not in use, the endoscope is wrapped in sterile towels to avoid contamination.

RESULTS

The duration of endoscopy was 1-5 min in 53 cases, 5-10 min in 29, and more than 10 min in nine. Positive findings were noted in 60 of the 91 patients (66%), which consisted of intimal shreds and atheromatous debris in 47, elevated or irregular intimal flaps in 25, thrombi in five, and stenosis of the vascular repair in three. In 26 cases (29%), the endoscopic findings were considered to be significant enough possibly to affect the eventual outcome of the reconstructions. Seventeen (40%) of 42 external carotid arteries examined had elevated distal intimal flaps. One of three aortic bifurcation grafts examined following thrombectomy revealed a large thrombus tightly adherent to the graft wall that could not be removed by a Fogarty balloon catheter. Following visualization, the thrombus was extracted with a Randall stone forceps.

The endoscope was too large to insert into the artery in eight patients (9%) and cumbersome to use because of its size in 15 others (17%). There were no infections. The only apparent vessel injury produced by the insertion and intraarterial manipulation of the endoscope was a 1-cm linear tear in the intima of the internal iliac artery which produced no problem after operation. There were no neurological defects related to the use of the endoscope during carotid endarterectomy.

In over 120 patients in whom vascular endoscopy has been performed, no infections have occurred. Endoscopy permits immediate correction of any visualized defect prior to closure of the suture line and avoids reoperation or, at least, reopening of the suture line if problems develop after flow is restored. Instrumentation currently available was not designed for use in vascular endoscopy. The choledochoscope is too large to insert into small vessels and the arthroscope with the right-angle attachment is too bulky for convenient use. Endoscopy would be facilitated by decreasing the size of the endoscope for use in small vessels. Manipulation of the vascularscope would be less cumbersome if the angle between the viewing and exploring lenses were increased to 120°.

CONCLUSIONS

Vascular endoscopy is an alternative to operative arteriography for the intraoperative evaluation of vascular repairs. It provides a three-dimensional view of the reconstructed segment. It takes less time than arteriography and allows correction of defects prior to restoration of blood flow. Endoscopy adds a new dimension to vascular surgery permitting more precise repair, which should improve the results of vascular reconstruction. Further, technical refinements need to be made so that endoscopy can be useful in the evaluation of medium and small vessels.

REFERENCES

1. Towne JB, Bernhard VM: Vascular endoscopy: Useful tool or interesting toy. Surgery 82:415-419, 1977.
2. Vollmer JF, Storz LW: Vascular endoscopy. Surg Clin North Am 54:111, 1974.
3. Towne JB, Bernhard BM: Vascular endoscopy—An adjunct to carotid surgery. Stroke 8:569-571, 1977.
4. Tanabe T, Yokota A, Surgie S: Cardiovascular fiberoptic endoscopy: Development and clinical application. Surgery 87:375-379, 1980.
5. Mose KM, Shure D, Harrell JH, Tulamello J: Angioscopic visualization of pulmonary emboli. Chest 77:198-201, 1980.
6. Litvack F, Grundfest WS, Lee ME, Carroll RM, Foran R, Chaux A, Berci G, Rose HB, Matlott JM, Forrester JS: Angioscopic visualization of blood vessel interior in animals and humans. Clin Cardiol 8:65-70, 1985.
7. Itoh T, Motokazu H: Vascular endoscopy of major vascular reconstruction—experimental and clinical studies. Surgery 93:391-396, 1983.
8. Shure D, Moser KM, Harrell JH II, Hartman MT: Identification of pulmonary emboli in the dog: Comparison of angioscopy and perfusion scanning. Circulation 64:618-621, 1981.
9. Bernhard VM, Ray LF, Towne JB: The reoperation of choice for aortofemoral graft occlusion. Surgery 82:867-874, 1977.
10. Towne JB, Bernhard VM: Technique of intraoperative endoscopic evaluation of occluded aortofemoral grafts following thrombectomy. Surg. Gynecol Obstet 148:87-89, 1979.

19

Intraoperative Assessment of Bowel Viability

ALLAN R. PASCH
University of Illinois
  College of Medicine at Chicago
Chicago, Illinois

INTRODUCTION

In 1979, 32,000 persons were discharged from short-stay hospitals in the United States with a diagnosis of mesenteric vascular insufficiency (1). In these patients, a major problem in surgical decision-making is the intraoperative determination of bowel viability and the need for concomitant resection of intestine. Similar difficulties in assessment of bowel viability arise in the treatment of abdominal trauma, strangulation obstruction, necrotizing enterocolitis, and occasionally during elective resections of intestine.

Assessment of bowel viability is not only a guide to the extent of intestinal resection, but may also determine the necessity of mesenteric revascularization. For example, standard treatment of mycotic aneurysms of the superior mesenteric artery is excision of the aneurysm and ligation of the artery (2). Since collateral blood supply to the intestine gradually develops during growth of the aneurysm, only a few patients do not require revascularization. Assessment of bowel viability would be helpful in determining which patients require restoration of mesenteric blood flow. A second example is ligation of the portal vein after penetrating injury; assessment of intestinal viability could guide the need for portal decompression (3). A more common problem is the 2% incidence of colon ischemia following abdominal aortic reconstruction (4,5). Intraoperative identification of patients with colon ischemia who need inferior mesenteric reimplantation could lessen the occurrence of this complication, and reduce overall mortality from aortic surgery.

Clearly, intraoperative assessment of intestinal viability is an important issue for both the vascular and general surgeon. In this chapter we will review those maneuvers that may aid the surgeon in determining the viability of intestine while in the operating theatre.

DETERMINATION OF INTESTINAL VIABILITY

Clinical Criteria

Historically, the decision to resect intestine of indeterminate viability has been a clinical judgment based upon bowel color, peristaltsis, bleeding from the cut edge of intestine, and the presence of palpable pulsations in the mesentery. The high mortality after treatment of acute mesenteric ischemia make retrospective evaluation of the accuracy of clinical criteria difficult. However, numerous experimental and several prospective clinical studies have confirmed the inadequacy of clinical judgment. Overall accuracy is 58-89%, with sensitivity of 50-78% and specificity of 74-91% (6-8).

Second-Look Procedures

The unreliability of clinical judgment led Shaw in 1959 and Zuidema in 1964 to propose planned abdominal reexploration 24 hr after mesenteric revascularization (9,10). There has not been great enthusiasm for this approach, and clinical data on the utility of second-look procedures is equivocal. In a series from the University of Rochester, 17 planned rexplorations contributed to survival in only three patients (11). Ottinger reported on 15 patients at Massachusetts General with planned reexploration (12). Eight required repeat resection of bowel, yet only a single patient ultimately survived.

A specific role of second-look procedures in the management of ischemic bowel secondary to acute mesenteric venous thrombosis has been proposed, since propagation of thrombus causes recurrent intestinal infarction in one-third of patients in the perioperative period (13). However, the efficacy of second-look procedures in this setting has not been demonstrated, and anticoagulation is probably as effective in preventing recurrent ischemia (14).

Routine use of second-look procedures might partially compensate for false-negative errors in clinical judgment, i.e., failure to resect nonviable bowel at the initial laparotomy. However, second-look procedures do not resolve the dilemma of unnecessarily resecting viable bowel. Furthermore, second-look operations do not obviate the need for a reliable method of determining bowel viability, since at reoperation the surgeon is again required to determine bowel viability. Though no direct morbidity has been attributed to reexploration, physicians are hesitant to subject very ill patients to a reoperative procedure with questionable yield, and its overall impact on the management of ischemic bowel has been slight.

Miscellaneous Methods

There have been numerous attempts to develop an objective method of determining bowel viability (15-26), reflecting the clinical magnitude of this problem. Advances in knowledge of the electrical physiology of the gut have led to the experimental use of electromyography to determine bowel viability (15-17). Normally the intestine exhibits two types of electrical activity: quick spikes, which are the action potentials of intestinal muscle and correspond with peristaltsis, and a slow baseline pattern that is independent of mechanical activity of the intestine. Ischemia eliminates both electrical patterns, but after revascularization the slow pattern will reappear in bowel that is viable. Despite encouraging experimental results, clinical application of electromyography has been scant. Subserosal placement of an electrode is required, and clinicians may be reluctant to transgress the bowel wall.

Other experimental methods have included measurement of serosal pH or CO_2 or the transserosal potential difference; staining with Trypan Blue, patent blue V, or bromphenol blue; tetrazolium analysis of mucosa; thermography; and the use of radioactive microspheres. Determination of serosal pH has not been predictive of intestinal viability (18), whereas measurement of the transserosal electric potential difference is more accurate but requires an enterotomy for lead placement (19). Tetrazolium analysis of mucosa requires intestinal biopsies, which may be impractical (17,20). Measurement of the increase in bowel temperature, based on the phenomenon of reactive hyperemia seen in viable bowel after revascularization, has yielded equivocal results (16,21-23). Scintiscanning after aortic injection of radioactive microspheres or injection of dye into the superior mesenteric artery have also been useful in experimental settings. However, the technical problems in performing most of these tests has led to little clinical application. In contrast, intravenous injection of dyes (24,25) is fairly simple to perform. Refinement of this technique using fluorescein has emerged as a useful tool.

Fluorescein

First described as a test of bowel viability in 1942 (26), fluorescein subsequently received little utilization in general surgery, but was applied in retinal arteriography, in the assessment of skin flaps, and in evaluating peripheral vascular disease (27-30).

After injection into a peripheral vein, fluorescein freely distributes into the extracellular space. In animal studies, most is excreted unchanged in the urine and a small amount is conjugated in the liver (31). Peak serum concentrations occur in approximately 10 min, and then decrease according to first-order elimination kinetics as equilibration in extracellular body fluids occurs (32). With standard room light sources, tissues appear grossly yellow for 12 hr whereas urine remains colored for 36 hr. When exposed to ultraviolet light with a wavelength of 3900 Angstroms, the dye emits a strong gold-green fluorescence. The fluorescence reflects accumulation of dye in interstitial fluid, since intracellular penetration by fluorescein is minimal. Though the fluorescence does not directly correlate with blood flow, the amount of fluorescence appears to be a rough indicator of local perfusion (33).

Fluorescein testing for bowel viability is easily and safely performed. After injecting 20 cc of a 5% solution (i.e., 15 mg/kg) into a peripheral vein, a Wood's (ultraviolet) light is held above the bowel and the fluorescent pattern observed. If a permanent record of the fluorescence is desired, instant photography can be employed using minor modifications of Polaroid equipment (34-36). In addition to the ease of performance, fluorescein is quite safe. Though 0.6% of conscious patients undergoing retinal arteriography experience urticaria, nausea, or vomiting (37), anaphylactoid reactions are rare (38,39). In patients under general anesthesia, the safety of using fluorescein can be increased by first injecting a test dose of 0.5 cc.

The modern application of fluorescein to the determination of bowel viability was developed by Stolar in 1978 (40). In an experimental model involving ischemia with subsequent restoration of flow, viable intestine exhibited either bright

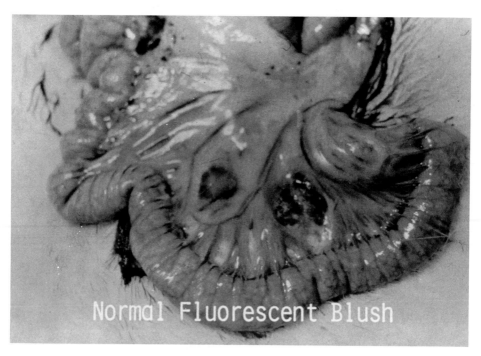

Figure 1   Green-gold fluorescence seen in normal intestine after intravenous injection of fluorescein. (From Ref. 23.)

fluorescence, or in some cases a more reticular pattern. Animals with patchy areas of nonfluorescence were reexplored 24 hr later. If the dye had cleared by that time, two-thirds of the segments of bowel survived. In contrast, bowel with fluorescein still visible at 24 hr was uniformly nonviable. Thus, at the initial laparotomy fluorescein was 100% sensitive in identifying nonviable bowel, but a second-look procedure was required to increase specificity and avoid resecting segments of viable bowel.

An example of the evenly distributed green-gold fluorescence seen in normal bowel is illustrated in Figure 1, whereas Figure 2 demonstrates the reticular pattern. The latter is often seen after restoration of flow to ischemic bowel, and indicates viability. The third pattern, nonfluorescence (Fig. 3) is easily detected by gross inspection.

The potential for false-positive results (i.e., resection of viable bowel) with the fluorescein method has been confirmed by other investigators, with specificity ranging from 75 to 100% in the literature (7,8,41-44). While the unnecessary resection of viable bowel is certainly undesirable, failure to resect nonviable bowel due to

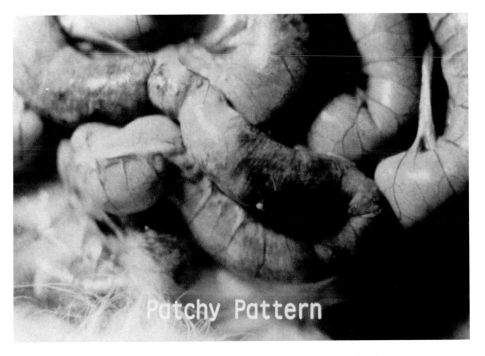

Figure 2 Reticular pattern seen after temporary ischemia in viable intestine. (From Ref. 23.)

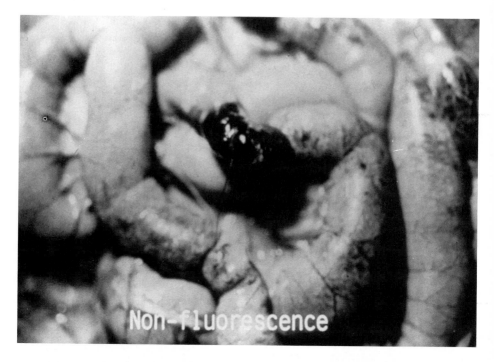

Figure 3 Nonfluorescent and nonviable intestine. (From Ref. 23.)

false-negative results will undoubtedly have more serious clinical consequences and is of greater concern.

Unfortunately, there is a wide variation in the reported sensitivity of fluorescein in determining bowel viability. Numerous studies have demonstrated sensitivity of 95-100% (7,8,40,44,45), yet Carter, Silverman, and Lanzafame found sensitivity of only 11%, 40%, and 90%, respectively (41-43).

In an attempt to increase the accuracy of fluorescein, Silverman has quantified fluorescence using a perfusion fluorometer (42,43). In this method, a lower dose of fluorescein (2 mg/kg) is administered. Repeated quantification of fluorescence at frequent intervals and measurement of fluorescein excretion as well as uptake enables construction of fluorometric curves. In animal studies, two fluorescent patterns, hypofluorescence and hyperfluorescence with slow clearing of dye, indicated nonviable bowel. However, nonviable bowel with a hyperfluoremetric pattern appeared normal in the standard fluorescein test. As a result, in this experimental model sensitivity was 11% and accuracy 64% for qualitative fluorescein, versus 100% for the quantitative method.

The wide divergence in the experimental accuracy of fluorescein is cause for concern. Certainly the use of different species and models of ischemia and the need for subjective interpretation of the fluorescent pattern have contributed to the variability in results. Quantification of fluorescein may eventually prove more accurate, but this requires additional equipment that is not readily available in all hospitals. The standard (qualitative) fluorescein test retains the attributes of simplicity and availability, and has been proven accurate in clinical trials.

Doppler Ultrasound

Doppler ultrasound is a useful means of perioperative assessment of blood flow in the extremities. In 1975, Wright and Hobson first described the application of Doppler ultrasound to assessment of intestinal blood flow (46). In this technique, a gas-sterilized 9-MHz, pencil-shaped Doppler probe is positioned at the antimesenteric border of the intestine, using water-soluble coupling gel. Arterial flow signals are easily heard in viable bowel, but are absent in bowel of questionable viability.

In animals with experimental mesenteric ischemia and revascularization, Wright and Hobson found Doppler examination more accurate than clinical judgment. In subsequent experimental work, Cooperman confirmed the accuracy of Doppler in predicting bowel viability (47). In 20 animals with intestinal ischemia, bowel was histologically viable at the location of the last audible Doppler signal. In a second part of this study, ischemic bowel was resected and primary anastomosis of the remaining bowel performed. Anastomoses located within 1 cm of the last Doppler signal healed, while 67% of anastomoses performed 2 cm or more from the signal developed leaks or stricture.

The above experiments all involved a mixed model of arterial and venous insufficiency. In separate investigation of experimental mesenteric venous insufficiency, the presence of Doppler signals after relief of venous obstruction also accurately predicted bowel viability (48).

On the basis of laboratory evidence, Doppler has been successfully applied to clinical practice (49,50). In a series of 23 patients with intestinal ischemia of diverse etiologies, Doppler was 100% accurate in predicting bowel viability, and prevented 10 false-negative and 2 false-positive results that would have occurred if clinical criteria had been used to assess bowel viability (51). Cooperman, who clearly has the most experience with this technique, has also utilized Doppler ultrasound to guide elective resections of small intestine and colon (52,53).

Both fluorescein and Doppler are more accurate than clinical judgment, and have gained acceptance by the surgical community. Three studies have attempted to compare the two methods directly. In an experimental study, Doppler was 75% sensitive for venous occlusion, but only 0% and 14% sensitive for arterial and arteriovenous models of ischemia, respectively, while fluorescein achieved overall sensitivity and specificity of 95% and 53%, respectively (44). Fluorescein specificity was 83%, 0%, and 75%, respectively, for arterial, venous, and mixed ischemic models. In another experimental study, Gorey evaluated 64 segments of intestine. Sensitivity and specificity of Doppler were 57% and 89%, versus 96% and 95%, respectively, for fluorescein (45). In a prospective, controlled study of 28 patients with 71 segments of bowel needing evaluation, fluorescein exhibited 100% accuracy, compared with a 64% sensitivity and 88% specificity for Doppler (7).

Both methods are safe and easily performed with equipment available in most hospitals. However, in comparative studies, the Doppler method appears to be relatively insensitive, and when used alone, may result in failure to recognize nonviable bowel.

New Methods

A new and relatively untested method of assessing bowel viability is the transserosal measurement of the partial pressure of oxygen. This technique involves placement of a small oxygen electrode on the bowel serosa with continuous measurement of PO_2 in the underlying serosa. In contrast to other methods, surface oximetry not only reflects intestinal blood flow, but also the arterial PO_2 as well as tissue oxygen consumption. In the only study to date, Shoemaker demonstrated excellent experimental accuracy of surface oximetry in predicting anastomotic healing (54). However, unlike fluorescein or Doppler, a major problem is the current unavailability of electrodes for use on bowel.

A second relatively new and experimental method of assessing bowel viability is external gamma counting after intraperitoneal injection of Xenon-133 (55). Like quantitative fluorescence, this test utilizes the slow washout of xenon as an indication of diminished perfusion and hence nonviability. However, relatively sophisticated and expensive equipment is required, and the potential role of this modality is not yet clear.

COLON ISCHEMIA AND ABDOMINAL AORTIC RECONSTRUCTION

A very common problem facing the vascular surgeon is ischemia of the left colon after abdominal aortic reconstruction. Though the clinical incidence of this complication is only 1-2% (4,5), prospective studies utilizing colonoscopy reveal a 6% incidence (56). More importantly, mortality is well over 50% (57-59).

Blood to the descending and sigmoid colon normally emanates from the left colic and sigmoidal branches of the inferior mesenteric artery (IMA), while the rectum is nourished by the superior hemorrhoidal artery from the IMA as well as the middle and inferior hemorrhoidal branches of the internal iliac arteries (60). Thrombosis of the IMA occurs in 40-78% of patients with abdominal aortic aneurysms and 48% of patients with aortoiliac occlusive disease, in which case the left colon receives its blood supply from anastomoses with the middle colic artery (61-63).

Patients with thrombosis of the IMA rarely develop symptoms of colon ischemia, since the gradual nature of the occlusion allows formation of collateral pathways. However, if IMA flow is acutely reduced by ligation, colon ischemia may result. Ligation of the IMA is a standard technique during aneurysmectomy; in contrast, during aortobifemoral bypass for occlusive disease IMA ligation is not required and IMA patency may be maintained by retrograde iliac blood flow. Thus, patients with a patent IMA who undergo resection of abdominal aortic aneurysms represent a group at higher risk for colon ischemia.

When the IMA is patent, many surgeons routinely ligate the IMA during aneurysmectomy, while a few routinely reimplant the vessel into the aortic graft to avoid colon ischemia. In contrast to these two approaches, a selective policy is feasible. Ernst described a method of cannulating the orifice of the IMA and measuring the stump pressure, which reflects collateral flow (64). In his study, no patient with a stump pressure greater than 40 mmHg developed ischemic colitis. Alternatively, Hobson described the diminution of left colon Doppler signals when the IMA is clamped as a reliable indicator of left colon ischemia and the need for IMA reimplantation (65,66). One advantage of the Doppler technique is its applicability to aortic reconstruction for occlusive disease, in which case the IMA is not easily cannulated to measure back pressure.

For completeness, the possibility of small intestinal ischemia during aortic surgery should be mentioned (67,68). Early in the course of the laparotomy, the IMA should be palpated. A large IMA may indicate occult occlusive disease of the superior mesenteric artery, with collateral flow from the IMA supplying the midgut. In this case, IMA reimplantation is indicated to prevent small bowel ischemia.

In summary, both measurement of the IMA stump pressure and evaluation of mesenteric Doppler signals are useful in assessing the left colon during aortic reconstruction. With these tools, routine reimplantation of the IMA is not indicated. Rather, a policy of selective reimplantation can hopefully lower the incidence of colon ischemia.

SUMMARY AND CONCLUSIONS

Determination of bowel viability is a ubiquitous problem in general and vascular surgery. Reliance on visual inspection of the bowel has proven unsatisfactory. The benefits of second-look procedures are not readily apparent, and surgeons are reluctant to utilize this approach. Two methods of intraoperative assessment of intestinal viability, fluorescein and Doppler, have been useful in experimental and clinical testing. Both are easily and inexpensively performed. In several direct comparisons, the fluorescein method was more accurate than Doppler. However, a major drawback of qualitative fluorescein is the need to determine fluorescence subjectively, and as a result, disparate experimental results have been reported in the literature. Preliminary experimental data using a quatitative fluorescein technique shows promise for increasing the accuracy of fluorescein. However, apparatus for this is not widely available. The qualitative fluorescein method, which is clearly more accurate than Doppler, is presently the method of choice for intraoperative assessment of bowel viability.

The particular problem of left colon ischemia during aortic reconstruction can be avoided by selectively implanting the IMA into the aortic graft, guided by Doppler assessment of collateral flow to the descending and sigmoid colon or by direct measurement of the IMA stump pressure.

REFERENCES

1. United States Department of Health and Human Services, Public Health Service, Office of Health Research Statistics: Detailed Diagnosis and Surgical Procedures for Patients Discharged from Short-Stay Hospitals, United States, 1979, Hyattsville, Maryland, 1982.
2. Stanley JC, Thompson NW, Fry WJ: Splanchnic artery aneurysms. Arch Surg 101:689, 1970.
3. Mattox KL: Abdominal venous injuries. Surgery 91:498, 1982.
4. Ottinger LW, Darling RC, Nathan MJ, Linton RR: Left colon ischemia complicating aorto-iliac reconstruction. Arch Surg 105:841, 1972.
5. Johnson WC, Nabseth DC: Visceral infarction following aortic surgery. Ann Surg 180:312, 1974.
6. Zarins CK, Skinner DB, Rhodes BA, James AE Jr.: Prediction of the viability of revascularized intestine with radioactive microspheres. Surg Gynecol Obstet 138:576, 1974.
7. Bulkley GB, Zuidema GD, Hamilton SR, O'Mara CS, Klacsmann PG, Horn SD: Introperative determination of small intestinal viability following ischemic injury. Ann Surg 193:628, 1981.
8. Marfuggi RA, Greenspan M: Reliable intraoperative prediction of intestinal viability using a fluorescent indicator. Surg Gynecol Obstet 152:33, 1981.
9. Shaw RS, Rutledge RH: Superior mesenteric artery embolectomy in the treatment of massive mesenteric infarction. N Engl J Med 252:595, 1957.
10. Zuidema GD, Reed D, Turcotte JG, Fry WJ: Superior mesenteric embolectomy. Ann Surg 159:548, 1964.
11. Sachs SM, Morton JM, Schwartz SI: Acute mesenteric ischemia. Surgery 92:646, 1982.
12. Ottinger LW: The surgical management of acute occlusion of the superior mesenteric artery. Ann Surg 188:721, 1978.
13. Khodadadi J, Rozencwajg J, Nacasch N, Schmidt B, Feuchtwanger MM: Mesenteric vein thrombosis: The importance of a second-look operation. Arch Surg 115:315, 1980.

14. Jona J, Cummins GM Jr, Head HB, Govostis MC: Recurrent primary mesenteric venous thrombosis. J Am Med Assoc 227:1033, 1974.
15. Schamaun M: Electromyography to determine viability of injured bowel segments: An experimental study with preliminary clinical observations. Surgery 62:899, 1967.
16. Bussemaker JB, Lindeman J: Comparison of methods to determine viability of small intestine. Ann Surg 176:97, 1972.
17. Katz S, Wahab A, Murray W, Williams LF: New parameters of viability in ischemic bowel disease. Am J Surg 127:136, 1974.
18. Myers MB, Cherry G, Gesser J: Relationship between surface pH and pCO2 and the vascularity and viability of intestine. Surg Gynecol Obstet 134:787, 1972.
19. Gurll NJ, Braxton G: Potential difference as an estimate of intestinal viability. J Surg Res 20:231, 1976.
20. Carter K, Halle M, Cherry G, Myers MB: Determination of the viability of ischemic intestine. Arch Surg 100:695, 1970.
21. Laufman M, Method H: The role of vascular spasm in recovery of strangulated intestine. Surg Gynecol Obstet 85:675, 1947.
22. Moss AA, Kressel HY, Brito AC: Use of thermography to predict intestinal viability and survival after ischemic injury: A blind experimental study. Invest Radiol 16:24, 1981.
23. Papachristou D, Fortner JG: Prediction of intestinal viability by intra-arterial dye injection: A simple test. Am J Surg 132:572, 1976.
24. Meyers MB, Cherry G: Use of vital dyes in the evaluation of the blood supply of the colon. Surg Gynecol Obstet 128:97, 1969.
25. Dineen P, Goulian D Jr, McSherry CK: A method of demonstrating intestinal viability. Am J Gast 45:335, 1966.
26. Herrlin JO Jr., Glasser ST, Lange K: New methods for determining the viability of bowel. Arch Surg 45:785, 1942.
27. Novotny HR, Alvis DL: A method of photographing fluorescence in circulating blood in the human retina. Circulation 24:82, 1961.
28. Myers MB: Prediction of skin sloughs at the time of operation with the use of fluorescein dye. Surgery 51:158, 1962.
29. McCraw JB, Myers B, Shanklin KD: The value of fluorescein in predicting the viability of arterialized flaps. Plast Reconstr Surg 60:710, 1977.
30. Lowry K Jr, Kirkpatrick JF Jr, Thoroughman JC: Evaluation of peripheral vascular disease using intra-arterial fluorescein. Am Surg 30:35, 1964.
31. Webb JM, Fonda M, Brouwer EA: Metabolism and excretion patterns of fluorescein and certain halogenated fluorescein dyes in rats. J Pharmacol Exper Ther 137:141, 1962.
32. Crisman JM, Fuhrman FA: Studies on gangrene following cold injury, IV. The use of fluorescein as an indicator of local blood flow: Distribution of fluorescein in body fluids after intravenous injection. J Clin Invest 26:259, 1947.
33. Lanzafame RJ, Naim JO, Francis M, Tomkiewicz ZM, Voytek A, Hinshaw JR: Prediction of blood flow in and viability of ischemic small bowel: Fluorescein versus radiolabelled microspheres. Curr Surg 40:286, 1983.

34. Lanzafame RJ, Naim JO, Blackman JR, Hinshaw JR: Streamlined fluorescein photography. Surg Gynecol Obstet 160:357, 1985.
35. Lanzafame RJ, Naim JO, Blackman JR, Welch E, Hinshaw JR: Fluorescein photography. Curr Surg 39:310, 1982.
36. Lanzafame RJ, Naim JO, Blackman JR, Welch E, Hinshaw JR: A method of documentation of tissue perfusion using instant photography. Surg Gynecol Obstet 156:749, 1983.
37. Stein MR, Parker CW: Reactions following intravenous fluorescein. Am J Ophthalmol 72:861, 1971.
38. LaPiana FG, Penner R: Anaphylactoid reaction to intravenously administered fluorescein. Arch Ophthalmol 79:161, 1968.
39. Cunningham EE, Venkataraman B: Cardiac arrest following fluorescein angiography. J Am Med Assoc 242:2431, 1979.
40. Stolar CJH, Randolph JG: Evaluation of ischemic bowel viability with a fluorescent technique. J Ped Surg 13:221, 1978.
41. Lanzafame RJ, Naim JO, Tomkiewicz ZM, Hinshaw JR: The accuracy of predicting intestinal viability with fluorescein: Experimental observations. Curr Surg 40:292, 1983.
42. Silverman DG, Hurford WE, Cooper HS, Robinson M, Brousseau DA: Quantification of fluorescein distribution to strangulated rat ileum. J Surg Res 34:179, 1983.
43. Carter MS, Fantini GA, Sammartano RJ, Mitsudo S, Silverman DG, Boley SJ: Qualitative and quantitative fluorescein fluorescence in determining intestinal viability. Am J Surg 147:117, 1984.
44. Wheaton LG, Strandberg JD, Hamilton SR, Bulkley GB: A comparison of three techniques for intraoperative prediction of small intestinal injury. JAAHA 19:897, 1983.
45. Gorey TF: The recovery of intestine after ischemic injury. Br J Surg 67:699, 1980.
46. Wright CB, Hobson RW II: Prediction of intestinal viability using Doppler ultrasound techniques. Am J Surg 129:642, 1975.
47. Cooperman M, Pace WG, Martin EW Jr., Pflug B, Keith LM Jr., Evans WE, Carey LC: Determination of viability of ischemic intestine by Doppler ultrasound. Surgery 83:705, 1978.
48. Cooperman M, Martin EW, Carey LC: Determination of intestinal viability by Doppler ultrasonography in venous infarction. Ann Surg 191:57, 1980.
49. Shah SD, Anderson CA: Prediction of small bowel viability using Doppler ultrasound. Ann Surg 194:97, 1981.
50. O'Donnell JA, Hobson RW: Operative confirmation of Doppler ultrasound in evaluation of intestinal ischemia. Surgery 87:109, 1980.
51. Cooperman M, Martin EW Jr, Carey LC: Evaluation of ischemic intestine by Doppler ultrasound. Am J Surg 139:73, 1980.
52. Cooperman M, Martin EW Jr, Keith LM, Carey LC: Use of Doppler ultrasound in intestinal surgery. Am J Surg 138:856, 1979.
53. Cooperman M, Martin EW Jr, Evans WE, Carey LC: Assessment of anastomotic blood supply by Doppler ultrasound in operations upon the colon. Surg Gynecol Obstet 149:15, 1979.

54. Locke R, Hauser CJ, Shoemaker WC: The use of surface oximetry to assess bowel viability. Arch Surg 119:1252, 1984.

55. Bulkley GB, Gharagozloo F, Alderson PO, Horn SD, Zuidema GD: Use of intraperitoneal xenon-133 for imaging of intestinal stragulation in small bowel obstruction. Am J Surg 141:128, 1981.

56. Hagihara PF, Ernst CB, Griffen WO Jr.: Incidence of ischemic colitis following abdominal aortic reconstruction. Surg Gynecol Obstet 149:571, 1979.

57. Kalman PG, Johnston KW, Lipton IH: Prevention of severe intestinal ischemia following reconstruction of the abdominal aorta. Can J Surg 26:634, 1981.

58. Kim MW, Hundahl SA, Dang CR, McNamara JJ, Strachley CJ, Whelan TJ Jr: Ischemic colitis after aortic aneurysmectomy. Am J Surg 145:392, 1983.

59. Young JR, Humphries AW, DeWolfe VG, LeFeore FA: Complications of abdominal aortic surgery. Arch Surg 86:51, 1963.

60. Basmajian JV: The marginal anastomoses of the arteries to the large intestine. Surg Gynecol Obstet 99:614, 1954.

61. Ernst CB, Hagihara PF, Daugherty ME, Sachatello CR, Griffen WO Jr: Ischemic colitis incidence following abdominal aortic reconstruction. Surgery 80:417, 1976.

62. Bell DD, Gaspar MR: Routine aortography before abdominal aortic aneurysmectomy. Am J Surg 144:191, 1982.

63. Baur GM, Porter JM, Eidemiller LR, Rosch J, Keller F: The role of arteriography in abdominal aortic aneurysm. Am J Surg 136:184, 1978.

64. Ernst CB, Hagihara PF, Daugherty ME, Griffen WO Jr: Inferior mesenteric artery stump pressure: A reliable index for safe IMA ligation during abdominal aortic aneurysmectomy. Ann Surg 187:641, 1978.

65. Hobson RW III, Wright CB, O'Donnell JA, Zamil A, lamberth WC, Najem Z: Determination of intestinal viability by Doppler ultrasound. Arch Surg 114:165-168, 1979.

66. Hobson RW II, Wright CB, Rich NM, Collins GJ Jr: Assessment of colonic ischemia during aortic surgery by Doppler ultrasound. J Surg Res 20:231, 1976.

67. Connolly JE, Stemmer EA: Intestinal gangrene as the result of mesenteric arterial steal. Am J Surg 126:197, 1973.

68. Perler BA, Brewster DC: Massive small bowel infarction: An unusual complication of abdominal aortic surgery. Am Surg 50:402, 1984.

Part III

POSTOPERATIVE METHODS

20

Early and Late Postoperative Monitoring of Extremity Graft Function

SPENCER F. GOODSON and JAMES J. SCHULER
University of Illinois College of Medicine at Chicago
Chicago, Illinois

The objective of reconstructive arterial surgery of the lower extremities is to improve the limb hemodynamics sufficiently to relieve disabling claudication or prevent limb loss secondary to severe ischemia. Certainly graft occlusion, whether early or late, represents failure and is usually attended by a prompt recurrence of claudication or limb-threatening ischemia. A patent graft, however, does not necessarily insure improved flow and hemodynamic failure frequently predates occlusion (1-4). Careful follow-up incorporating noninvasive hemodynamic measurements allows the surgeon to identify hemodynamically failed or "failing" grafts and salvage a significant number of grafts prior to complete occlusion.

The subjective assessment of the success of an arterial reconstructive procedure is based upon the disappearance of preoperative symptoms and the physical signs of ischemia. When severe claudication or rest pain recurs, when ulcers fail to improve, or gangrene advances, graft failure is obvious. In some instances however, physical examination and the evaluation of symptoms do not reliably indicate a failed graft. Clearly, early failure may go unrecognized in the postoperative setting when only symptomatic evaluation and the clinical appearance of the foot or pulse determinations are made (5). O'Mara and colleagues reported 5 of 34 postoperative patients with improved symptoms and 7 with either a palpable or Doppler detectable pulse in the immediate postoperative period whose increase in ankle pressure index showed little, if any, improvement (6). Arteriography demonstrated the cause of hemodynamic failure in each case.

Delayed failure can be even more difficult to detect on the basis of recurrence of symptoms or physical signs. Berkowitz found this to be true in evaluating 30 vein graft stenoses, of which 77% presented within the first year of follow-up. He detected 17 proximal anastomotic strictures, 10 midgraft fibrotic valve strictures, and 6 involving the distal anastomosis. Of the 30 stenotic vein grafts, Berkowitz found that 57% presented with normal pulses and a like number were asymptomatic. Forty percent were *both* asymptomatic and had intact distal pulses. He concluded that the noninvasive laboratory ". . . becomes of primary importance in diagnosing the conditions of patients who are asymptomatic and reinforces clinical judgment when presenting symptoms are not overwhelming" (1). In 27 patients reported by O'Mara with late failure (average 2.5 years), symptoms were variably present and when present were uniformly less severe than preoperatively (6). All grafts were patent but angiographically showed pronounced host disease progression or graft stenosis. The initial postoperative improvement in segmental pressures and indices returned to preoperative levels (or worse, if distal disease progression was the cause).

In general, it has been shown that observer variability in the assessment of occlusive vascular disease is considerable. A word of caution is especially needed in assessing diabetics. The arteries most often involved are the tibio-peroneal vessels where claudication symptoms are at best variable and peripheral neuropathy masks ischemic rest pain. Because of this, distal reconstructions in diabetics require more objective surveillance than clinical evaluation alone affords (7).

Graft performance, then, cannot reliably be judged with conventional observation alone unless findings obviously indicate occlusion. More accurate physiologic and anatomic data can be gathered using either noninvasive or invasive studies. These studies include Doppler segmental lower extremity pressure measurements and indices, pulse volume recordings, waveform analyses, and contrast angiography. The goal in graft follow-up is to secure safe and accurate data that enables the clinician objectively to define both occlusive and hemodynamic failures within a time frame that optimizes chances for secondary salvage. Prompt intervention, instigated by failing hemodynamics significantly increases the salvage rate of patent but failing grafts. The final common pathway in the management of failures is in almost every case angiography. Obvious shortcomings, however, exist in the too frequent use of angiography during follow-up. Angiography not only carries a well-defined risk but is considerably more costly than noninvasive methods of assessing graft function. Clinical renal failure is variably implicated in 5-10% of cases. Bleeding, thrombosis, and embolus may threaten the integrity of previous vascular repairs or create new problems needing operative intervention. Furthermore, the anatomic data provided by angiography does not always accurately indicate the functional significance of lesser degrees of stenosis. In combination with hemodynamic screening and better resolution in the use of computer imaging, intravenous digital subtraction angiography may well represent the ideal postoperative surveillance as indicated by the work of Turnipseed and Acher (8).

THE ETIOLOGY OF GRAFT FAILURE

There are a host of causes of graft failure. Early graft failure (within 30 days) is usually technical or the result of an underestimation of the severity of inflow or outflow disease. Technical or judgmental errors were chiefly responsible for seven of O'Mara's early failures (6). Such errors as anastomotic narrowing, use of small ex situ (less than 4 mm) veins, kinks and twists, excessive graft length, poor routing, and the presence or persistence of small residual platelet thrombi accounted for 18% of failed grafts in an additional study group of 109 (9).

Secondary reconstruction for early failure has in many series lead to a poorer eventual outcome: 20% 1-year patency in a series of 48 patients (10), 55% patency at 5 years (11), 54% limb salvage at 4.5 years (9). These results compare to those for all secondary reconstructions regardless of the timing of failure. Technical mistakes are costly. The incidence of early failures can be minimized by the combination of intraoperative arteriography and intraoperative ankle pressure measurements. It makes sense that the same vigilance is necessary in the early postoperative setting to detect as quickly as possible the failure of a graft. This minimizes the propagation of distal clot and increases the chances of successful reoperation. Such vigilance should ideally be objective and noninvasive.

Delayed graft failure also has a multiplicity of etiologies, ranging from technical (rare) to degenerative changes within the graft itself to host disease progression. When failure occurs within the first year, it is frequently due to problems within the graft itself. Such problems include neointimal thickening, vein valve cusp stenosis, fibrotic stenoses, or intimal hyperplasia at the anastomosis. Failures seen later than 1 year postoperatively generally imply progression of host atherosclerosis (9, 12). Mozersky stresses that ankle indices always worsen when occlusive failure is caused by new host disease whereas the earlier failures secondary to changes within the reconstruction itself show ankle pressures nearly identical or slightly better than those present prior to operation (13).

As mentioned by Whittemore, lesions causing failure with the first year after bypass were most often intrinsic to the bypass graft itself (9). Seventy-seven percent of 33 vein graft stenoses presented in the first year of follow-up in Berkowitz's series (1). Vein graft stenosis can arise from valve cusps of arterialized saphenous veins as shown by Whitney (12), who observed that valves actually worked in the arterialized reversed saphenous vein segment and postulated that the turbulence caused by the working valve caused injury which progressed to later fibrosis and occlusion. Down found six valvular stenoses in 14 conduits and three went on to occlude the graft (2). A case example is presented below:

Case example: The patient is a 65-year-old diabetic hypertensive man who presented in August 1983 with complaints of left rest pain and left foot arterial ulcer. Indices (Fig. 1A) were consistent with severe ischemia, and

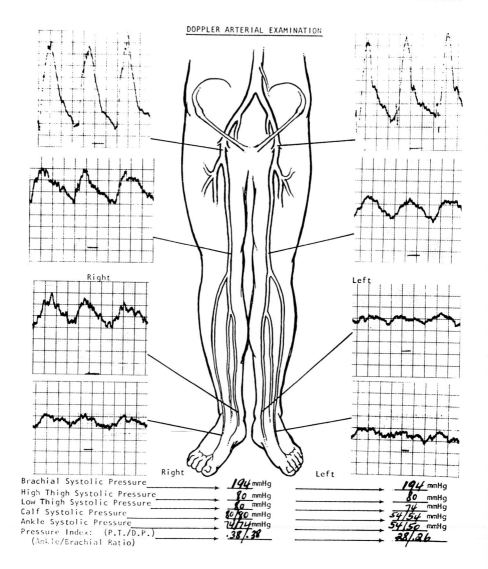

Figure 1a Preoperative arterial blood flow examination.

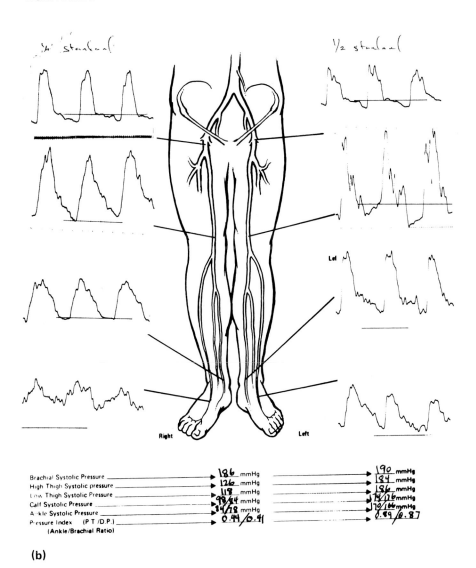

(b)

Figure 1b Postoperative arterial blood flow examination.

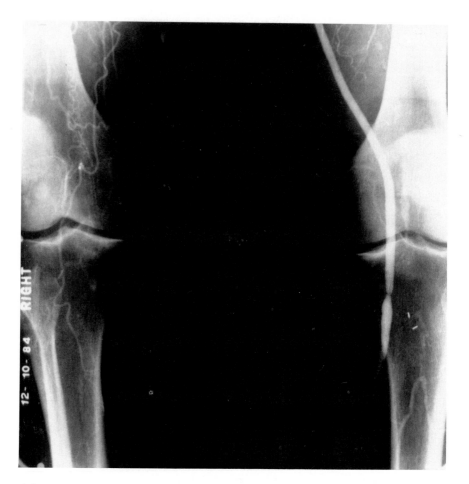

(c)

Figure 1c Arteriographic demonstration of vein graft stenosis.

angiography demonstrated a superficial femoral artery occlusion with severe trifurcation disease and a single posterior tibial vessel runoff. Ac-
cordingly, after intraoperative papaverine testing demonstrated sufficient
inflow, a left femoro-posterior tibial reverse saphenous vein bypass was
performed with an ankle/brachial index greater than 1.0 intraoperatively
and 0.89 at discharge (Fig. 1b). Routine blood flow studies 14 months
postoperatively showed dropping low thigh and ankle indices despite a
lack of symptoms. This led to arteriography and the discovery of a vein
graft stenosis (Fig. 1c). At exploration, a valve cusp stenosis (Fig. 1d, e)

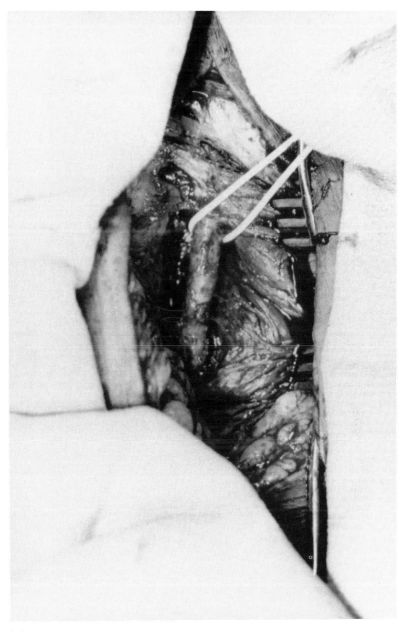

(d)

Figure 1d   Valve cusp stenosis at operation.

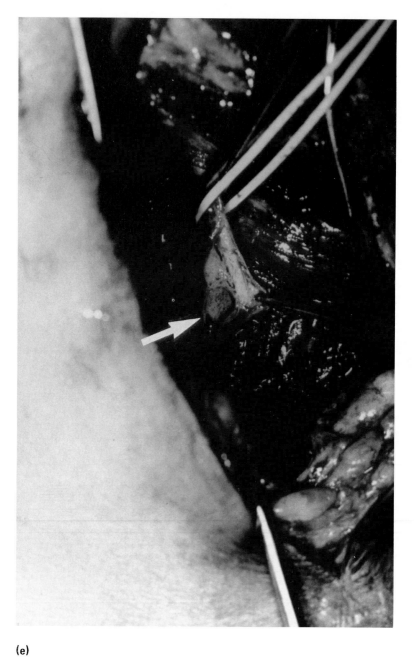

(e)

Figure 1e   Valve cusp stenosis (arrow) after arteriotomy.

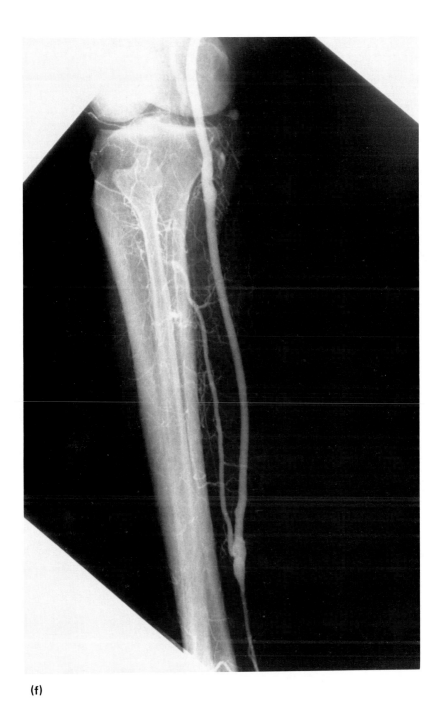

(f)

Figure 1f Intraoperative angiogram after patch angioplasty of valve cusp stenosis.

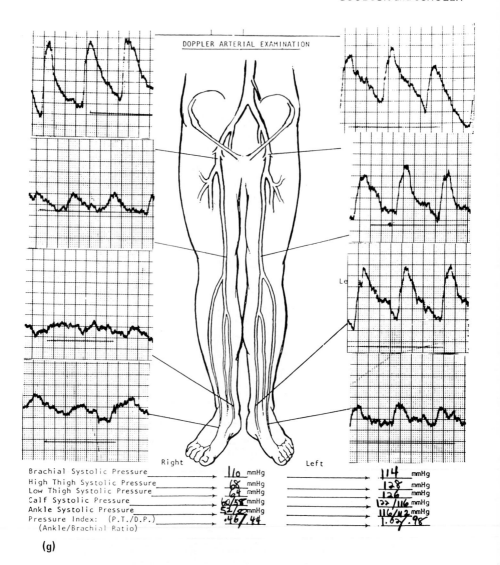

DOPPLER ARTERIAL EXAMINATION

Right   Left

	Right		Left	
Brachial Systolic Pressure	110	mmHg	114	mmHg
High Thigh Systolic Pressure	68	mmHg	128	mmHg
Low Thigh Systolic Pressure	64	mmHg	126	mmHg
Calf Systolic Pressure	60/58	mmHg	122/116	mmHg
Ankle Systolic Pressure	52/50	mmHg	116/112	mmHg
Pressure Index: (P.T./D.P.)	.46/.44		1.62/.98	
(Ankle/Brachial Ratio)				

(g)

Figure 1g   Arterial blood flow examination after "salvage" surgery.

was isolated and repaired with Goretex patch angioplasty (Fig. 1f) returning the ankle index to greater than 1.0 (Fig. 1G).

Vein graft stenoses can also arise from areas of previous injury where side branches were ligated too closely to the vein graft, where clamps were applied, in veins with previously undetected phlebitis, in veins overdistended during preparation, and perhaps where the adventitia was disrupted during harvest. The use of small vein grafts (less than 4 mm for ex situ reconstructions and less than 2 mm for in situ reconstructions) and the use of cephalic vein more often leads to early degenerative changes, stenoses, and occlusion. Veins graded as fair to poor based on varices, fibrotic valves, and sclerosis in Szilagyi's 1979 study of autogenous vein grafting had "disastrous" effects on patency rates (patency half-life of good to excellent veins was 10.5 years compared with 0.5 years for poor quality veins) (14).

We have noted a particularly intriguing use for noninvasive segmental Doppler pressures in detecting subtle hemodynamic compromise caused by the development of AV fistulae in in situ femoral distal grafts. When dropping segmental pressures are noted, the simple use of a hand-held Doppler probe along the graft may identify an area suspicious for increased flow and turbulence. Palpation may reveal a thrill or even warm, hyperemic overlying skin. Compression distal to the suspicious area produces a persistent, even "noisier" flow disturbance occupying the entire cardiac cycle. It has allowed simple and timely repair in a host of these grafts. Truly this graft's refractoriness to thrombosis, even at very low flow rates, will see its role expanded in treating distal disease permitting a significant number of salvaged grafts to be included in very good long-term patency rates.

Of all failures presenting later than 1 year from reconstruction, the majority are due to host disease progression affecting outflow rather than inflow. Forty-seven percent of the 21 patients who showed disease progression in Mozersky's group did so distal to their original lesion (13). Forty-eight percent of O'Mara's 27 late failures and 60% of Whittemore's failures later than 1 year postoperatively were due to progression of distal host disease (6,9).

The progression of inflow disease is more rare. In infrainguinal surgery it is variably implicated in the failure of 6-19% of grafts (9,11,15). In Down's series of postoperative angiograms on autogenous vein grafts, 13% showed progressive proximal disease though only two were occluded (2). It is important to identify inflow progression early since it is more easily and successfully treated than progression of outflow occlusive disease.

In procedures such as aortofemoral bypass, inflow problems are, of course, more rare. However, stenosis of a donor iliac artery is instrumental in the failure of femoro-femoral bypass. In such situations, preocclusive inflow failure eludes diagnosis with simple pulse palpation. O'Mara and associates salvaged two of their femoro-femoral grafts simply by demonstrating flow reversal with directional Doppler—a sure sign of preocclusive hemodynamic failure (6).

Probably underestimated in the genesis of infrainguinal graft failure is the frequency of athero-embolism from proximal sources. In Flinn's report in 1981, athero-embolism was the cause of early graft failure in 10 patients and late failure in 5 patients (16). Salvage surgery restored patency to 10 of these 15 patients, at which time thrombotic debris was recovered and no other technical problems or significant host disease progression was discovered.

Anastomotic intimal hyperplasia may be related to flow disturbances that produce local vessel injury according to Imparato (17). There is some question whether this lesion has a particular predilection for polytetrafluoroethylene (PTFE) grafts. Oblath and colleagues presented evidence that aspirin and dipyridamole may attenuate progression of this lesion in experimental arterial grafts as reported in a review by Vieth (5).

The two entities frequently affecting the distal femoral anastomoses of Dacron inflow procedures are neointimal thickening and pseudoaneurysmal disease. Neo-intimal build-up consists of a compacted fibrin layer remodelled to fit the flow dynamics of the anastomosis. Moore writes that the fibrin layer, itself thrombogenic, can eventually encroach upon the lumen sufficiently to cause hemodynamic failure and graft thrombosis (18). Pseudoaneurysmal disease has a predilection for high-flow anastomoses whose turbulence and sheer forces cause host arterial degeneration and suture line disruption. Sequelae include distal athero-emboli, progressive stenosis, spontaneous thrombosis, or rupture.

POSTOPERATIVE SURVEILLANCE

Obviously, despite the array of noninvasive procedures available, there remains a timeless role for careful clinical observation. Though palpable pulses do not always indicate normal hemodynamics, a once-palpable pulse subsequently lost certainly heralds the need for further investigation. The detection of a bruit or thrill over an in situ graft explains in advance the decreasing postoperative segmental limb pressures. Dampened femoral pulses or conversely, bounding broad pulses identify preocclusive lesions of aortobifemoral grafts and femoral pseudoaneurysms respectively. A sensitive clinician who tempers his eagerness for his patients to have good results can pick up subtle complaints of recurring claudication or deteriorating activity tolerance.

Astute clinical skills notwithstanding, the role of the vascular laboratory is no longer a debatable issue. What specific roles then do the various noninvasive studies play in the early and late monitoring of extremity graft function?

THE VASCULAR LABORATORY

The ankle systolic blood pressure, as measured by a Doppler probe and standard bladder cuff, is the most reliable and reproducible of all segmental measurements

(19). It forms the basis for most modes of follow-up, especially in infrainguinal reconstructive surgery. When indexed with the brachial blood pressure both at rest and after standard treadmill exercise or reactive hyperemia, it is invaluable in assessing single and multiple significant stenoses or occlusions. Pressures can easily be performed by ICU and ward nursing personnel and can, therefore, form the basis for intelligent postoperative monitoring.

Doppler-derived velocity waveforms complement the segmental pressure measurements. The phases of the Doppler waveform correspond to forward flow in systole followed rapidly and transiently be reversed flow and then by a slight component of forward flow in diastole. Triphasic waveforms usually indicate that flow proximal to the site of examination is normal. Waveforms distal to stenotic lesions become monophasic or biphasic losing their reverse component. The waveforms distal to occlusion, in addition to monophasicity, are slower in acceleration and deceleration. The unreliability of upper thigh pressures in detecting significant iliac disease is well known and the abnormal waveforms in particular supplement the inflow evaluation. They may often lead the examiner to more appropriate inflow evaluation including exercise responses and pharmacologic vasodilatation with papaverine when necessary. The value of waveform evaluation is limited somewhat in early postoperative surveillance (by wound edema, hematoma, and scar tissue, all of which causes a falsely abnormal waveform) but is an integral part of longterm follow-up. Pulse volume recordings are often used instead of waveform analysis. They are essentially the plethysmographic equivalent of direct Doppler-derived arterial waveforms.

The timing of postoperative surveillance is crucial and should encompass high-risk periods. We recommend that noninvasive measurements begin in the operating room and complement post-bypass angiography.

FOLLOW-UP OF INFLOW PROCEDURES

In suprainguinal bypass surgery, the thigh/brachial index should increase by at least 0.15 over the preoperative level and be maintained throughout the postoperative course (unless, of course, the operation is done to correct subcritical aortoiliac stenosis that potential infrainguinal surgery will be based upon, in which case the resting thigh/brachial index may be normal to start with). Ankle indices should increase commensurate with the amount of distal occlusive disease remaining, but time should be allowed immediately postoperatively to maximize the effect of collateralization, resolving hypothermia, and corrected hypovolemia. With suprainguinal inflow reconstruction, the ankle index immediately postoperatively may be too easily influenced by the vagaries of postoperative physiologic changes to be used as strict criteria for reexploration. In general, however, an ankle index unchanged from preoperative levels several hours after surgery, despite physiologic equilibration of fluid and temperature, arouses suspicion that a technical flaw exists or there is need for infrainguinal reconstruction. More accurate prediction of successful bypass utilizes preoperative hemodynamic criteria that are especially helpful if direct-puncture, common femoral pressure is known. This method, described by Flanigan et al. (20,21), postulates that successful reconstruction restores systemic pressure to the site of the distal anastomosis, and more distal segmental pressures thus increase in proportion to the gradient measured preoperatively.

$$\frac{\text{Predicted pressure index}}{\text{(level of interest)}} = \frac{\text{Preoperative pressure index (level of interest)}}{\text{Preoperative pressure index (site of distal anastomosis)}}$$

When this method errs, it does so in most cases by underestimating the predicted values, allowing some margin of error to the surgeon in assessing the ankle index and the need for further investigation (Figs. 2, 3).

Again, caution should be used in applying this method too rigidly following aortoiliofemoral surgery since time is needed to equilibrate the aforementioned affects of anesthesia, temperature, and volume. Yao recommends following ankle pressures up to 6 hr and if no improvement is noted to consider reoperation (19).

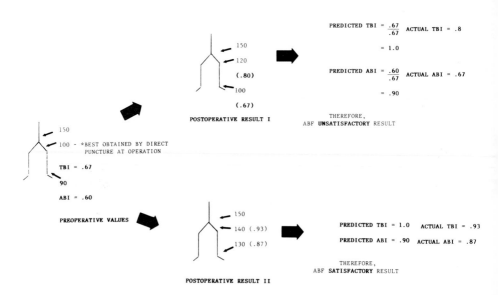

Figure 2 Application of predictive pressure index for aortobifemoral bypass.

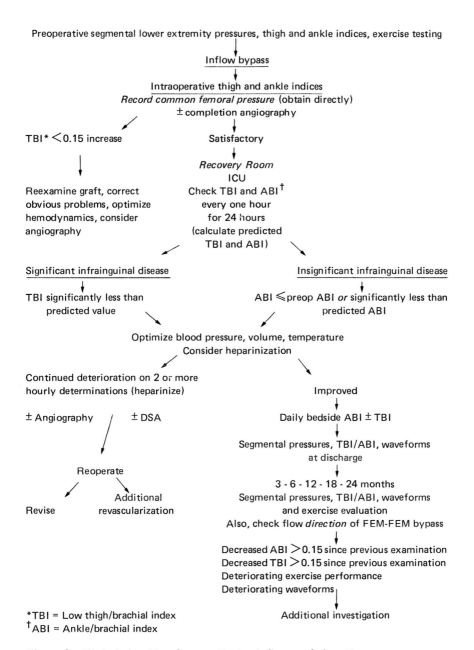

Preoperative segmental lower extremity pressures, thigh and ankle indices, exercise testing

Inflow bypass

Intraoperative thigh and ankle indices
Record common femoral pressure (obtain directly)
± completion angiography

TBI* <0.15 increase   Satisfactory

Reexamine graft, correct   *Recovery Room*
obvious problems, optimize   ICU
hemodynamics, consider   Check TBI and ABI[†]
angiography   every one hour
                                              for 24 hours
                                              (calculate predicted
                                              TBI and ABI)

Significant infrainguinal disease   Insignificant infrainguinal disease

TBI significantly less than   ABI ≤ preop ABI *or* significantly less than
predicted value   predicted ABI

Optimize blood pressure, volume, temperature
Consider heparinization

Continued deterioration on 2 or more
hourly determinations (heparinize)   Improved

± Angiography   ± DSA   Daily bedside ABI ± TBI

                                             Segmental pressures, TBI/ABI, waveforms
                                             at discharge

Reoperate   3 - 6 - 12 - 18 - 24 months
                                             Segmental pressures, TBI/ABI, waveforms
              Additional   and exercise evaluation
Revise   revascularization   Also, check flow *direction* of FEM-FEM bypass

                                             Decreased ABI >0.15 since previous examination
                                             Decreased TBI >0.15 since previous examination
                                             Deteriorating exercise performance
                                             Deteriorating waveforms

*TBI = Low thigh/brachial index   Additional investigation
†ABI = Ankle/brachial index

Figure 3 Clinical algorithm for monitoring inflow graft function.

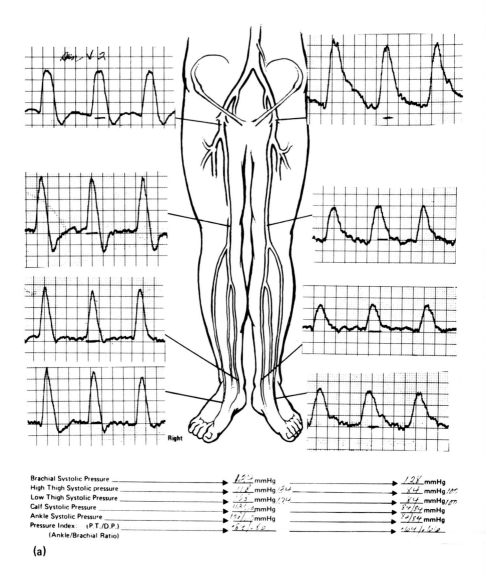

Brachial Systolic Pressure _____ ➤ _____mmHg   ➤ _128_mmHg
High Thigh Systolic pressure _____ ➤ _____mmHg   ➤ _84_mmHg
Low Thigh Systolic Pressure _____ ➤ _____mmHg   ➤ _84_mmHg
Calf Systolic Pressure _____ ➤ _____mmHg   ➤ _84/84_mmHg
Ankle Systolic Pressure _____ ➤ _____mmHg   ➤ _80/84_mmHg
Pressure Index: (P.T./D.P.) _____ ➤ _____   ➤ _.64/.60
      (Ankle/Brachial Ratio)

(a)

Figure 4a Preoperative arterial blood flow examination.

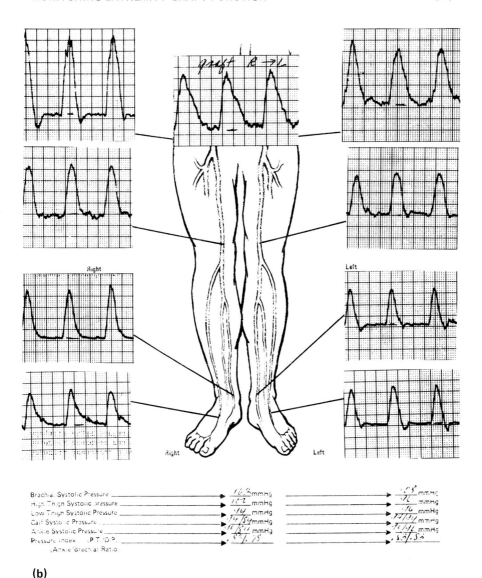

Brachial Systolic Pressure	→ _16.3_ mmHg	→ _16.5_ mmHg
High Thigh Systolic Pressure	→ _162_ mmHg	→ _16_ mmHg
Low Thigh Systolic Pressure	→ _14_ mmHg	→ _16_ mmHg
Calf Systolic Pressure	→ _14_/_84_ mmHg	→ _14_/_14_ mmHg
Ankle Systolic Pressure	→ _16_/_84_ mmHg	→ _16_/_14_ mmHg
Pressure Index (P.T./D.P.)	→ _84_/_.15_	→ _.83_/_.82_
(Ankle/Brachial Ratio)		

(b)

Figure 4b Improvement after femoral-femoral bypass. [Note that the thigh-brachial index improved by approximately 0.25 (0.65 →0.90).]

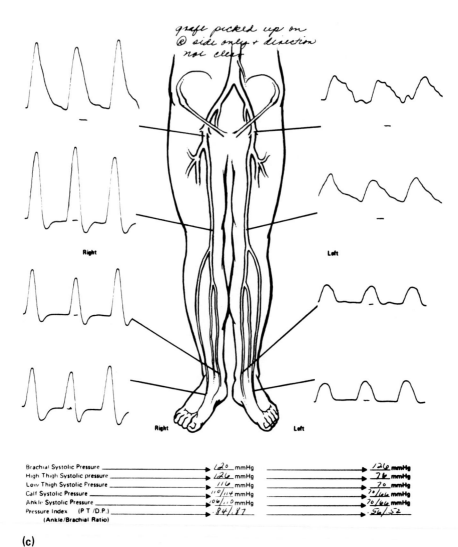

Figure 4c Marked deterioration of ABI on follow-up arterial blood flow examination.

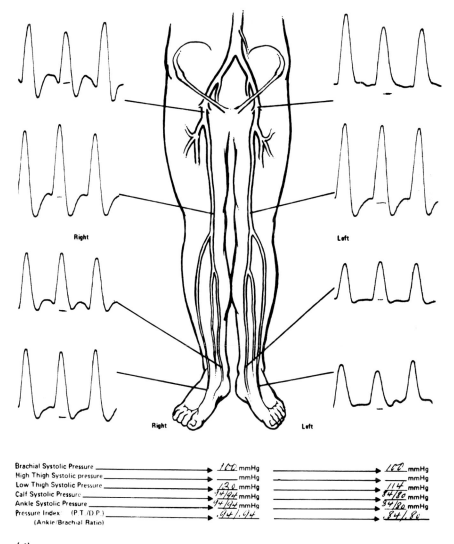

Brachial Systolic Pressure	*100* mmHg		*100* mmHg
High Thigh Systolic pressure	mmHg		mmHg
Low Thigh Systolic Pressure	*130* mmHg		*114* mmHg
Calf Systolic Pressure	*94/94* mmHg		*84/80* mmHg
Ankle Systolic Pressure	*94/94* mmHg		*84/80* mmHg
Pressure Index (P.T./D.P.)	*.94/.94*		*.84/.80*
(Ankle/Brachial Ratio)			

(d)

Figure 4d Improved indices after definitive aorto-bifemoral inflow reconstruction.

Our practice is to perform hourly indices in the first 24 hr and reexplore when predicted ankle pressures drop consecutively on two or more measurements. Heparin should be given at the first sign of suspected deterioration to prevent clot propagation distally (Fig. 3).

Long-term follow-up of inflow procedures should include segmental limb pressures, with thigh/brachial and ankle/brachial indices, and waveform analysis. Exercise testing is important for claudicants who should have regained normal exercise response. Those with multilevel disease should experience a significant increase in exercise time and faster recovery times (Fig. 3). Again, simple directional Doppler analysis of femoral-femoral crossover grafts may discover a failed though pulsatile graft (6). Hemodynamic failure in femoro-femoral grafts can result from a "steal" syndrome in which donor iliac artery stenosis precludes effective flow to either limb. The donor limb may experience progressive femoropopliteal disease, which is easy to identify on serial noninvasive studies. Both situations are amenable to corrective surgery. A case is presented below illustrating the vascular laboratory's role in identifying failure of inflow grafts allowing subsequent reconstruction.

> Case example: A 54-year-old man with severe coronary artery disease and angina presented with left buttock, thigh, and calf claudication. Preoperative blood flow studies demonstrated abnormal pressures and waveforms at all locations with an ankle/brachial index of 0.66 (Fig. 4a). Angiography confirmed left iliac artery stenosis. He underwent femoro-femoral bypass with 8 mm PTFE. His postoperative index improved (Fig. 4b). He returned 3.5 years later with sudden complaints of recurrent but less severe claudication. Blood flow studies showed a marked deterioration in pressures and waveforms and the ankle/brachial index dropped by 0.27 (Fig. 4c). His graft had occluded. Reexploration found a right femoral psuedoaneurysm and a thrombosed graft that was replaced and stayed patent for 7 months, at which time the patient returned with rest pain and an occluded graft. He underwent eventual aorto-femoral bypass and currently has both a satisfactory life style and improved indices (Fig. 4d).

As with other inflow procedures, axillo-femoral grafts should show at least 0.15 increase in thigh/brachial index. Again, ankle hemodynamics may not reflect true failure in those with concomitant infrainguinal atherosclerosis.

FOLLOW-UP OF INFRAINGUINAL BYPASS

Immediate postoperative surveillance of infrainguinal arterial surgery is crucial to pick up graft thrombosis at a time when most early failures occur, usually due to technical errors or inadequate graft flow because of severe distal disease. Preventing the changes that lead to rethrombosis demands prompt intervention. It has been shown that early thrombectomy and revision achieve patency rates that justify an

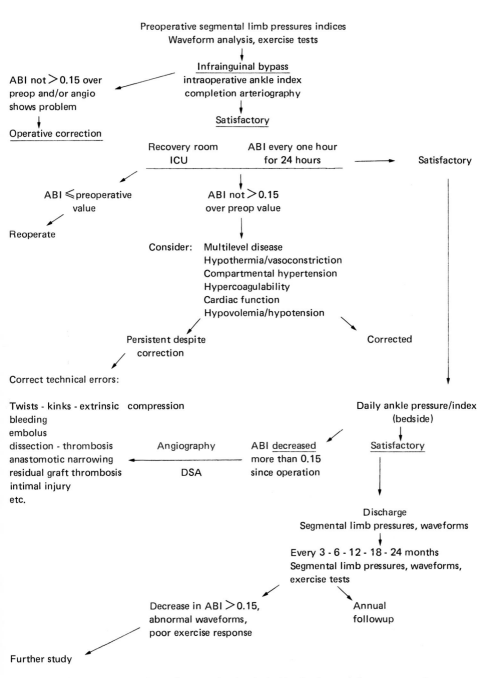

Figure 5 Clinical algorithm for monitoring infrainguinal arterial reconstructions.

aggressive posture to reoperation (9,22). Vieth adds that simple thrombectomy allows a significant number of PTFE grafts to be salvaged (5).

Ankle pressures should be assessed hourly in the postanesthetic recovery period for the first 24 hr and then every few days prior to and at discharge. Immediate reoperation is indicated for ankle pressures lower than or equal to preoperative levels. The aforementioned predictive index is extremely useful and when the actual index is less than predicted by an amount greater than 0.15, then further follow-up studies are warranted. Short of reoperation, further investigation can include measurement of compartment pressures (especially in reconstruction done for acute ischemia and trauma), search for missed AV fistulae with in situ graft bypasses, and a general assessment of the patient's cardiac status.

The first year of follow-up requires frequent evaluation because of hemodynamic failures detected, most are salvageable situations and usually require rather straightforward surgical solutions on the conduit or the anastomosis. Thereafter, reoperations are very often for progressive distal disease and surgical options are more demanding and certainly less rewarding. In addition, two-thirds of graft failures will usually have occurred by 1 year (1,9,22). The role of the vascular laboratory in late follow-up has been most clearly defined by Berkowitz. Only 26% of the patients in his series presented with unequivocal clinical evidence of graft stenosis. Fifty-seven percent were asymptomatic and 57% in addition had normal "distal pulses" (1). Moreover, hemodynamically failed but patent grafts have a significantly higher rate of salvage than those presenting with occlusion as documented by various studies (1, 4, 6, 13). The overall salvageability of grafts not thrombosed approaches 80%.

The three most important noninvasive parameters in postoperative surveillance are simple measurements of ankle pressures, exercise testing, and waveform analysis. In general, most authorities state that a decrease in ankle index by more than 0.15 indicates a new lesion. Occluded grafts return ankle indices to the preoperative level, or worse. Waveform analyses alert the clinician to flow changes that may or may not be associated with significant pressure changes, and are especially helpful in detecting inflow abnormalities. Exercise testing is important to document subcritical stenoses in claudicants. Despite multilevel disease, successful bypass should improve or normalize the exercise response. When it does not, further consideration should be given to additional reconstruction (Fig. 5).

RESULTS OF SECONDARY RECONSTRUCTION

Though somewhat beyond the intention of this chapter, the issue of vigilant postoperative monitoring is moot unless secondary procedures extend the functional life of bypass grafts and improve limb salvage. Several reports in the literature support reoperative surgery, which in general achieves a 50-60% 5-year limb salvage rate (8,9,11,22-24). When patent grafts have failed functionally, the salvage rate increases to 75-85% (1,6,8,9). Berkowitz stresses an exciting role for percutaneous transluminal angioplasty to correct stenotic vein grafts prior to thrombosis (1). Though a discreet number of failed repetitive revascularizations elevate the subsequent amputation to above the knee, the gains made in limb salvage ". . . far outweigh the risks of failure and the combined results were far superior to the outcome in comparable patients undergoing primary amputation" (25).

SUMMARY

The monitoring of lower extremity arterial reconstructive surgery should document hemodynamic improvement, not just graft patency. Symptomatic evaluation and careful examination of the vascular system is invaluable in the postoperative surveillance of patients but is not foolproof and may occasionally be misleading. Noninvasive blood flow studies play an integral role in the early and late follow-up of bypass surgery providing accurate physiologic assessment of graft performance. Segmental limb pressures, Doppler waveform analysis, and exercise testing form the basis for follow-up. Such studies can identify early postoperative failures (usually caused by flaws in technique or judgement), lesions intrinsic to the bypass conduit itself (seen commonly within a year or so after reconstruction), and those failures caused by host disease progression (usually seen later than 1 year after surgery). Since over two-thirds of failures are seen within 1 year from surgery, postoperative surveillance should be particularly intensive during this critical period. Moreover, failures identified during this time have a higher rate of salvage. The overall success of secondary revascularization procedures justifies an aggressive approach toward identifying and reconstructing failed grafts, especially if occlusion has not yet attended failed hemodynamics.

REFERENCES

1. Berkowitz HD, Hobbs CL, Roberts B, Freiman D, Oleaga J, Ring E: Value of routine vascular laboratory studies to identify vein graft stenosis. Surgery 90: 971, 1981.
2. Downs AR, Morrow IM: Angiographic assessment of autogenous vein grafts. Surgery 72:699, 1972.
3. Szilagyi ED, Elliot JP, Hageman JH, Smith RF, Dall'Olmo CA: Biologic fate of autogenous vein implants as arterial substitutes. Ann Surg 178:232, 1973.
4. Sumner DS, Strandness DE: Hemodynamic studies before and after extended bypass grafts to the tibial and peroneal arteries. Surgery 86:442, 1979.
5. Vieth F, Gupta SK: Thrombosis of infrainguinal grafts. In F Vieth (ed): Critical Problems in Vascular Surgery, Appleton-Century-Crofts, New York, pp. 159, 1982.

6. O'Mara CS, Flinn WR, Johnson ND, Bergan JJ, Yao JST: Recognition and surgical management of patent but hemodynamically failed arterial grafts. Ann Surg 193:467, 1980.

7. Marinelli MR, Beach KW, Glass MJ, Primozich JF, Strandness DE: Noninvasive testing versus clinical evaluation of arterial disease. J Am Med Assoc 249: 2031, 1979.

8. Turnipseed WD, Acher CW: Postoperative surveillance: An effective means of detecting correctable lesions that threaten graft patency. Arch Surg 120:324, 1985.

9. Whittemore AD, Clowes AW, Couch NP, Mannick JA: Secondary femoropopliteal reconstruction. Ann Surg 1:35, 1981.

10. Craver JM, Ottinger LW, Darling RC, Austen WG, Linton RR: Hemorrhage and thrombosis as early applications of femoropopliteal bypass grafts. Surgery 74:839, 1973.

11. Flinn WR, Harris JP, Rudo ND, Bergan JJ, Yao JST: Results of repetitive distal revascularization. Surgery 91:566, 1982.

12. Whitney DG, Kahn EM, Estes JW: Valvular occlusion of the arterialized saphenous vein. Am Surg 42:879, 1976.

13. Mozersky DJ, Sumner DS, Strandness DE: Disease progression after femoropopliteal surgical procedures. Surg Gynecol Obstet 135:700, 1977.

14. Szilagyi DE, Hageman JH, Smith RF, Elliott JP, Brown F, Dietz P: Autogenous vein grafting in femoropopliteal atherosclerosis: The limit of its effectiveness. Surgery 86:836, 1979.

15. Schuler JJ, Flanigan DP: Alternate inflow for repeated failure of femorodistal grafts. In JJ Bergan and JST Yao (ed): Reoperative Arterial Surgery, Grune & Stratton, Inc, Orlando, Florida, 1986.

16. Flinn WR, Harris JP, Rudo ND, Bergan JJ, Yao JST: Atheroembolism as cause of graft failure in femoral distal reconstruction. Surgery 90:698, 1981.

17. Imparato AM, Bracco A, Kim GE, Zeff R: Intimal and neointimal fibrous proliferation causing failure of arterial reconstructions. Surgery 72:1007, 1972.

18. Moore WS: Thrombosis of aortofemoral, axillofemoral, or femorofemoral grafts. In Frank Vieth (ed): Critical Problems in Vascular Surgery, Appleton-Century-Crofts, New York, pp. 445, 1982.

19. Yao JST, Nicolaides AN: Ultrasound in the management of lower limb ischemia. In AN Nicolaides and JST Yao (ed): Investigation of Vascular Disorders, Churchill Livingstone, New York, pp. 249, 1981.

20. Flanigan DP, Williams LR, Schuler JJ: Perioperative and intraoperative assessment of limb revascularization. In JJ Bergan and JST Yao (ed): Treatment of Upper and Lower Extremity Circulatory Disorders, Grune & Stratton, Orlando, Florida, pp. 135, 1984.

21. Flanigan DP, Ryan TJ, Williams LR, Schwartz JA, Gray B, Schuler JJ: Aortofemoral or femoropopliteal revascularization? A prospective evaluation of the papaverine test. J Vasc Surg 1:215, 1984.

22. Brewster DC, LaSalle AJ, Robison JG, Strayhorn EC, Darling RC: Femoropopliteal graft failures: Clinical consequences and success of secondary reconstructions. Arch Surg 118:1043, 1983.

23. Sladen JG, Gilmour JL: Vein graft stenosis: Characteristics and effect of treatment. Am J Surg 141:549, 1981.
24. Painton JF, Avellone JC, Plecha FR: Effectiveness of reoperation after late failure of femoropopliteal reconstruction. Am J Surg 135:235, 1978.
25. Raviola CA, Nichter L, Baker JD, Busuttil RW, Barker WF, Machleder HI, Moore WS: Femoropopliteal tibial bypass: What price failure? Am J Surg 144:115, 1982.

GENERAL REFERENCES

1. Corson JD, Johnson W, LoGerfo FW, Bush HL, Menzoian JO, Krimaki DJ, Nabseth DC: Doppler ankle systolic blood pressure: Diagnostic value in vein bypass grafts of the lower extremity. Arch Surg 118:932, 1978.
2. Fuchs JCA, Mitchener JS, Hagen P-O: Postoperative changes in autologous vein grafts. Ann Surg 188:1, 1978.
3. Sumner DS, Strandness DE: Aortoiliac reconstruction in patients with combined iliac and superficial femoral arterial occlusion. Surgery 84:348, 1978.
4. Root JA, Giustra PE: "Spoon bowl" deformity of proximal femoral bypass vein graft: A cause of late graft failure on four occasions. Arch Surg 112:166, 1977.
5. Strandness DE: Abnormal exercise responses after successful reconstructive arterial surgery. Surgery 59:325, 1966.
6. Taylor RS, Fox ND: Ultrasonic prediction of graft failure. J Cardiovas Surg 18:309, 1977.
7. Szilagyi DE, Elliott JP, Smith RF, Hageman JH, Sood RK: Secondary arterial repair: The management of late failures in reconstructive arterial surgery. Arch Surg 110:485, 1975.
8. Tyson RR, Grosh JD, Reichle FA: Redo surgery for graft failure. Am J Surg 136:165, 1978.
9. Sumner DS, Strandness DE: The hemodynamics of the femorofemoral shunt. Surg Gynecol Obstet 134:629, 1972.
10. Ascer E, Veith FJ, Morin L, White-Flores SA, Scher LA, Samson RH, Weiser RK, Rivers S, Gupta SK: Quantitative assessment of outflow resistance in lower extremity arterial reconstructions. J Surg Research 37:8, 1984.
11. Dolgin C, Collins R, Martin E, Voorhees AB, Nowygrod R: The prognostic value of the noninvasive vascular laboratory in autologous vein bypasses of the lower extremities. J Cardiovasc Surg 24:231, 1983.
12. Crawford ES, Bomberger RA, Glaeser DH, Saleh SA, Russell WL: Aortoiliac occlusive disease: Factors influencing survival and function following reconstructive operation over a twenty-five year period. Surgery 90:1055, 1981.
13. Malone JM, Goldstone J, Moore WS: Autogenous profundoplasty: The key to long-term patency in secondary repair of aortofemoral graft occlusion. Ann Surg 88:817, 1978.
14. Reidy SC, Walden R, Abbott WA, Greenfield SJ, L'Italien G, Megerman J: Anatomic localization of atherosclerotic lesions by hemodynamic tests. Arch Surg 116:1041, 1981.

21

Early and Late Evaluation of Postoperative Carotid Restenosis and Occlusion

ANDRIS KAZMERS
University of Washington and
Seattle Veterans Administration
 Medical Center
Seattle, Washington

D. EUGENE STRANDNESS, Jr.
University of Washington
 School of Medicine
Seattle, Washington

INTRODUCTION

Carotid endarterectomy is currently the most frequently performed peripheral vascular surgical procedure (1). The immediate results of this operation are variable, with many centers reporting a 2% or less stroke rate; an occasional report describes a rate that exceeds 10% (2-10). These complications are frequently due to technical problems occurring at the time of the procedure (6-7,11-17). Intraoperative detection and immediate correction of these technical defects, therefore, should reduce the incidence of perioperative neurologic complications (11-12,15, 18-20). Such intraoperative evaluation of the immediate results of carotid endarterectomy is also necessary for differentiation of truly recurrent from persistent postendarterectomy carotid stenosis. The latter distinction is mandatory for precise evaluation of the late results of carotid endarterectomy and for the determination of the natural history of recurrent carotid stenosis.

Serial clinical evaluation and postoperative noninvasive carotid testing are the current practices following carotid endarterectomy at our center. Through such routine postoperative noninvasive testing, the incidence of hemodynamically significant carotid restenosis following endarterectomy has been found to be much higher than anticipated (5,21-24). The incidence of carotid restenosis depends upon the method of postoperative noninvasive testing used for detection of this problem (22). Studies based on postoperative Duplex scanning suggest that from 10.2 to 22% of patients will develop recurrent hemodynamically significant carotid stenosis or occlusion following endarterectomy (5,21-24). Though these recurrent stenotic lesions are usually asymptomatic, delayed neurologic complications are not rare following endarterectomy (2,9,21,24-30). These problems suggest that proper management of patients with extracranial arterial disease should not end at the time of discharge from the hospital following carotid endarterectomy. This chapter will review our current approach to the early evaluation of the results of carotid endarterectomy, both during and immediately after surgery, and our current approach to the late evaluation of patients following carotid endarterectomy.

INTRAOPERATIVE ASSESSMENT

Evaluation of the results of carotid endarterectomy should begin in the operating room, since intraoperative detection and correction of technical errors should reduce the frequency of neurologic complications (11-12,15,18-20). Visual inspection and palpation of the carotid following endarterectomy are inadequate to detect such errors (31). Subjective interpretation of the audible signals generated by direct interrogation of the exposed carotid arteries using a continuous-wave Doppler has been used intraoperatively, as has indirect testing using the supraorbital Doppler technique (32). Other direct methods of intraoperative assessment include intraoperative B-mode imaging, which requires considerable training and experience before one is skilled at interpretation of the images (33-34). One group that uses intraoperative B-mode imaging has advocated the addition of a pulsed Doppler in order to increase the accuracy of this technique (33).

Intraoperative Angiography

Vascular surgeons are familiar with completion angiography following extremity revascularization, but are not as likely to use this technique to evaluate the results of carotid surgery. Blaisdell reported startling results from the routine use of carotid completion angiography following endarterectomy (11). Arterial narrowing greater than 30% was present in 26% of the patients in that series. Correction of these technical defects, sometimes requiring multiple revisions, was performed in 25% of the patients undergoing carotid endarterectomy in that original series (11). The need for carotid revision, as determined by intraoperative angiography, is currently less than 10% (12,15,20,31). One recent large series reported that only 2.5% of carotid endarterectomies required immediate revision (15).

The technique of intraoperative angiography has been described in detail elsewhere in this volume (20). An occasional report describes the potential complications that may result from carotid completion angiography (35). The experience at centers that routinely perform carotid completion angiography indicates that such complications are very rare, thus rendering the technique suitable for routine use (12,20). Minimal experience is required before one obtains consistently good-quality films that are easy to interpret (Fig. 1). However, since the angiograms

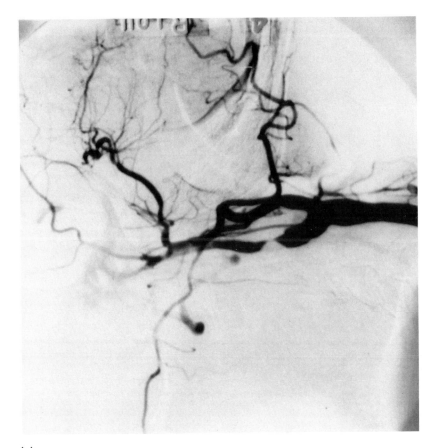

(a)

Figure 1 (a) Preoperative angiogram. This patient had recurrent symptomatic carotid restenosis over 7 years following previous endarterectomy. (b) This intraoperative completion angiogram shows a satisfactory result following repeat endarterectomy and vein patch angioplasty.

reveal only one plane of the carotid system, a mild stenosis might be missed, but a high-grade stenosis, significant intimal flap, or carotid thrombosis would be readily detected (18).

Intraoperative Pulsed Doppler with Spectral Analysis

At our center, completion angiography is combined with intraoperative pulsed Doppler examination to assess the immediate results of carotid endarterectomy. The technique of evaluation of carotid arterial flow using a pulsed Doppler and

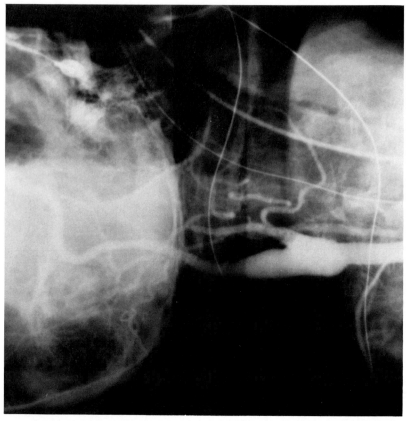

(b) (Figure 1, continued)

spectral analysis has been outlined elsewhere in this volume (18-20). Velocity changes from the center of the artery flowstream are inspected visually and permanently recorded proximal to, within, and distal to the endarterectomy site before arterial clamping and following arterial closure once the endarterectomy has been completed. Lack of improvement or worsening of the spectra following endarterectomy suggest a technical problem (18-20). Patients with flow-reducing carotid stenoses noted prior to endarterectomy should experience reductions of peak systolic frequencies following endarterectomy (Fig. 2). An increase in peak systolic frequency or an increase in spectral broadening from the preendarterectomy baseline each suggest a technical problem. The intraoperative pulsed Doppler technique is extremely sensitive for detecting residual defects, with the sensitivity ranging from 94 to 100%, with a 100% negative predictive value noted in one study

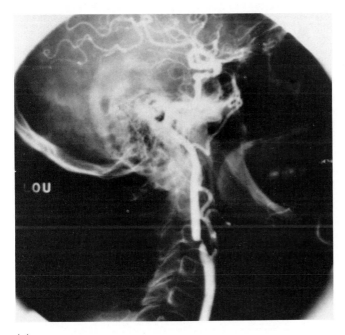

(a)

Figure 2 These studies were obtained from a patient who had presented with right amaurosis fugax. (a) Patient's preoperative angiogram. (b) These spectra were obtained prior to endarterectomy using the 20-MHz pulsed Doppler. The internal carotid artery spectra show increased peak frequencies (much greater than 20 KHz) with marked spectral broadening. (c) The completion angiogram shows minor irregularities but no major area of stenosis. (d) The internal carotid artery shows a clear reduction in peak frequencies and decreased spectral broadening after endarterectomy.

(18-20). Unfortunately, some patients will exhibit no significant spectral improvement despite satisfactory operative arteriographic results (19). A normal intraoperative pulsed Doppler study strongly suggests the absence of a technical problem, but flow disturbances may persist despite satisfactory operative results (19). These false-positive results are thought to be due to irregularities of the carotid luminal surface following endarterectomy, but this requires further study (19).

Combined Approach

The pulsed Doppler detects flow disturbances but, unlike angiography, cannot define the morphology of the responsible lesion. Intraoperative carotid angiography

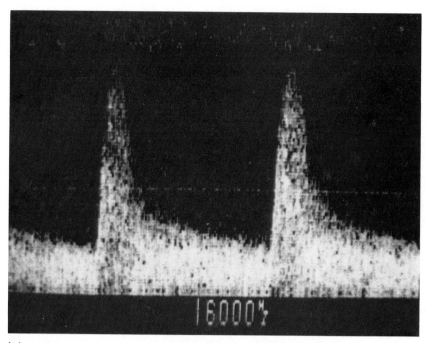

(b)

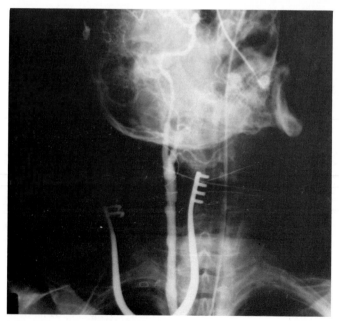

(c) (Figure 2, continued)

362

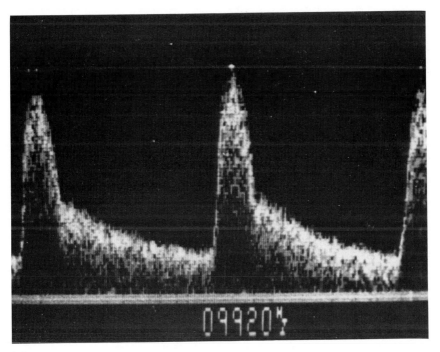

(d)

is able to evaluate the entire ipsilateral carotid artery system, not just the surgically exposed carotid endarterectomy site. Using these techniques, 7% of carotid endarterectomies have required immediate revision (20). Angiographic defects that are accompanied by deterioration of the pulsed Doppler exam, as shown in Figure 3, should be repaired. It remains to be determined which minor defects justify reopening the carotid artery, since revision of the endarterectomy is not an innocuous endeavor. The carotid artery has the potential to remodel following endarterectomy, but this is not a predictable occurrence and should not be used to justify acceptance of suboptimal technical results of endarterectomy (12,14,36). At present, minor angiographic irregularities are not revised in the absence of abnormalities of the pulsed Doppler examination.

Correction of technical errors at the time of carotid endarterectomy should reduce, but will not eliminate, the chance of developing a perioperative stroke (12,15). Cerebral embolization may occur during operative dissection of the carotid artery or during shunt manipulation (6,7). Further, postoperative carotid thrombosis can occur in the absence of any identifiable technical problems (6,17). Correction of technical errors should also reduce the incidence of *persistent* postendarterectomy carotid artery stenosis. The clinical significance of persistent carotid

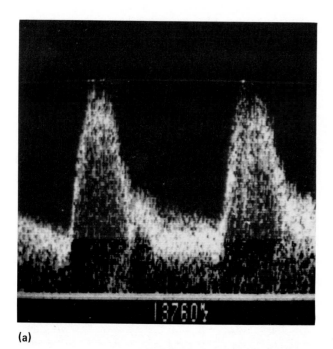

(a)

Figure 3 (a) Intraoperative internal carotid artery spectra taken prior to carotid endarterectomy. Peak frequency is 13,760 Hz with moderate spectral broadening. (b) Initial operative results by angiography indicating residual carotid stenosis. (c) Spectra from same location in internal carotid artery following endarterectomy. Note the increase in peak frequency to 19,840 Hz and the increase in spectral broadening suggesting a technical problem. (d) Repeat angiogram following vein patch angioplasty revealing correction of the stenosis. (e) Improvement in pulsed Doppler exam following revision. Note the reduction in peak frequencies to 6800 Hz.

stenosis is unclear at present. It is only through the use of intraoperative evaluation that the etiology and natural history of postoperative carotid stenoses can be defined. Although the issue remains unsettled, the natural history of a persistent postoperative carotid stenosis may be different from those stenoses that develop in the postoperative period.

POSTOPERATIVE EVALUATION

Clinical Assessment

Early (Immediate Perioperative Period)

The immediate results of carotid endarterectomy are quite variable from one center to another. Reported perioperative stroke rates range from less than 1% to

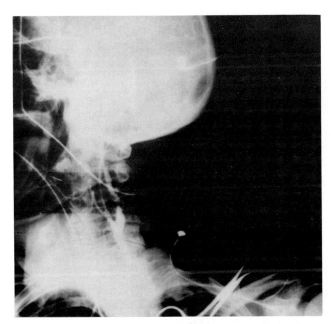

(b)

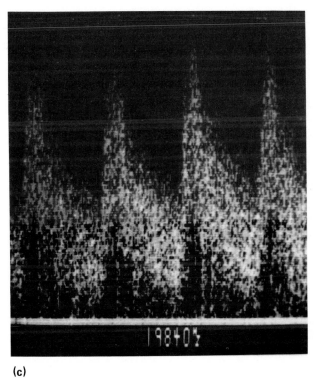

(c)

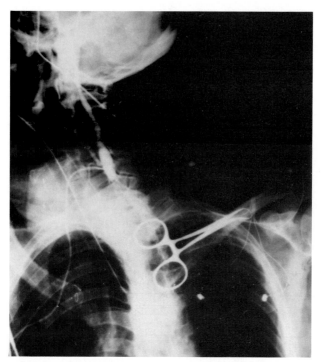

(d)

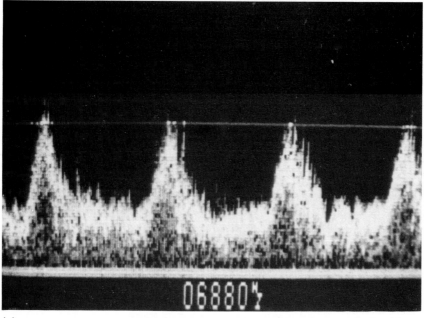

(e)

(*Figure 3, continued*)

14.5% (2-10). The indication for carotid endarterectomy has significant impact on the immediate stroke rate. The frequency of perioperative stroke is significantly higher in those undergoing endarterectomy for a previous stroke as compared with those patients undergoing a prophylactic procedure (25). The reported frequency of transient perioperative neurologic deficits is also quite variable, ranging from less than 1% to 15% (2-10,26). Reported operative mortality rates have ranged from less than 1% to 6.6% (2-10). Operative mortality rates of 1-2% or less and operative stroke rates of 3% or less have been achieved in community hospitals as well as in training centers (2-10).

Clinical evaluation is critically important in the immediate postoperative period. If a patient awakens without neurologic deficit and remains neurologically intact following carotid endarterectomy, the patient is discharged without any further in-hospital studies. Duplex studies are not usually performed unless clinically warranted in the immediate postoperative period.

If a patient who was neurologically intact upon emergence from anesthesia following endarterectomy subsequently developed a neurologic deficit appropriate to the endarterectomized artery within the first few hours of surgery, the patient would immediately be returned to the operating room for carotid reexploration at our center (6,37-38). Such a neurologic deficit could result from cerebral embolism, thrombosis, or a combination thereof. Although carotid reexploration would not be helpful for the embolus itself, it might be possible to remove the source of embolism. The possibility that such a deficit resulted from an acute perioperative carotid thrombosis is such an overriding concern that returning the patient to the operating room for reexploration is justified. If the carotid artery is indeed found to be occluded at reexploration, and the patient has been returned to the operating room within 2 hr of the onset of the neurologic deficit, the artery should be reopened and repaired since a good outcome is possible (37-38). The management of such a patient who develops a neurologic deficit after being normal upon emergence from anesthesia and is found to have a patent carotid artery at reexploration is less clear. In such an unusual circumstance, decisions to accept the technical results of surgery or to revise the carotid artery have been based on intraoperative angiographic findings at reexploration.

Management of the patient who awakens with a neurological deficit is equally controversial, as is management of the clinically silent postoperative carotid occlusion (38). Our tendency is to reexplore the carotid artery of those who awaken with a neurologic deficit, but our approach to this problem is dependent upon the findings of intraoperative testing done during the original endarterectomy. If the results of intraoperative testing were satisfactory, and the carotid system was proven to be normal by an emergent Duplex exam, reexploration might be avoided. Given our approach to the patient following carotid endarterectomy, clinically silent postoperative carotid occlusions would not ordinarily be detected in the immediate postoperative period. Others have advocated that patients undergo noninvasive testing (OPG-Gee) in the recovery room to detect silent perioperative carotid occlusions

(38a). Such problems would best be detected and repaired in the operating room. The treatment of an asymptomatic postoperative carotid occlusion diagnosed postoperatively remains to be determined. Surgeons have limited experience managing patients with these difficult problems, so their proper treatment is still in evolution. Firm guidelines are not yet available and treatment of these difficult clinical conditions should be individualized.

Late

Though late postoperative ipsilateral stroke has occasionally been reported to be a rare event, one series indicated as many as 1.6% new strokes per year occur ipsilateral to previous carotid endarterectomy (29,39). It is of interest that both immediate and late postoperative stroke rates are dependent on the indications for endarterectomy (25). In one study, the incidence of stroke 5 years after endarterectomy ranged from 6.3 to 8.7% in those undergoing surgery for asymptomatic carotid stenosis or TIAs, respectively, compared with a 23.3% stroke rate for those with a prior stroke as their indication for operation (25).

Clinical evaluation suggests the incidence of recurrent TIAs following carotid endarterectomy may be as high as 10-23% (25-28a). However, the incidence of TIAs in patients with documented recurrent carotid stenosis is less than 5% (1,5, 21-24,30,40-55). Thus, recurrent carotid stenosis is common, but the development of symptoms secondary to these lesions is relatively uncommon (48).

Late mortality following carotid endarterectomy is most commonly due to myocardial infarction, whereas neurologic complications are frequently the next most common cause of death (2,9-10,25-26). Thompson reported that 13.4% of late deaths following carotid endarterectomy were due to stroke (9). Another more recent series reported that 9.6% of late deaths were due to stroke (25).

Postoperative Angiographic Assessment

In one series, standard cerebral angiography performed within 2 weeks of carotid operation revealed that 33% of carotid arteries had some degree of stenosis (13). A separate angiographic study has confirmed these findings (14). Because of the short time interval after operation, it is likely that most of these stenoses were persistent and not recurrent in nature. Intravenous digital subtraction angiography (IVDSA) in the very early postoperative period (1-6 days postendarterectomy) revealed a 2.0% incidence of significant carotid stenosis following carotid reconstruction, a 17% incidence of slight to moderate carotid stenosis, and a 2.0% incidence of carotid occlusion (56). Thus, a total of 21% of patients had residual carotid abnormalities found using early postoperative intravenous digital subtraction angiography. This radiographic technique tends to underestimate the severity of carotid disease, and is not more accurate than Duplex scanning in determining the degree of carotid stenosis (57).

It would appear that the routine use of early postoperative angiography is not justified. Detection of technical problems should be done at the time of endarterectomy, when they can be most easily repaired. Cerebral angiography is an invasive procedure with a variety of potential complications, it is expensive, and it is not suitable for serial followup. Much information about the status of the carotid vessels that was provided only by angiography in the past can now be obtained by noninvasive testing. Cerebral angiography is certainly justified for investigation of the etiology of recurrent neurologic symptoms following endarterectomy, whether early or late.

Noninvasive Assessment—Duplex Scanning after Carotid Endarterectomy

Improvements in noninvasive testing have made it possible to monitor more objectively the long-term technical results of carotid endarterectomy. The accuracy of direct carotid examination techniques such as duplex scanning is superior to the accuracy of indirect noninvasive techniques such as oculoplethysmography (58-61). The duplex scanner is able to assess accurately the degree of narrowing in the atherosclerotic carotid artery (57). In addition, duplex evaluation of the operated carotid has a sensitivity of 94% in predicting greater than 50% internal carotid diameter reduction or total internal carotid artery occlusion (62).

Duplex scanning combines B-mode ultrasound imaging and pulsed Doppler flow detection (5,21-24,59,62-64). The B-mode ultrasound displays the carotid artery anatomy and serves as a template for placing the sample volume of the pulsed Doppler system at any desired point in the artery. A digital fast Fourier transform spectrum analyzer provides a continuous display of the Doppler shift frequency and amplitude of the velocity signals. The frequency resolution is 100 Hz and allows a total frequency display of 10 kHz (7 KHz forward, 3 kHz reverse). Normal centerstream velocity patterns exhibit a narrow band of frequencies reflecting normal laminar flow. When a stenosis is present, the red cells distal to the lesion move in random directions with varying velocities giving rise to spectral broadening. Flow within the stenosis itself is associated with an increase in the peak systolic frequency.

With a 5-MHz duplex system, internal carotid arteries normally have a peak systolic frequency of less than 4 kHz without spectral broadening. Mild diameter reductions of 1-15% have spectral broadening only in the deceleration phase of systole, but peak systolic frequencies are less than 4 kHz. A 16-49% diameter reduction has spectral broadening throughout the pulse cycle. When the stenosis exceeds a 50% diameter reduction, the peak systolic frequency exceeds 4 kHz (63). Recently, it has been noted that end-diastolic frequencies greater than 4.5 kHz are associated with a greater than 80% internal carotid artery stenosis (65,65a). Thus, it is now possible to classify high-grade stenoses into either a 50-79% or 80-99%

diameter category. Internal carotid occlusion is detected by the absence of detect-able flow in the internal carotid artery associated with flow in the common caro-tid artery going to zero (63).

At our center, duplex carotid scanning and clinical evaluation are generally performed within 1 month of carotid endarterectomy, then every 3 months during the first postoperative year, and then at 6-month intervals during the second post-operative year if there is no evidence of neurologic symptoms or hemodynamically significant carotid restenosis. If the patients have no such problems during the first 2 postoperative years, continued annual duplex scanning and clinical assessment are recommended.

Using these techniques Zierler reported a persistent postoperative carotid re-stenosis rate of 19% (24). Most of these restenoses occurred within the first year following endarterectomy (24). All of the patients had intraoperative angiography, so it was possible to eliminate technical errors as the etiology for the observed rate of postoperative stenosis. Subsequent studies have reported varying rates of hemo-dynamically significant carotid restenosis, ranging from 9 to 17%, based on postop-erative duplex scanning (5,21-23,25,40). If one combines the number of postoper-ative carotid occlusions with the number of hemodynamically significant restenoses found using the duplex scanner, the total incidence of such significant postopera-tive problems ranges from 10.2 to 22% (21-25). It is apparent that the incidence of postoperative carotid restenosis will be above 10%. Despite claims to the con-trary, it is clear there is a substantial risk of developing a recurrent postoperative carotid stenosis (45). Fortunately, the risk of developing recurrent neurologic symptoms secondary to these restenotic lesions has been quite small (24,48).

MANAGEMENT OF POSTOPERATIVE CAROTID RESTENOSES

Symptomatic

Patients who develop recurrent cerebrovascular symptoms following carotid en-darterectomy should undergo careful clinical, noninvasive, and arteriographic eval-uation. In the last 6 years, only 11 patients have undergone repeat operation ipsi-lateral to previous carotid endarterectomy for recurrent neurologic symptoms and recurrent carotid stenoses at the Seattle V.A. Hospital (48). Only 1.3% of the pa-tients undergoing carotid endarterectomy at our center since 1974 ultimately re-quired carotid reoperation for symptomatic carotid restenoses. Most (64%) patients presented with neurological symptoms similar to those prompting the initial pro-cedure. Seven patients presented with focal TIAs, one with a stroke followed by repetitive TIAs, and three with vertebrobasilar insufficiency. Two of the 11 pa-tients had early symptomatic restenoses at 8 and 9 months after previous endart-erectomy, whereas nine had late symptomatic restenoses prompting reoperation at a mean interval of 57.4 months after the previous endarterectomy.

Eight patients underwent repeat carotid endarterectomy and carotid patch angioplasty, two patients underwent patch angioplasty without endarterectomy, and the remaining patient underwent internal carotid artery replacement with a saphenous vein graft. Repeat endarterectomy with patch angioplasty was the preferred operative approach. Patch angioplasty alone is thought to be adequate treatment for patients with uncomplicated smooth stenoses due to myointimal hyperplasia when development of an endarterectomy plane is difficult. It has been stated that repeat endarterectomy is often not possible in patients with myointimal hyperplasia (44). It is our impression that repeat endarterectomy is the treatment of choice when a mural thrombus is adherent to the hyperplastic lesion (48). Those reporting the largest series of carotid reoperations agree that an endarterectomy plane can usually be developed regardless of the underlying pathology of the recurrent carotid lesion (48,54). In the rare case when repeat endarterectomy is not possible, but appears indicated due to the severity or nature of the recurrent arterial disease, carotid replacement with a saphenous vein graft should be considered. Using these techniques, there were no perioperative TIAs or strokes during the carotid reoperations performed at our center (48). There was one permanent vocal cord palsy postoperatively. There were no persistent or recurrent symptoms referable to the reoperated carotid arteries during followup (mean 16.6 months, range 1-65 months). Carotid reoperation is technically demanding, but acceptable surgical results have been reported by many others (42,45,47,54,55).

Our series of patients requiring carotid reoperation was too small to draw any firm conclusions regarding the nature of the risk factors responsible for the development of carotid restenoses. Others suggest the following factors may be important: (a) women appear to be at greater risk for carotid restenosis; (b) cigarette smoking may be a contributing factor; (c) antiplatelet therapy or anticoagulation do not appear to prevent restenoses; and (d) hyperlipidemia may be a risk factor (5,42,46). In our series of reoperations, 11 patients had smoked prior to the previous carotid endarterectomy, and only one patient stopped. Eight had received aspirin and/or persantine. There were no apparent technical problems clearly responsible for the symptomatic carotid restenoses (48). The most significant area of carotid restenosis occurred in the proximal internal carotid artery, presumably within the previous endarterectomy site in all but one of these 11 patients.

It has been suggested that the most common cause of early carotid restenosis (within the first 2 years) following endarterectomy is myointimal hyperplasia, whereas late (over 2 years postoperatively) recurrence is most frequently due to atherosclerosis (55). This is an oversimplification. It is true most early recurrent lesions are due to myointimal hyperplasia, but symptomatic carotid restenosis due to myointimal hyperplasia has prompted reoperation as late as 85 months following endarterectomy. Late recurrent lesions may be due to atherosclerosis, myointimal hyperplasia, or to hybrid lesions which contain both atherosclerosis and myointimal hyperplasia (42,48).

A recent report suggested that mural thrombosis may additionally play a very important role in the pathogenesis of recurrent carotid stenosis (66). A separate pathologic study suggests that some degree of mural thrombosis is uniformly present immediately following carotid endarterectomy (36). B-mode imaging done within the first few days after endarterectomy was thought to confirm this finding, indicating that "soft," presumably thrombotic deposits are regularly present lining the new arterial lumen (67). B-mode imaging studies performed 6 months or longer following endarterectomy, however, suggest a very low incidence of intraplaque hemorrhage associated with the recurrent carotid stenosis (51). The low incidence of ulceration or hemorrhage in these recurrent plaques was thought to be responsible for their usual lack of associated symptoms (51). In our small series of patients who underwent reoperation for symptomatic recurrent carotid artery stenosis, mural thrombus was present in 50% of the cases where the endarterectomy specimen was available for pathologic review. The clinical importance of mural thrombosis in the early and late postoperative period requires further clarification.

Asymptomatic

Given the likelihood that recurrent carotid stenoses infrequently lead to the development of symptoms, a conservative course is recommended for asymptomatic patients with postoperative carotid stenoses (5,21,24,48). Although it is our current practice to prescribe antiplatelet therapy for patients who have undergone carotid endarterectomy, the efficacy of this approach in preventing carotid restenosis is unproven. Zierler reported that the degree of postoperative carotid stenosis regressed in 41% of cases that developed hemodynamically significant stenoses and were studied serially following endarterectomy (24). Only 4.5% of these restenotic internal carotid arteries went on to complete carotid occlusion (24). It has been suggested that not only are the carotid restenoses usually asymptomatic, but the postoperative carotid occlusions are usually asymptomatic as well (21). In contrast, another group has reported that 17% of patients who develop a recurrent stenosis, as detected by oculopneumoplethysmography, will present with a stroke (30). The very high stroke rate reported in that small series has not been confirmed by other studies.

Because most patients with restenosis have a benign clinical course, it is our current approach to follow patients with frequent clinical examination and serial duplex testing. If a patient becomes symptomatic, arteriography is indicated. At present, reoperation is recommended only for those patients who develop recurrent symptoms appropriate to the restenotic carotid artery. A policy of routine reoperation for asymptomatic postoperative hemodynamically significant (>50%) carotid restenoses, as recommended by others, cannot be supported by existing data (30,54). The group with the largest experience with carotid reoperation suggests reoperation is justified for those with greater than 75% recurrent carotid stenosis, even if they are asymptomatic (54). Although we frequently recommend carotid endarterectomy for asymptomatic patients with greater than 80% *atherosclerotic* carotid narrowing, we do not feel justified in recommending a similar approach to those patients with high-grade recurrent carotid stenosis. No study as yet has clearly documented the risk of stroke in those with carotid restenoses, and it is inappropriate to assume that these recurrent lesions will behave like standard atherosclerotic lesions (62).

CONCLUSIONS

The assessment of the results of carotid endarterectomy should begin in the operating room. The combination of completion carotid arteriography and intraoperative pulsed Doppler studies is currently preferred. Although it is unknown how many neurologic complications have been prevented by the routine use of these techniques, it is probable that some of the patients requiring immediate revision of their endarterectomy may have suffered a perioperative neurologic event without such correction. Without objective assessment of the technical results of carotid endarterectomy, it is impossible to define the true incidence of recurrent carotid stenosis. Postoperative detection of recurrent carotid stenosis is best accomplished with duplex scanning. There is a substantial risk of developing a carotid restenosis following carotid endarterectomy, but the risk of developing a symptomatic recurrent stenosis requiring reoperation is acceptably low, being less than 2.5% (45). Despite the fact that it is such a common problem, the management of those with asymptomatic carotid restenosis is controversial, since the natural history of the lesion has not been adequately defined. We currently favor nonoperative management for those with asymptomatic postoperative carotid restenosis. The management of those with symptomatic carotid restenosis is less ambiguous. In the small population of patients with carotid restenosis and resultant neurologic symptoms, carotid reoperation can be performed safely with the expectation that these recurrent symptoms will be relieved (48).

REFERENCES

1. Callow AD: Recurrent stenosis after carotid endarterectomy. Arch Surg 117: 1082-1085, 1982.
2. DeWeese JA: Long-term results of surgery for carotid artery stenosis. In Bergan JJ and Yao JS (eds): Cerebrovascular Insufficiency, Chapter 33, Grune & Stratton, New York, 1983, pp. 507-518.
3. Easton JD and Sherman DG: Stroke and mortality rate in carotid endarterectomy: 228 consecutive operations. Stroke 8:565-568, 1977.

4. Hertzer NR, Beven EG, Modic MT, O'Hara PJ, Vogt DP, and Weinstein MA: Early patency of the carotid artery after endarterectomy: Digital subtraction angiography after two hundred sixty-two operations. Surgery 92:1049-1057, 1982.

5. Nicholls SC, Phillips DJ, Bergelin RO, Beach KW, Primozich JF, and Strandness DE, Jr: Carotid endarterectomy. Relationship of outcome to early restenosis. J Vasc Surg 2:375-381, 1985.

6. Rosenthal D, Zeichner WD, Lamis PA, Stanton PE, Jr: Neurologic deficit after carotid endarterectomy: Pathogenesis and management. Surgery 94:776-780, 1983.

7. Steed DL, Peitzman AB, Grundy BL, and Webster MW: Causes of stroke in carotid endarterectomy. Surgery 92:634-641, 1982.

8. Swenson WM, Gunflach WJ: Carotid endarterectomy in a community hospital. In Bergan JJ and Yao JST (eds): Cerebrovascular Insufficiency, Grune & Stratton, New York, pp. 497-504.

9. Thompson JE, Austin DJ, and Patman RD: Carotid endarterectomy for cerebrovascular insufficiency: Long-term results in 592 patients followed up to thirteen years. Ann Surg 172:663-679, 1971.

10. Thompson JS and Talkington CM: Carotid endarterectomy. Ann Surg 184:1-15, 1976.

11. Blaisdell FW, Lim R Jr, and Hall AD: Technical result of carotid endarterectomy. Arteriographic assessment. Am J Surg 114:239-246, 1967.

12. Corbier R, Jausseran JM, Reggi M, Bergeron P, Formichi M, and Ferdani M: Peroperative carotid arteriography. In Greenhalgh RM (ed): Diagnostic Techniques and Assessment Procedures in Vascular Surgery, Chapter 11, Grune & Stratton, New York, pp. 111-121, 1985.

13. Diaz FG, Patel S, Boulos R, Mehta B, and Ausman JI: Early angiographic changes after carotid endarterectomy. Neurosurgery 10:151-161, 1982.

14. Holder J, Binet EF, Flanigan S, and Ferris EJ: Arteriography after carotid endarterectomy. Am J Radiol 137:483-487, 1981.

15. Jernigan WR, Fulton RL, Hamman JL, Miller FB, and Mani SS: The efficacy of routine completion operative angiography in reducing the incidence of perioperative stroke associated with carotid endarterectomy. Surgery 96:831-838, 1984.

16. Baker WH: Management of stroke during and after carotid surgery. In Bergan JJ and Yao JST (eds): Cerebrovascular Insufficiency, Chapter 31, Grune & Stratton, New York, pp. 481-495, 1983.

17. Treiman RL, Cossman DV, Cohen JL, Foran RF, and Levin PM: Management of postoperative stroke after carotid endarterectomy. Am J Surg 142:236-238, 1981.

18. Bandyk DF, Zierler RE, and Thiele BL: Detection of technical error during arterial surgery by pulsed Doppler spectral analysis. Arch Surg 119:421-428, 1984.

19. Zierler RE, Bandyk DF, Berni GA, and Thiele BL: Intraoperative pulsed Doppler assessment of carotid endarterectomy. Ultrasound Med Biol 9:65-71, 1983.

20. Zierler RE, Bandyk DF, and Thiele BL: Intraoperative assessment of carotid endarterectomy. J Vasc Surg 1:73-83, 1984.

21. Glover JL, Bendick PJ, Dilley RS, Jackson VP, Reilly MK, Dalsing MC, and Robison RJ: Restenosis following carotid endarterectomy. Arch Surg 120: 678-684, 1985.

22. Keagy BL, Edrington RD, Poole MA, Johnson G: Incidence of recurrent or residual stenosis after carotid endarterectomy. Am J Surg 149:722-725, 1985.

23. Thomas M, Otis SM, Rush M, Zyroff J, Dilley RB, and Bernstein EF: Recurrent carotid artery stenosis following endarterectomy. Ann Surg 200:74-79, 1984.

24. Zierler RE, Bandyk DF, Thiele BL, and Strandness DE Jr: Carotid artery stenosis following endarterectomy. Arch Surg 117:1408-1415, 1982.

25. Bernstein EF, Humber PB, Collins GM, Dilley RB, Devin JB, and Stuart SH: Life expectancy and late stroke following carotid endarterectomy. Ann Surg 198:80-86, 1982.

26. DeWeese JA, Rob CG, Satran R, Marsh DO, Joynt RJ, Summers D, and Nichols C: Results of carotid endarterectomies for transient ischemic attacks— five years later. Ann Surg 178:258-264, 1973.

27. Edwards WS, Wilson TAS, and Bennett A: The long-term effectiveness of carotid endarterectomy in prevention of strokes. Ann Surg 168:765-770, 1968.

28. Fields WS, Maslenikov V, Meyer JS, Hass WK, Remington RD, and MacDonald, M: Joint study of extracranial arterial occlusion. J Am Med Assoc 211: 1993-2003, 1970.

28a. Owens ML, Atkinson JB, and Wilson SE: Recurrent transient ischemic attacks after carotid endarterectomy. Arch Surg 115:482-486, 1980.

29. Norrving B, Nilsson B, and Olsson J-E: Progression of carotid disease after endarterectomy: A Doppler ultrasound study. Ann Neurol 12:548-552, 1982.

30. Salvian A, Baker JD, Machleder HI, Busuttil RW, Barker WF, and Moore WS: Cause and noninvasive detection of restenosis after carotid endarterectomy. Am J Surg 146:29-34, 1983.

31. Rosental JJ, Gaspar MR, and Movius HJ: Intraoperative arteriography in carotid thromboendarterectomy. Arch Surg 106:806-808, 1973.

32. Barnes RW: Intraoperative assessment of arterial reconstruction by Doppler ultrasound. Surg Gynecol Obstet 146:896-890, 1978.

33. Lane RJ and Appleberg M: Real-time intraoperative angiosonography after carotid endarterectomy. Surgery 92:5-9, 1982.

34. Sigel B, Coelho JC, Flanigan DP, Schuler JJ, and Spigos DG: Ultrasonic imaging during vascular surgery. Arch Surg 117:764-767, 1982.

35. Andersen CA, Collins GJ Jr, and Rich NM: Routine operative arteriography during carotid endarterectomy: A reassessment. Surgery 83:67-71, 1978.

36. French BN and Rewcastle NB: Sequential morphological changes at the site of carotid endarterectomy. J Neurosurg 41:745-754, 1974.

37. Kwaan JH, Connolly JE, and Sharefkin JB: Successful management of early stroke after carotid endarterectomy. Ann Surg 190:676-678, 1979.

38. Novick WM, Mullili JJ, and Neimer P: Management of acute postoperative thromboses following carotid endarterectomy. Arch Surg 120:922-925, 1985.

38a. Ortega G, Gee W, Kaupp HA, and McDonald KM: Postendarterectomy carotid occlusion. Surgery 90:1093-1098, 1981.

39. Lord RSA: Late survival after carotid endarterectomy for transient ischemic attacks. J Vasc Surg 1:512-519, 1984.

40. Baker WH, Hayes AC, Mahler D, and Littooy FN: Durability of carotid endarterectomy. Surgery 94:112-115, 1983.

41. Cantelmo NL, Cutler BS, Wheeler HB, Herrmann JB, and Cardullo PA: Noninvasive detection of carotid stenosis following endarterectomy. Arch Surg 116:1005-1008, 1981.

42. Clagett GP, Rich NM, McDonald PT, Salander JM, Youkey JR, Olson DW, and Hutton JE Jr: Etiologic factors for recurrent carotid artery stenosis. Surgery 93:313-318, 1983.

43. Cossman D, Callow AD, Stein A, and Matsumoto G: Early restenosis after carotid endarterectomy. Arch Surg 113:275-278, 1978.

44. Cossman DV, Treiman RL, Foran RF, Levin PM, and Cohen JL: Surgical approach to recurrent carotid stenosis. Am J Surg 140:209-211, 1980.

45. Das MB, Hertzer NR, Ratliff NB, O'Hara PJ, and Beven EG: Recurrent carotid stenosis. A five-year series of 65 reoperations. Ann Surg 202:28-35, 258-264, 1985.

46. French BN, and Rewcastle NB: Recurrent stenosis at site of carotid endarterectomy. Stroke 8:597-605, 1977.

47. Hertzer NR, Martinez BD, and Beven EG: Recurrent stenosis after carotid endarterectomy. Surg Gynecol Obstet 149:360-364, 1979.

48. Kazmers A, Zierler RE, Huang T, Pulliam CW, Radke HM: Reoperative carotid surgery (submitted for publication).

49. Kremen JE, Gee W, Kaupp HA, McDonald KM: Restenosis or occlusion after carotid endarterectomy. A survey with ocular pneumoplethysmography. Arch Surg 114:608-610, 1979.

50. McBride K, and Callow AD: Recurrent stenosis after carotid endarterectomy—a limited survey. In Bernhard VM and Towne JB (eds): Complications in Vascular Surgery, Grune & Stratton, New York, pp. 259-273.

51. O'Donnell TF Jr, Callow AD, Scott G, Shepard AD, Hegerrick P, and Mackey WC: Ultrasound characteristics of recurrent carotid disease: Hypothesis explaining the low incidence of symptomatic recurrence. J Vasc Surg 2:26-41, 1985.

52. Palmaz JC, Hunter G, Carson SN, and French SW: Postoperative carotid restenosis due to neointimal fibromuscular hyperplasia. Radiology 148:699-702, 1983.

53. Pierce GE, Iliopoulos JI, Holcomb MA, Rieder CF, Hermreck AS, and Thomas JH: Incidence of recurrent stenosis after carotid endarterectomy determined by digital subtraction angiography. Am J Surg 148:848-854, 1984.

54. Rapp J and Stoney R: Recurrent carotid stenosis. In Bernhard VM and Towne JB (eds): Complications in Vascular Surgery, Chapter 43, Grune & Stratton, New York, pp. 763-771, 1985.

55. Stoney RJ and String ST: Recurrent carotid stenosis. Surgery 80:705-710, 1976.

56. Raithel D, Schweiger H, Gentsch HH, Serferth W, and Zietler E: Digital transvenous angiography in follow-up examination after carotid reconstruction: Early results. J Cardiovasc Surg 25:400-403, 1984.

57. Glover JL, Bendick PJ, Jackson VP, Becker GJ, Dilley RS, and Holden RW: Duplex ultrasonography, digital subtraction, angiography, and conventional angiography in assessing carotid atherosclerosis. Arch Surg 119:664-669, 1984.

58. Blackshear WM, Thiele BL, Harley JD, Chikos PM, and Strandness DE Jr: A prospective evaluation of oculoplethysmography and carotid phonoangiography. Surg Gynecol Obstet 148:201-205, 1979.

59. Keagy BA, Pharr WF, Thomas D, and Bowes DW: Comparison of oculoplethysmography/carotid phonoangiography with Duplex scan/spectral ananlysis in the detection of carotid artery stenosis. Stroke 13:43-45, 1982.

60. Lynch TG, Hobson RW, and Berry SM: The role of real-time B-mode ultrasonography and ocular pneumoplethysmography following carotid endarterectomy. Am Surgeon 49:31-36, 1983.

61. Otis SM, Smith RA, Dalessio DJ, Kroll AD, Rush M, and Dilley RB: Ineffectiveness of the Doppler ophthalmic test (DOT) in post-endarterectomy evaluation. Stroke 10:396-399, 1979.

62. Roederer GO, Langlois Y, Chan ATW, Breslau P, Phillips DJ, Beach KW, Chikos PM, and Strandness DE Jr: Postendarterectomy carotid ultrasonic Duplex scanning concordance with contrast angiography. Ultrasound Med Biol 9:73-78, 1983.

63. Zierler RE, Roederer GO, and Strandness DE Jr: The use of frequency spectral analysis in carotid artery surgery. In Bergan JJ and Yao JST (eds): Cerebrovascular Insufficiency, Grune & Stratton, New York, pp. 137-163, 1983.

64. Sumner DS: Pitfalls of noninvasive cerebrovascular testing and angiography. In Complications in Vascular Surgery, Chapter 41, Grune & Stratton, New York, pp. 663-703, 1985.

65. Roederer GO, Langlois YE, Jager KA, Lawrence RJ, Primozich JF, Phillips DJ, and Strandness DE Jr: A simple spectral parameter for accurate classification of severe carotid disease. Bruit 8:174-178, 1984.

65a. Roederer GO, Langlois YE, Jager KA, Primozich JF, Beach KW, Phillips DJ, and Strandness DE Jr: The natural history of carotid arterial disease in asymptomatic patients with cervical bruits. Stroke 15:605-613, 1984.

66. Clagett GP, Robinowitz M, Youkey JR, Fisher DF Jr, Fry RE, Myers SI, Collins GJ, and Virmani R: Morphogenesis and clinicopathologic characteristics of recurrent carotid disease. Abstract presented at 33rd Annual Meeting, North American Chapter, International Society for Cardiovascular Surgery, p. 18, 1985.

67. Marosi L, Chringer H, Piza F, and Wagner O: Early postoperative morphology
    of the carotid artery following endarterectomy: Systemic prospective stud-
    ies with a high-resolution ultrasound Duplex real time imaging system. In
    Greenhalgh RM (ed): Diagnostic Techniques and Assessment, Procedures in
    Vascular Surgery, Chapter 15, Grune & Stratton, New York, pp. 161-173,
    1985.

Index